Global Mental Health Ethics

Allen R. Dyer • Brandon A. Kohrt
Philip J. Candilis
Editors

Global Mental Health Ethics

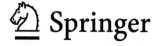

Editors
Allen R. Dyer
Department of Psychiatry and Behavioral
Sciences
The George Washington University
Washington, DC
USA

Brandon A. Kohrt
Division of Global Mental Health
George Washington University
Washington, DC
USA

Philip J. Candilis
Department of Behavioral Health
Saint Elizabeths Hospital
Washington, DC
USA

ISBN 978-3-030-66298-1   ISBN 978-3-030-66296-7   (eBook)
https://doi.org/10.1007/978-3-030-66296-7

This Springer imprint is published by the registered company Springer Nature Switzerland AG
The registered company address is: Gewerbestrasse 11, 6330 Cham, Switzerland

Preface

Global mental health is at heart an ethical enterprise. The global mental health movement emerges in the twenty-first century from the recognition of inequities in access to mental health care, which adversely impact the quality of life of millions (actually billions) of people across the globe, particularly in lower and middle income countries (LMICs). But in truth, inadequate care for mental health and substance misuse is a problem around the globe, even in otherwise well-resourced areas. As the slogans remind us: There is no health without mental health. And in mental health, everywhere is a developing country.

The World Health Organization (WHO) definition of health famously includes mental health. In the preamble to the UN Constitution, WHO defined "health" as the "state of complete physical, mental and social well-being and not merely the absence of disease or infirmity" (WHO, 1948). Although this definition was adopted in the wake of the massive social disruptions of the first half of the twentieth century, it was largely ignored in the latter half of the twentieth century. The understanding of "global" in global mental health is usually understood to mean around the planet, but harkening back to the wisdom of the original WHO definition of health, "global" may best be understood as "comprehensive," the "state of complete physical, mental, and social well-being."

This volume is intended to address a gap in existing textbooks of global mental health—of which there are now several excellent ones—by focusing explicitly on ethical considerations that are often implicit in discussions of health policy. The subtitle "Ethical Principles and Best Practices" links principle and practice, theory and application. What makes a practice good, or better, or best? In suggesting a visual metaphor, the lens of ethics, we look both closely (microscopically) and also from a distance (telescopically) at ethical issues, conflicts, and dilemmas, which often get translated into legal issues, economic issues, or political issues.

This volume may differ from similar texts in one important regard. In order to bring ethical values into focal awareness, the authors were invited to not only state their conclusions, but also to state how they reached their conclusions. While many textbooks report on what are considered to be already established facts, this one considers what should be, and what might be. It looks forward explicitly as well as tacitly. The first person accounts and narratives give nuance to the theories and link theory to practice.

There is a tension that runs throughout work in the field of global mental health—field understood here as both location where the work is done and also as the discipline(s) studying (and reflecting on) what goes on. That tension might best be represented by the tension between anthropology, the discipline that studies cultures in a detached way, but that also applies those understandings to alleviate human suffering, and psychiatry and related disciplines that treat mental disorders, but also try to understand the social and cultural context in which they occur. The authors of this textbook represent an array of disciplines, including anthropology, psychiatry, and psychoanalysis, forensic psychiatry, child psychiatry, sociology, ethics, philosophy, theology, educational psychology, and law.

This text is designed to be accessible to and useful for students in various health and mental health disciplines such as psychiatry, psychology, social work, and nursing, those in public health and public policy as well as professionals and academics, and those working in health ministries, health departments, and NGOs. It is of sufficient depth and length to be used as a primary text in a one-semester undergraduate or professional level course.

Many of the chapters come from the Global Mental Health program at the George Washington University and our colleagues around the world. We are grateful for all their contributions. We would like to acknowledge especially the second-year residents in our global mental health seminar, who read most of the chapters, offered helpful critiques and suggestions, and in several cases noticed significant gaps in the text and offered chapters to fill those gaps.

The reader of this book might raead chapters selectively from regions of particular interest, or from approaches or themes. Weaving the various disciplines represented by the more than two dozen authors, there are four chapters in particular that serve as pillars on which the structure is built: my own introductory chapter on the lens of ethics and Brandon A. Kohrt's chapter on the history of the global mental health movement, Kelso Cratsley and colleagues' chapter on human rights, and Philip Candilis' concluding synoptic chapter (another visual metaphor) on arriving at the ethics of global mental health.

Focusing on underlying ethical principles sharpens the understanding of best practices, not just in terms of best conventions but the ethical warrants for best policies. The ethics lens is one way to look at particulars from a broader perspective, but also can help sharpen the focus of that broader perspective by elucidating the guiding principles, particularly justice. What can professionals do? What can governments do? What can NGOs do? And significantly, what is the role of communities?

As this book goes to press, the world is under lockdown, a global quarantine, to protect the lives of as many of its citizens as possible. As we self-isolate, we look for novel ways to remain socially and spiritually connected, even as we are physically distanced. There is no longer an us-and-them. There is no longer here and there. We are all in the same boat, or at least in the same storm. If there is any opportunity in the danger, it may be that we may begin to learn together how to face problems that affect everyone. Contagions know no national boundaries. A pandemic is a global problem. Just as global climate change affects the entire planet, not just isolated corners, rising tides of oceans and disease affect east and west, north and south equally without discrimination. And while less resourced people and regions may be most affected, most vulnerable, global mental health and well-being are universal concerns.

Washington, DC, USA   Allen R. Dyer

Contents

Contributors

Nilanga Abeysinghe Faculty of Graduate Studies, University of Colombo, Colombo, Sri Lanka

Amir A. Afkhami Department of Psychiatry and Behavioral Sciences, The George Washington University, Washington, DC, USA

George David Annas Forensic Psychiatry Consulting, LLC, Syracuse, NY, USA

Elizabeth Berger Department of Psychiatry and Behavioral Sciences at the George Washington University School of Medicine and Health Sciences, Washington, DC, USA

Philip J. Candilis Department of Behavioral Health, Saint Elizabeths Hospital, Washington, DC, USA

Department of Psychiatry and Behavioral Sciences, The George Washington University, Washington, DC, USA

Kelso R. Cratsley Department of Philosophy & Religion, American University, Washington, DC, USA

Allen R. Dyer Department of Psychiatry and Behavioral Sciences, The George Washington University, Washington, DC, USA

Evangeline S. Ekanayake Faculty of Graduate Studies, University of Colombo, Colombo, Sri Lanka

Javad John Fatollahi Department of Psychiatry and Behavioral Sciences, The George Washington University, Washington, DC, USA

James L. Griffith Department of Psychiatry and Behavioral Sciences, The George Washington University, Washington, DC, USA

Samah Jabr Department of Psychiatry and Behavioral Sciences at the George Washington University School of Medicine and Health Sciences, Washington, DC, USA

Palestinian Ministry of Health, Ramallah, Palestine

Marie Grâce Kagoyire Historical Trauma and Transformation, Stellenbosch University, Stellenbosch, South Africa

Bonnie N. Kaiser University of California San Diego, Department of Anthropology and Global Health Program, La Jolla, CA, USA

Andrew Wooyoung Kim Center for Global Health, Massachusetts General Hospital, Boston, MA, USA

Brandon A. Kohrt Division of Global Mental Health, George Washington University, Washington, DC, USA

Janet L. Lewis University of Rochester, Penn Yan, NY, USA

Sana Loue Case Western Reserve University, Department of Bioethics, Cleveland, OH, USA

Tim K. Mackey Department of Anesthesiology and Division of Global Public Health, School of Medicine, University of California San Diego, San Diego, CA, USA

Rida Malick Department of Psychiatry and Behavioral Sciences, The George Washington University, Washington, DC, USA

Emily Mendenhall School of Foreign Service, Georgetown University, Washington, DC, USA

Byamah B. Mutamba Butabika Hospital, Kampala, Uganda

Community Mental Health, YouBelong Uganda, Kampala, Uganda

Samuel O. Okpaku President, Center for Health, Culture, and Society, Nashville, TN, USA

Clinical Professor, George Washington University, Washington, DC, USA

Maya Prabhu Yale School of Medicine, New Haven, CT, USA

Megan Quinn Department of Biostatistics and Epidemiology, College of Public Health, East Tennessee State University, Johnson City, TN, USA

Rajkaran Sachdej, MD Department of Psychiatry and Behavioral Sciences, George Washington University, Washington, DC, USA

Jeremy Safran Child and Adolescent Psychiatry Fellow at Children's National Hospital, The George Washington University School of Medicine, Washington, DC, USA

Suzanne Shanahan Kenan Institute for Ethics, Duke University, Durham, NC, USA

Suzan J. Song, MD, MPH, PhD Department of Psychiatry and Behavioral Sciences, George Washington University, Washington, DC, USA

Edith Stein, MD, MMSc Department of Global Health and Social Medicine, Harvard Medical School, Boston, MA, USA

William M. Timpson School of Education, Colorado State University, Fort Collins, CO, USA

Vanessa Torres-Llenza George Washington University Hospital, Washington, DC, USA

Marisha N. Wickremsinhe Ethox Centre and Wellcome Centre for Ethics and Humanities, University of Oxford, Oxford, UK

Maggie Zraly Mental Health and Psychosocial Support (MHPSS) Collective, Copenhagen, Denmark

Part I
Background

Global Mental Health Through the Lens of Ethics

Allen R. Dyer

The term "global" in global mental health is usually understood to mean around the planet, designing strategies for less resourced areas, lower middle-income countries (LMIC). But harkening back to the wisdom of the original WHO definition of health, "global" may best be understood as "comprehensive," the "state of complete physical, mental, and social well-being." What does comprehensive mean in the context of global health and mental health? How is equity to be achieved in a fair and just manner? How are scarce resources best allocated? What does this mean from culture to culture, from place to place, and from time to time? These are value propositions that create tensions and even conflicts that may be political, legal, economic, or personal. The lens of ethics is a way of looking at such value conflicts in a manner of ordering priorities to mitigate, if not resolve, conflict, by reasoned reflection, realizing that there may be strong emotions that are not always recognized and may be difficult to articulate. Ethics itself is a product of culture. Ethics involves both reason and emotion in dynamic tension, the forces that motivate behavior in tension with the forces that constrain it. The lens of ethics can be a way of observing the outside world – or it may be turned inward as a way of understanding oneself.

Morality is often used synonymously with ethics, but in global context it is useful to distinguish *morality* as the social norms of a particular culture or group that one learns by living in that environment from *ethics* as the discipline that attempts to clarify issues of right and wrong. Ethics may be the attempt of persons trying to be moral, but it also may be used as a point of reference to judge the behavior of others as unethical or immoral.

Philosophers generally distinguish two approaches to ethics, rule-based ethics (called *deontological*) or end-based or principle-based ethics (called *teleological*, from the Greek *telos*, or end) [6]. Rules imply duties upon us; principles are

A. R. Dyer (✉)
Department of Psychiatry and Behavioral Sciences, The George Washington University, Washington, DC, USA
e-mail: allen.r.dyer@gmail.com

© Springer Nature Switzerland AG 2021
A. R. Dyer et al. (eds.), *Global Mental Health Ethics*,
https://doi.org/10.1007/978-3-030-66296-7_1

aspirational, what we aspire to. Rules are prescriptive, "cast in stone," such as the Code of Hammurabi or the Ten Commandments. Ethics in the deontological perspective is a matter of adherence or conformity to the rules, which are more or less given (by a higher source) and thus immutable. Principles require an internal process of interpretation. Principles are inherently ambiguous; they tacitly give us direction in application to particular situations. Teleological ethics is sometimes disparagingly called "situation ethics" or "contextual ethics," but it should not be understood as (culturally or philosophically) relative, but rather implies a direction (moral compass), with the context being the terrain which must be navigated. *Utilitarianism* is a form of contextual ethics: the greatest good for the greatest number, where utility implies value or happiness, as described by Mill, Bentham, and Aristotle, and the utilitarian assessment invites a calculation of the envisioned trade-offs (which ultimately cannot be measured).

How does one learn social norms by living in a culture? Initially this may be understood behaviorally as a stimulus-response exercise. Children learn to anticipate the smiles or frowns (rewards or punishments) of the parents or caretakers in their environment. Parents, teachers, or authority figures "reinforce" behaviors they find desirable, not necessarily in a conscious reflective way. As social skills and cognitive development become more complex, so does the complexity of navigating the moral terrain. Psychologists from Piaget to Kohlberg [11, 15] see ethics in terms of *moral development.* The child seeks to avoid punishment, adolescents learn to live by the rules they perceive to be operative in their group, and adults (some adults) try to live by principles to guide them in navigating complex realities.

Piaget observed that children at different ages employed progressively more complex reasoning to assess the right or wrong of particular situations. For example, one boy accidentally breaks ten of his mother's teacups; another boy recklessly plays with a ball in the dining room after being told not to, but he breaks only one teacup. Which boy is the more blameworthy? Younger children tend to assess the amount of damage, but are less likely to factor the motives. Kohlberg also posed dilemmas, such as Heinz and the drug. Heinz's wife has cancer. A pharmacist has developed a drug that will cure her but refuses to sell the drug at a price Heinz can afford. Should Heinz steal the drug? In assessing moral development, the answer doesn't matter as much as the reasoning that one uses to come to the decision. Was it fair of the pharmacist not to make the drug available at a price Heinz could afford? Isn't stealing always wrong? What would happen if everyone stole what they wanted or needed?

Kohlberg identified three levels of moral development, each with two stages (Table 1.1). Kohlberg's stages of moral development are based on Piaget's concepts of cognitive development [11, 15]. Cognitive theory is about how one thinks and reasons. Cognitive theory also involves how one behaves and what one does; it involves *both* feelings *and* emotions – feelings and emotions that may or may not be consciously reflected. Freud's developmental theory incorporates the unconscious or unacknowledged thoughts and emotions. His *structural theory of the mind* – super-ego, ego, id – postulates the ego as the agency of reason, mediating between the impulses of the id (playful, sexual, destructive) and the prohibitions of the

Table 1.1 Stages of moral development

Preconventional level, a child's sense of morality is externally controlled. Children accept and believe the rules of authority figures, such as parents and teachers, and they judge an action based on its consequences.
    Stage 1 – Obedience and punishment orientation
    Stage 2 – Instrumental orientation (what's in it for me?)

Conventional level, an individual's sense of morality is tied to personal and societal relationships. Children continue to accept the rules of authority figures, but this is now because they believe that this is necessary to ensure positive relationships and societal order.
    Stage 3 – Good boy, nice girl orientation
    Stage 4 – Law-and-order orientation

Postconventional level, a person's sense of morality is defined in terms of abstract principles and values. People now believe that some laws are unjust and should be changed or eliminated.
    Stage 5 – Social-contract orientation
    Stage 6 – Universal ethical principle orientation

super-ego [20]. Feelings such as shame and guilt, often seen as "neurotic" vestiges to be dispelled, in fact serve as regulators of morality, helping the developing child learn the boundaries of what is acceptable in a particular family, community, and culture [4].

Looking at global mental health through the lens of ethics brings together the approaches of several disciplines to bear on the conflicts of global interactions. Rules-based and principle-based approaches may seem to be discrete alternatives, but at heart they are not mutually exclusive. The absolutist is concerned that principles may be relative and nothing really matters. The consequentialism wants to assure that ethics is grounded in a particular context. Recognition of cultural pluralism is a third pole that gives rise to other ethical considerations and values, diversity, inclusiveness, and recognition of otherness, seeing a problem from someone else's point of view. Pluralism invites a deeper investigation, reflection, and conversation [13]. The recognition of pluralism brings in the perspective of culture, and culture involves a developmental component.

The development of moral reasoning presumes growing up in a stable culture. One learns the rules of a culture by living them. How does this happen? And how does one adapt to a new reality, where the things one had tacitly understood to be right or wrong no longer obtain? Imagine that one moves from one culture to another, as may happen, for example, in going off to school or taking a job somewhere else or being forced (displaced) from home by natural disaster or political conflict.

These "snowmen" diagrams (Fig. 1.1) of structures of the individual mind are contained in larger spheres of family, community, and society/culture, the outside world.

Historically it may be instructive to look at ethical theory as a developmental progression from more fixed codes, such as the Code of Hammurabi or the Ten Commandments, to a set of broad principles as articulated by the Hippocratic Oath, to more abstract universals, such as Immanuel Kant's categorical imperative – *act*

Fig. 1.1 Dynamic social contract

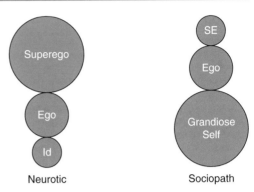

Neurotic   Sociopath

only according to that maximum which you would will to be a universal law. To speak of inalienable rights, "held to be self-evident," as in the US Declaration of Independence, is to speak of the inspiration of a nation yearning to be free of arbitrary constraints of a foreign power. "Yearning to be free" is an ongoing theme of persons everywhere in repressive regimes. Enshrining those ideals as a universal declaration of human rights is a recognition that these same ideals are ideals for everyone, everywhere – and they are fragile aspirations that are all too frequently viciously suppressed. This was vividly and poignantly expressed by a Greek surgeon on the island of Lesvos. He was looking across the water to the hills of Turkey, from where so many Syrian (and Iraqi and Afghanistan and African) refugees had made the perilous crossing, many losing their lives, after having already given up their homes, homeland, and possessions: "It is tragical," he said, "this desire for more democracy" (personal communication, 2017).

Cast in Stone

The Code of Hammurabi (Table 1.2) is often seen in retrospect as draconian: an eye for an eye, a tooth for a tooth. Of greater significance historically is the emergence of a systematic code and one that established the principle of proportional punishments, implicit in the 282 precepts. Let the punishment fit the crime, but not exceed it. The Code of Hammurabi was divinely inspired. At the top of the stele is a thumbnail carving of the deity approaching the young king in a dream (Table 1.2). (Iraqi friends tell me that it wasn't clear to them growing up whether it was the king or the deity who was seated. Apparently, the king remained seated, approached by the deity; it was the king's dream.) Imagine, almost 4000 years ago, the emergence of urban life and every conflict brought to the king for adjudication. What a divine inspiration and an administrative relief it must have been to the young king to have everything spelled out so explicitly!

Table 1.2 Code of Hammurabi and Oath of Hippocrates

The Stele of Hammurabi (eighteenth century BCE)

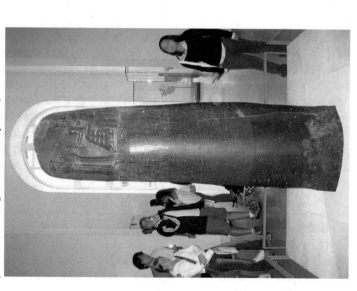

282 laws carved in stone, governing prices, wages, payment of loans, marriage contracts, property, slaves, and medical practice, all divinely inspired to maintain justice, peace, and prosperity. Originally in Babylon, it is now in Louvre, Paris. (Photo by A. Dyer)

Oath of Hippocrates (fifth century BCE)

1. I swear by Apollo Physician and Asclepius and Hygieia and Panaceia and all the gods and goddesses, making them my witnesses, that I will fulfil according to my ability and judgment this oath and this covenant:

2. To hold him who has taught me this art as equal to my parents and to live my life in partnership with him, and if he is in need of money to give him a share of mine, and to regard his offspring as equal to my brothers in male lineage and to teach them this art – if they desire to learn it – without fee and covenant; to give a share of precepts and oral instruction and all the other learning to my sons and to the sons of him who has instructed me and to pupils who have signed the covenant and have taken an oath according to the medical law, but no one else

3. I will apply dietetic measures for the benefit of the sick according to my ability and judgment; I will keep them from harm and injustice

4. I will neither give a deadly drug to anybody who asked for it, nor will I make a suggestion to this effect. Similarly, I will not give to a woman an abortive remedy. In purity and holiness, I will guard my life and my art

5. I will not use the knife, not even on sufferers from stone, but will withdraw in favor of such men as are engaged in this work

6. Whatever houses I may visit, I will come for the benefit of the sick, remaining free of all intentional injustice, of all mischief and in particular of sexual relations with both female and male persons, be they free or slaves

7. What I may see or hear in the course of the treatment or even outside of the treatment in regard to the life of men, which on no account one must spread abroad, I will keep to myself, holding such things shameful to be spoken about

8. If I fulfil this oath and do not violate it, may it be granted to me to enjoy life and art, being honored with fame among all men for all time to come; if I transgress it and swear falsely, may the opposite of all this be my lot

Interestingly for health professionals, 53 of the 282 precepts spell out rewards and punishments for physicians based on outcomes, ranging from payments in gold to death.

More recently (approximately 2500 years ago), the Oath of Hippocrates (Table 1.2) articulated a set of principles, *beneficence, justice, confidentiality, and non-maleficence* (a neologism for "First, Do no harm," which is in the Hippocratic writings, but not the oath itself). The Hippocratic principles have, more or less, off and on, guided the behavior of physicians for centuries and are considered to be "sacred" for the invocation of the gods Hygeia and Panacea and all the gods and goddesses in the Greek pantheon. Hippocrates is an interesting figure historically because he straddled science and spirituality. The Asklepion at Kos, where he taught his students and healed his patients, is at once a temple with niches for each of the gods and goddesses, but also a clinic, where people went to heal, and a "laboratory." Hippocrates based his recommendations on observations of the natural history of illnesses and the importance of diet and environment in healing. On a hillside overlooking the sea, Kos is a place of abundant sunshine and "warm breezes."

Notable in the Hippocratic Oath is the second paragraph, in which we see the origins of professional organization, the swearing "to give a share of precepts and oral instruction and all the other learning to my sons and to the sons of him who has instructed me and to pupils who have signed the covenant and have taken an oath according to the medical law, but no one else" [5]. For all its anachronisms, such as "not cutting on the stone," requiring the swearing by a set of ethical principles has become paradigmatic of what it means to be a profession, and most occupational groups, from health professionals to lawyers to auto mechanics, and now humanitarian workers, attempt some organizational articulation of shared ethical standards of behavior [2, 4].

Professional organizations, such as the British Medical Association and the American Medical Association, usually organize themselves around some sort of oath or professional standards. Typically, these are broad principles, goal-based, not explicit rules. The AMA *Principles of Medical Ethics* states in its *Preamble* that the principles are "not laws, but standards of conduct which define the essentials of honorable behavior for the physician." In practice principles sometimes become ossified as rules. The distinction between principles and rules becomes an important aspect of professional judgment, where novel situations cannot be entirely anticipated and require the professional to integrate complex realities based on broad principles, which of necessity are open-ended.

IASC Guidelines

IASC Guidelines are illustrative of a practical approach to ethics that starts with principles, officers specific rules in certain situations, and recognizes that real persons acting as moral agents must make real decisions based on conscience in real situations, in real time, in real places. As the global community becomes increasingly aware of and responsive to an array of disasters transcending the local resources to respond, government and nongovernmental organizations become an important part of relief and rehabilitation as well as economic development.

For humanitarian organizations and humanitarian workers, the coordination and "professional" ethical specifications come under the IASC (Inter-Agency Standing Committee) Guidelines on mental health and psycho-social support (MHPSS) in emergency settings for dealing with large-scale disasters. The Inter-Agency Standing Committee [8] is the primary mechanism for inter-agency coordination of humanitarian assistance, organized by the United Nations. It is a unique forum involving the key UN and non-UN humanitarian partners. In disaster situations, many people, professionals, organizational staff, national (local) staff, and volunteers may be mobilized quickly in ways which might be uncoordinated and even chaotic. IASC Guidelines provide a basic, coordinated framework for diverse groups to function harmoniously and efficiently. Created in 1991 by the UN General Assembly, the IASC has expanded its guidelines to include not only mental health and psycho-social support (MHPSS) but also gender-based violence (GBV) and guidance for persons with disabilities.

IASC Guidelines outline essential practices for humanitarian response in emergencies, which are based on six articulated core principles (Table 1.3).

Most people in an emergency will not need the services provided by mental health professionals. Epidemiologically we know that most populations will include 1–2% with serious mental illnesses, such as schizophrenia or bipolar disorder [21]. These people may be overlooked in the immediate aftermath of a disaster where attention may be focused on the situation facing everyone. There is increasing recognition that depression is a large unmet need globally, and many people experience symptoms of post-traumatic stress from natural disasters, ongoing political conflict, or adverse childhood experiences (ACE) such as childhood abuse (Quinn, Chap. 11, this volume). It may be tempting to pathologize stress reactions as PTSD with the stigma associated with mental illness. Conversely, it may be useful and reassuring to remind people that these are *normal reactions to an abnormal situation*, rather than reinforce the idea that there is something wrong with them that requires medical intervention.

Following Maslow's hierarchy of needs [12], basic social services, food, shelter, and security are foundational for more complex interventions, strengthening family

Table 1.3 IASC Guidelines core principles

1. *Human rights and equity* for all affected persons ensured, particularly protecting those at heightened risk of human rights violations
2. *Participation* of local affected populations in all aspects of humanitarian response
3. *Do no harm* in relation to physical, social, emotional, mental, and spiritual well-being and being mindful to ensure that actions respond to assessed needs, are committed to evaluation and scrutiny, supporting culturally appropriate responses and acknowledging the assorted power relations between groups participating in emergency responses
4. *Building on available resources and capacities* by working with local groups, supporting self-help and strengthening existing resources
5. *Integrated support systems* so that MHPSS is not a stand-alone program operating outside other emergency response measures or systems (including health systems)
6. *Multilayered supports*, acknowledging that people are affected by crises in different ways and require different kinds of support. Multilayered supports are ideally implemented concurrently (though all layers will not necessarily be implemented by the same organization). These are commonly represented by the IASC "intervention pyramid" (Fig. 1.2) [8]

Intervention pyramid

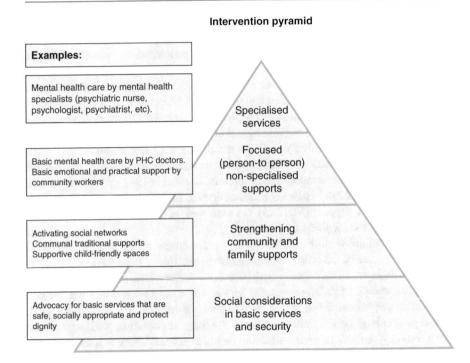

Fig. 1.2 IASC intervention pyramid

Table 1.4 IASC Guidelines do's and don'ts

Do's	Don'ts
Establish one overall coordination group on mental health and psychosocial support	Do not assume that everyone in an emergency is traumatized or that people who appear resilient need no support
Pay attention to gender differences	Do not use recruiting practices that severely weaken existing local structures
Build local capacities, supporting self-help and strengthening the resources already present in affected groups	Do not assume that methods from abroad are necessarily better or impose them on local people in ways that marginalize local supportive practices and beliefs
Establish effective systems for referring and supporting severely affected people	Do not focus solely on clinical activities in the absence of a multi-sectoral response

and community supports, and focused person-to-person interventions by community level workers, health providers and primary care personnel, nurses, doctors, trained in techniques such as Psychological First Aid (PFA) [17], compassionate listening, mindfulness techniques, and hope modules [7].

IASC Guidelines is at heart an ethical document. Organized around core ethical principles (teleological, goal-based), it goes on to offer specific do's and don'ts (deontological, rule-based) (Table 1.4). Some examples illustrate the application of specific recommendations to the core principles (Modified after [8]):

One of the key principles of global mental health has come to be known as "cultural competence," the recognition that not all cultures value the same things. Often, we become aware of cultural differences in situations of personal or cultural conflict (sometimes armed conflict between nations, or even wars). It is thus one of the tasks of ethics to try to understand those conflicts in order to mitigate them.

Western cultures (particularly since the latter half of the twentieth century) have tended to prioritize autonomy of the individual, the right to self-determination, as a key ethical precept. Individual autonomy is the basis for the requirement of informed consent for medical procedures or participation in research involving human subjects (Loue, this volume). But autonomy is often in tension with the principles of beneficence (beneficent paternalism) of traditional cultures, where decisions are more likely to be made by family or community elders. Such social cohesion may be a source of support and resilience, or it may be a source of constraint. Physicians in the Hippocratic tradition may adhere to the priority of the principle of beneficence, whereas philosophers and bioethicists often give priority to patient autonomy.

Of course, "Do No Harm" is important everywhere (principle of non-maleficence), but best intentions often have unintended consequences. Justice is often overlooked or misunderstood or taken for granted. Justice is sometimes understood as fairness, likes treated as likes, but the word "justice" may be used to signify punishment, vengeance, or getting even. Health disparities and inequities may be ways of calling into focus issues of justice and injustice.

Health professionals, those offering specialized care at the pinnacle of the IASC Pyramid (doctors, nurses, psychologists, and social workers) will be schooled in the ethical norms of their professional groups, codified in Hippocratic-like statements. These codes encompass the usual settings in which these professionals might work, such as hospitals, clinics, or offices. In emergency settings, these professionals may volunteer for short stints or be hired for longer assignments, working with multidisciplinary teams, in settings which are often beset with urgency and may in fact be chaotic. IASC Guidelines provide a useful framework and guidance.

Accountability in the IASC Guidelines shifts from the aspirational and idealistic goals of the individual professional or community worker to accountability of the organization employing them [3]. Recently the Interagency Standing Committee has issued a Common Framework for Monitoring and Evaluation (M&E) ([9]). The Common Framework has the goal of "reducing suffering and improving mental health and psycho-social wellbeing with specific outcomes for both Community-focused and Person-focused interventions." Individual practitioners/providers may be motivated by altruistic goals, but humanitarian organizations must be held accountable for delivering specific "deliverables," and they have a responsibility to hold the workers to standards that are clearly and explicitly identified.

Globalization and the Humanitarian Imperative

Global health, global mental health, and global well-being can only be imagined in the context of an increasingly interdependent world. Global mental health often implies an attempt to address the mental health needs of people in lower middle-income countries (LMIC) adapting approaches and understandings of more developed nations [10]. Embedded in this understanding are economic considerations of value that transcend national boundaries and national resources. Here we are using the hyphenated term inter-national to highlight issues that arise between nation-states using the term globalization as the more apt descriptor of what once was loosely described as "international." *Globalization* is used to describe the growing interdependence of the world's economies, cultures, and populations, brought about by cross-border trade in goods and services, technology, and flows of investment, people, and information [14]. Global disasters, both natural disasters such as earthquakes, hurricanes, and floods and human-made conflicts such as wars, impact persons, families, and communities – and nations – beyond the ability of local resources to sustain the needs of their populations. In such instances, others *from elsewhere* may feel moved to respond in whatever ways they can. This response may be in the form of economic assistance, or volunteer activities on the ground. Or it may be in more systematic policy responses at a national level (such as foreign assistance), international level (through nongovernmental organizations), or transnational level, such as through organizations like the United Nations or World Health Organization. These activities are inherently ethical in the recognition that human beings have certain needs simply by virtue of being human. These needs might be construed in ethical terms as rights, human rights, and it remains to be specified what these rights are and who will recognize them as ethical imperatives.

One might try to imagine the perfect economic system, where justice and fairness would assure people across the globe with at least a modicum of dignity and essential needs. Echoing Freud's *Civilization and its Discontents*, which suggested that our misery stems from the constraints that civilization imposes on us, economists of different stripes see the emergence of global economies as increasing human misery or deepening the gap between the very wealthy and the very poor. Nobel Prize-winning economist Joseph Stiglitz (*Globalization and its Discontents*) sees economic development in the so-called Third World as the path to the alleviation of human suffering [18]. Burbach et al. [1] in a book of the same title, *Globalization and its Discontents*, suggest that the solution lies in "post-modern socialisms," recognizing diversity, multiculturalism, plurality of religions, lifestyles, identities, and discourses. Notwithstanding general theories, greater attention is needed as to the particular needs of individuals, families, and communities. In an economic sense, globalization of trade between nations, however imperfect or inequitable, promotes stable markets and hence mitigates if not alleviates the likelihood of conflicts among nations.

Globalization is thus a recognition that nation-states may not meet the needs of their populations, or they may not be able to. Lack of resources, overpopulation, food insecurity, and climate inhospitality may all contribute to human suffering. Fragile states and authoritarian leaders may inflict suffering on their populations by self-dealing, grifting, economic deprivation, poverty, other forms of exploitation, as well as conflicts pitting one group against another, or one nation against another. The desire for freedom runs deep in the human spirit – basically economic development is seen as a path to freedom [16].

Development implies a trajectory from what is or was to what might or should become. In economic terms, development implies a trajectory from poverty and deprivation to sufficiency (not necessarily wealth). Development is also a psychological term, the trajectory from the psychological dependency to the psychological independence, freedoms of choice that accompany adult rationality. That adult autonomy is, of course, not unconstrained. It may be constrained by unconscious compulsions, conformity to the expectations of others, authority figures, or in a broader sense the norms of one's culture. But ultimately freedom is constrained by economic circumstances. "Global" mental health, focusing on lower middle-income countries (LMIC), uses economic metrics (particularly disease-adjusted life years, DALYs) to justify the humanitarian need for attention to mental suffering. The high rates of depression worldwide reduce economic productivity, and conversely poverty contributes to the high rates of depression. Thus, economic "freedom" and psychological "autonomy" are inextricably linked. They are both ways of talking about fundamental human values.

Human Rights, the Rights That Accompany Being Human

Human rights are "those rights which are inherent to the human being." The modern human rights movement developed after the Second World War with the adoption by the United Nations in 1948 of the Universal Declaration of Human Rights. Negatively inspired by the horrific injustices of the Second World War – extreme violations of human rights – the UN Declaration of Human Rights is an affirmative statement that was intended to be transnational, going beyond the laws of politics of individual nations. The UN Declaration of Human Rights led to the adoption of treaties and other sources of law "protecting individuals and groups against actions which interfere with fundamental freedoms and human dignity." Human rights encompass civil, cultural, economic, political, and social rights. Structuring human rights through a legal framework means that governments (national state entities) have an affirmative moral and legal obligation to respect, protect, and fulfill human rights. The obligation means that governments must not interfere, directly or indirectly, with individuals' enjoyment of human rights. The obligation to protect human rights is understood to mean that a government has a duty to prevent third parties from interfering with individuals' enjoyment of human rights. This obligation requires governments to adopt legal, budgetary, and other measures to ensure that individuals' human rights are fully realized.

Although relatively modern in institutional and inter-national terms, the concept of rights has theological roots that can be traced to various religious precepts and texts. English constitutional law, for example, incorporates rights of citizens, and the US Declaration of Independence speaks of inalienable (or unalienable) rights, rights that people are endowed with by their Creator, rights that are held to be "self-evident." Among these are life, liberty, and the pursuit of happiness, and the Bill of Rights (the first ten amendments to the US Constitution) identifies others including political participation, freedom of speech, freedom of religion, separation of church and state, and protections of persons and property.

Human rights statements are of necessity broad and sometimes vague, idealistic and aspirational, often not realized, particularly when it comes to issues of health and especially mental health, and controversial in many areas such as reproductive

Table 1.5 Human rights declarations for physicians

Nuremberg Code (Trials of War Criminals, 1949) voluntary consent is essential using human subjects in research
World Medical Association *Declaration of Geneva* (1948) similar to Hippocratic Oath
World Medical Association *Declaration of Helsinki* (1964) concerns biomedical research involving human subjects
WPA *Declaration of Hawaii* (1977) concerns the political "abuse" of psychiatry, using psychiatric facilities to detail political dissenters
Declaration of Madrid (1996) euthanasia, torture, death penalty, sex selection, organ transplantation
World Psychiatric Association *Declaration of Hamburg* (1999) genetic research and counseling, discrimination on ethnic or cultural grounds, psychiatrists addressing the media

freedom or reproductive health. However, particular nation-states might choose to follow or avoid the enshrinement of human rights laws or treaties; the moral principles are transnational. That is to say, human rights are global. Table 1.5 lists important codes and declarations which articulate and specify guiding principles for physicians.

Global Health, Public Health, Global Psychiatry, and Mental Health: A Complex Inter-relationship

Issues of global mental health and well-being cannot be reduced to diagnostic categories and treatments. They are inextricably tied to issues of public health, human rights, and justice. Conversely mental health occupies a pivotal position between what we understand as "physical health" and public health. Social and economic determinants of health, poverty, health disparities, global pandemics, as well as wars, conflicts, natural disasters, and complex emergencies all have mental health etiological factors as well as impacts and outcomes. Psychiatry and mental health occupy a unique position between the physical and the cultural. Accordingly, they provide a bridging opportunity and reciprocally face unique challenges. First of all, there is a *paucity of resources* to enable and support psychiatric care abroad and a greater demand for psychiatric healthcare professionals. *Language barriers* may make understanding nuance more difficult. Psychological understandings may be shaped by spirituality or other belief systems. Longitudinal treatment is often an important part of psychological care, which often places more emphasis on care than cure. And finally, the effects of mental illness are often intangible.

Values held to be important in healthcare – such as autonomy, fairness, equity, compassion, honesty, freedom, solidarity, trust, and respect – seen from the perspective of the individual practitioner or professional organization map closely with the key ethical issues in public health: harm prevention, public good, and individual liberty, health promotion, health surveillance, and prevention.

Conclusion

The World Health Organization long ago recognized the importance of not only biological but also psychosocial factors in illness, when it offered its significant definition of health as "bio-psycho-social well-being, not just the absence of disease" [22]. Since the WHO declaration of 1946, humans have experienced an unrelenting series of emergencies: the dislocation of populations, the foundering of borders, the lowering of economic prospects, and the vanishing of the comforts of family and home, all the while discovering that their technical triumphs have now made an enemy of the sun. The experience does not discredit the affirmation of 1946, but calls for a deepening of the bond between the "bio-psycho-social" factors in human well-being. The artificial distinction between health and mental health obscures rather than clarifies the integral relationship of mind and body. There is no real difference between health and mental health. Health is health. The bio-psychosocial and spiritual approach is not just a good idea; it is a reality based on an increasing body of scientific evidence [19]. The challenge now is to apply that knowledge to practice in both resource-rich and resource-poor settings. "Global" health is not just about health somewhere else. "Global" in this sense means "comprehensive."

References

1. Burbach, R., Nuñez, O., & Kagarlitsky, B. (1997). *Globalization and its discontents*. London, Chicago: Pluto Press.
2. Candilis, P., Dyer, A. R., Noorani, F., Ghabra, M., May, C., Dhumd, S., & Kocher, E. (2018). *The Hippocratic Oath for humanitarian aid workers*. Pharos of Alpha Omega Alpha.
3. Cherepanov, E. (2018). *Ethics for global mental health: from good intentions to humanitarian accountability*. New York: Routledge.
4. Dyer, A. R. (1988). *Ethics and psychiatry: Toward professional definition*. Washington, DC: American Psychiatric Press, Inc.
5. Edelstein, L. (1943). The Hippocratic oath: Text, translation and interpretation, p. 56. ISBN 978-0-8018-0184-6.
6. Frankena, W. K. Ethics. 2nd ed. Published November 11th 1988 by Pearson (first published 1963). ISBN 0132904780 (ISBN13: 9780132904780).
7. Griffith, J. (2018). Hope modules: Brief psychotherapeutic interventions to counter demoralization from daily stressors of chronic illness. *Academic Psychiatry, 42*(1), 135–145. https://doi.org/10.1007/s40596-017-0748-7.
8. Interagency Standing Committee. (2007). *2007 IASC guidelines on mental health and psychosocial support in emergency settings*. Geneva: WHO.
9. IASC. (2019). Common framework for monitoring and evaluation.
10. Kaplan, J. P., Bond, T. C., Merson, M. H., Reddy, K. S., Rodriguez, M. H., Swankambo, M. K., & Wasserheit JN for the Consortium of Universities for global Health Executive Board. (2009). Towards a common definition of global health. *Lancet, 373*, 1993–1995.
11. Kohlberg, L. The philosophy of moral development: Moral stages and the idea of justice (Essays on moral development, volume 1) Published July 1st 1981 by Harper & Row. ISBN 0060647604 (ISBN13: 9780060647605).
12. Maslow, A. H. (1943). A theory of human motivation. *Psychological Review, 50*(4), 370–396. CiteSeerX 10.1.1.334.7586. https://doi.org/10.1037/h0054346.

13. May, W. F. (1992). The beleaguered rulers: The public obligation of the professional. *Kennedy Institute of Ethics Journal, 2*(1), 25–41.
14. Peterson Institute of International Economics. https://www.piie.com/microsites/globalization/what-is-globalization. Accessed 18 Nov 2020.
15. Piaget, J. The moral judgment of the child. Published December 16th 1997 by Free Press (first published 1932 Le jugement moral chez l'enfant) ISBN 0684833301 (ISBN13: 9780684833309).
16. Sen, A. (2000). *Development as freedom*. Oxford: Oxford University Press.
17. Snider, L. (2011). *Psychological first aid: Guide for field workers, World Health Organization, War Trauma Foundation and World Vision International*. Geneva: WHO.
18. Stiglitz, J. (2002). *Globalization and its discontents*. New York, London: Norton.
19. Tol ,W. A., Barbui, C., Galappatti, A., Silove, D., Betancourt, T. S., Souza, R., Golaz, A., & Van Ommeren, M. (2011). Mental health and psychosocial support in humanitarian settings: linking practice and research. *Lancet*. Author manuscript; available in PMC 2014 Apr 14. Published in final edited form as: *Lancet, 378*(9802):1581–91. Published online 2011 Oct 16. https://doi.org/10.1016/S0140-6736(11)61094-5. PMCID: PMC3985411 NIHMSID: NIHMS568164 PMID: 22008428.
20. Freud, Sigmund (1923). The Ego and the Id and Other Works. The Standard Edition of the Complete Psychological Works of Sigmund Freud. XIX. Hogarth Press.
21. Sorel, E. (2013) (Ed.) 21st Century Global Mental Health. Burlington, MA: Jones and Bartlett Learning.
22. World Health Organization. (2006). Constitution of the World Health Organization – Basic Documents, Forty-fifth edition, Supplement, October 2006, Geneva: World Health Organization.

Historical Origins of Global Mental Health

2

Brandon A. Kohrt

To understand the current ethical dilemmas in global mental health, it is important to have a historical perspective. There is a legacy of colonialism that has shaped power imbalances and contributed to the unethical practices that continue today in global mental health [111]. In this chapter, we explore global mental health's origins in colonialism and capitalism and the ramifications of those historical trajectories in today's practice. Global health is rooted in tropical medicine to support the British Empire and other Western powers and subsequent economic expansions and political control into the twenty-first century [73]. As Western powers expanded around the world, colonial administrations built asylums starting in the 1700s with some of these institutions continuing through the twentieth century. Many of the "Lunacy Acts" established during colonial governments have shaped mental health policy in low- and middle-income countries (LMIC) until today.

Within Europe, the end of the nineteenth century was a period of rapid growth and transformation in the fields of study that have led to modern psychiatry and neurology. Attention was focused on biological causes of mental and neurological conditions, and this was the era of German scientific leaders who have shaped much of the current practices. This included Kraepelin, Alzheimer, Nissl, and others [92]. However, the era was strongly rooted in perspectives of evolution and Social Darwinism at the time, with the populations in European colonies often characterized as being cognitively primitive.

During the centuries of colonialism, while there was no shortage of disparaging the behaviors and customs of colonized populations, most non-Western groups were considered not sufficiently evolved to have the privilege of suffering from mental illness [63]. A question that emerged at that period—and still has echoed today—is whether neuropsychiatric conditions are universal. In 1898, the British anthropologist Charles Seligman and physician-anthropologist W. H. R. Rivers were part of

B. A. Kohrt (✉)
Division of Global Mental Health, George Washington University, Washington, DC, USA
e-mail: bkohrt@email.gwu.edu

© Springer Nature Switzerland AG 2021
A. R. Dyer et al. (eds.), *Global Mental Health Ethics*,
https://doi.org/10.1007/978-3-030-66296-7_2

Cambridge University expedition to the Torres Strait between Papua New Guinea and Australia [63]. The pair studied cross-cultural differences in varied concepts ranging from kinship to perceptions of color to healing practices [88]. When Seligman tried to find signs of mental illness in this population, he concluded that it was absent in large part from the Torres Strait islanders. This interpretation shaped much of colonial psychiatry going forward by setting a foundation that continued through the twentieth century that "uncivilized" populations were less likely to manifest mental illness. Not all work at this time was dismissive of mental illness in non-European people. For example, Rivers drew upon his experience with traditional healers in the Torres Strait to influence his approach to treating British soldiers with neuropsychiatric conditions during World War I [52]. He demonsted that observing healing practices in other cultures has the potential to inform practices in Western biomedicine. In some way, Rivers foreshadowed current practices of adopting mindfulness, dialectical thinking, and other practices from non-Western groups to inform treatments that have become acceptable to biomedical psychiatry.

A contemporary of Rivers and Seligman was the German psychiatrist Emile Kraepelin. Although Kraepelin is widely known for establishing diagnostic practices that are still reflected in the Diagnostic and Statistical Manual of Mental Disorders (DSM) today, it is less commonly known that he was interested in and conducted cross-cultural work in mental health [44]. Prior to World War I, he visited a Dutch asylum in Jakarta. There he observed Javanese patients to determine if they demonstrated similar symptoms to persons with mental illness whom he studied in Germany. Kraepelin also traveled to North America after World War I, where he conducted cross-cultural psychiatry research with Caribbean, Native American, and African American populations. Although Kraepelin's own writings highlighted the role of social groups, he also maintained that different stages of modernization across societies influenced the presentation of mental illness.

Similarly, during the early twentieth century, anthropological research was often utilized as a tool for colonial management. Anthropology in the 1920–1930s supported colonial concepts of cognitive "primitivism," which was often a justification for political exploitation [12]. Lucien Lévy-Bruhl, a French anthropologist, described the "primitive mind," i.e., the "other" is deficient, in mentality and pre-logical thought. In contrast, Franz Boas, a leading figure in early American anthropology, suggested that these mental differences were culturally learned patterns of thought and not a reflection of biological differences in brain size or shape.

Another legacy of colonialism was efforts to characterize groups and nations as having a "modal personality," i.e., each culture has a particular constellation that could be used to predict general behavior of that group. These were often superficial external generalizations that one Native American tribe was more narcissistic and another more paranoid. This work grew, in part, in the first half of the twentieth century when psychiatrists and anthropologists also applied the work of Sigmund Freud and others in the psychoanalysis movement to understanding non-Western cultures. This field, "Culture and Personality," arose in the United States between World Wars I and II, as combination of psychoanalysis and anthropology [13, 60]. For example, in her book *Patterns of Culture*, Ruth Benedict [8] classified the modal personalities of different cultural groups as paranoid, megalomaniacal, Apollonian, and Dionysian. Benedict's discussion of "tradition" resembled Freud's discussion of culture as group neurosis. Freudian anxiety theories describe how anxiety motivates behaviors differently across cultures. His work contributed to the beginning of ethnopsychology, advancing the study of self, human nature, and motivation within particular cultural contexts [41].

There were also early studies that challenged Western cultural assumptions and drew upon the functioning of colonialized societies to reflect upon the colonizers' worldview and social norms. Margaret Mead's ethnography on gender and culture [66] examined how males and females were shaped by their societies and cultural ideals. Her work was instrumental in challenging normative assumptions around gender and sexuality. From a mental health perspective, this also introduced how gender norms could be a major contributor to psychological distress. The creation of gendered identities is a case in point, and Mead's book *Sex and Temperament in Three Primitive Societies* (1935) clearly illustrated gender variations [112].

One challenge to universalist assumptions was the Transcultural Psychiatry movement, which began in the 1950s with the work of Wittkower, Prince, the Murphys, and others at McGill University in Montreal [67, 68, 83, 101]. Some aspects of this group took Western psychiatric categories as a starting point, then critically evaluated their presentation and relevance in other cultural contexts and populations. The World Health Organization (WHO)'s *International Pilot Study on Schizophrenia* employed a similar framework, reaching a general conclusion that schizophrenia generally appears the same across all cultures, with similar findings identified in three successive studies, but noting differences in prognosis across cultures and settings [23, 42, 58, 89, 90, 102]. Medical anthropologists have criticized the study for downplaying the cultural differences in course, particularly the lower prevalence of chronic schizophrenia in non-industrial settings [49]. There has also been a critique that these cross-national studies have not led to refinement of diagnostic and conceptual models incorporating these global findings. This was in part due to methodological problems in the cross-national studies but also due to potential biases that Western presentations and prognosis are the norm and that other cultures represent deviations from the core European-American prototype [20, 30, 75].

The role of social, political, economic, and health institutions in shaping cultural expectations and subsequently professionalized clinical categories of mental illness has been important to research in medical anthropology and cultural psychiatry [61, 62]. Anthropologists examined the unconscious aspects both in the training of psychiatrists and their subjective cultural assumptions built into patterns of diagnosis and patient interaction. Anthropologists have critiqued the DSM suggesting that diagnostic categories are more driven by politics and economics—most notably by pharmaceutical companies more than by a neutral scientific march forward of knowledge. The critique of psychiatry as being blind to its own cultural assumptions and its use as an instrument of social control by a hegemonic state apparatus has a long intellectual history. These critiques of Western psychiatry grew out of postmodern scholars and the anti-psychiatry movement.

The French philosopher Michel Foucault critiqued how psychiatry was more focused on control than healing, with the structure of the asylum focused on creating a sense of ubiquitous observation—referred to as the *panopticon* [36]. Foucault's contemporaries, the Hungarian psychiatrist Thomas Szasz and British psychiatrist R.D. Laing, attacked conceptualizations of mental illness in the twentieth century [56, 57, 97]. As the anti-psychiatry movement burgeoned, the asylum movement was beginning to wane in the United States following President Kennedy's 1963 Community Mental Health Centers Act. Many institutions were closed or greatly reduced in size, and individuals went to live with families or back in the community. But the majority went to nursing homes, board and care centers, or jails and prisons, or they became homeless, as few resources were provided for deinstitutionalization [93]. One of the consequences of the anti-psychiatry movement is that it continued the same anti-intervention mode of colonial psychiatry. While anti-psychiatry proponents aspired to challenge the politicized nature of psychiatry, it did not advance approaches to reduce suffering around the world.

An alternative approach to the anti-psychiatry movement developed in Europe in the 1960s and 1970s through the Italian psychiatrist Franco Basaglia, who defined mental illness as a breach of values characterized by a functional disability to participate in social life [6]. He viewed mental illness from the perspective of social and living conditions. His work led to the closing of asylums in Italy and the development of a national community-based mental health system. Lovell and Scheper-Hughes [64] write that the Italian deinstitutionalization program was significantly different than the US one. The US model of deinstitutionalization was motivated by financial rather than ideological values; the government, as exemplified by then Governor Ronald Reagan's policies, shifted the economic burden onto families and communities freeing up state and national coffers. In contrast, Basaglia's model developed 24-hour community centers which were all voluntary and supported by local government. Ultimately, Lovell and Scheper-Hughes [64] state that deinstitutionalization did not fail in the US; "it was simply never really attempted" (p. 43).

The 1970s also witnessed the introduction of the *new cross-cultural psychiatry* developed by Arthur Kleinman, Byron Good, Mary-Jo Delvecchio Good, and colleagues trained through Harvard University's social medicine program [51, 53]. Kleinman explored the relationship of depression to somatic symptoms in the context of neurasthenia in China and Taiwan [54]. He explored conceptual models that framed somatic presentations in the context of social suffering, in particular experiences in the Cultural Revolution in China. Kleinman's subsequent work and collaborations focused on this issue of social origins of suffering, stigma, and morality, including the role of medical systems in shaping trajectories of suffering [50, 52]. Work on embodiment and how social suffering is manifest and expressed reflected similar interests [24]. The research on social suffering also built upon the Norwegian scholar Johan Galtung's writings on structural violence [39]. Ultimately, through the work of Kleinman's students Paul Farmer and Jim Kim, the importance of structural violence became a central focus in global health research [33, 34].

Anthropologists have also conducted ethnographies of the mentally ill in Western settings of Europe and North America. Nancy Scheper-Hughes [91] worked in Ireland combining techniques of basic and modal personality studies with historical ethnography examining the influence of Christian conversion in schizophrenia. Sue

Estroff [31] lived with the new populations of the mentally ill residing in commu-nity settings in the late 1970s. She found that the individuals were underserved and lived in contradictory worlds with altered time, space, and resources. Lorna Rhodes [87] documented the experience of patients and staff in a psychiatric emergency room. Allan Young [107] drew upon historical accounts to understand how the PTSD diagnosis originated in the 1970s in a process that retconned psychiatric models of trauma.

Tanya Luhrmann's [65] ethnography of a residency program outlines the death of psychodynamic psychiatry at the hands of managed care. Luhrmann also sug-gests that pharmacology reifies the categorical approach to psychiatry, and the phar-maceutical industry controls academic training including residency curriculums and professional society meetings. These works signal a move away from the distant accounts of psychiatrists and sociologists to experience-near ethnography, and it lays the groundwork for a transition from focusing on deviance to addressing suffer-ing. Their work also illustrates that Western psychiatry can be analyzed and decon-structed in the same fashion as folk psychiatries. Atwood Gaines [38] codifies this by defining the "new ethnopsychiatry" as a study which views all psychiatric and mental health classification and treatment systems as cultural constructions. There is increasing attention to the power of managed care in the US and pharmaceutical companies throughout the world in providing under- and overaccess to care. Including the role of pharmaceutical companies in frames of distress and recovery [48, 65]. Other anthropological critiques of Western psychiatry include Richard Grinker's descriptions of autism from a global perspective [40].

Other anthropologists critiqued the exportation of Western psychiatric labels and treatment in non-Western settings. It is argued that this exportation process is largely driven by the pharmaceutical industry in an attempt to "manufacture" illness to sell more medication. Others argue that it is unclear whether this gap represents a real need or simply an untapped market. Kirmayer [47] has examined the rapid rise in pharmaceutical use in Japan, which was preceded by much reticence to use or pre-scribe antidepressants. In response to this reticence, the idiom *kokoro no kaze* (cold of the soul) was used by pharmaceutical companies to reframe depression to fit into existing notions of self and illness. The influence of pharmaceutical companies in the development of psychiatric classifications, application of these labels, and gen-eration of "evidence" for treatment practices also has received considerable critical attention [4, 5, 9, 28, 29, 81].

For the majority of the twentieth century, Western institutions supported research on LMIC, often at the nexus of psychiatry and anthropology, but there was a glaring void in support and investment in mental health services and services research. It was acceptable to observe, but the moral imperative to engage, dialogue, and sup-port health systems and social change was mostly absent with the exception of ini-tiatives such as the WHO Primary Health Care (PHC) strategy adopted in 1978. The WHO attempted to raise awareness through a major report entitled "Mental Health Collaborative Study for Strategies on Extending Mental Health Care" [108]. This report proposed the integration of mental health activities into the duties of com-munity health workers. Similar WHO studies proposed the incorporation of traditional medical practitioners into PHC [109] although this idea was met with considerable critique. Attention to the scope of the global mental health problem was revived with the publication of *World Mental Health* [110].

A transformation in the field was signaled by the 2001 *World Health Report* entitled *Mental Health: New Understanding, New Hope*, which outlined the state of the mental health around the world and proposed key steps forward [103]. Other developments include the 2007 *Lancet* series *Global Mental Health* with the rallying call that there can be "no health without mental health" [82]. This was followed by a series of packages of care in *PLoS Medicine* [79]. In 2010, the WHO released the *mental health Gap Action Programme (mhGAP)-Intervention Guide* [105] which built upon some of the lessons learned from the work in the 1970s–1980s, but was more diagnostic-focused; it has now been disseminated in more than 90 countries [106].

In 2014, global mental health was defined as "an area for study, research and practice that places a priority on improving *mental* health and achieving equity in *mental* health for all people worldwide" [77]. Broadly, this global mental health movement has the mission to reduce the gap between the burden of mental illness and the availability of effective mental health services. This mission entails advocating for increased funding for mental health services and personnel, expanding research to develop evidence-based practices for LMICs and low-resource settings, developing government mental health policies, and advancing the rights of persons with mental illness [22, 27, 76, 105]. The global mental health field includes clinicians, government policy makers, public health researchers, mental health consumers, and members of development agencies and the World Health Organization (WHO). The formal Movement for Global Mental Health (MGMH) emerged from the 2007 *Lancet* call to action on scaling up global mental health.

MGMH practitioners and researchers emphasize the pressing need for improving access to mental health services in LMICs to address the shortage of 1.2 million healthcare providers needed to deliver adequate services [46]. This has led to support for the concept of *task sharing* as a mental healthcare delivery solution. Task sharing, also referred to as task shifting, is the process of training primary care and community health workers to assume some healthcare responsibilities traditionally delivered by specialists [104, 105]. The field of global mental health has largely utilized strategies in implementation, advocacy, policy development, and task shifting from the global public health approach to combating HIV/AIDS. This can be seen in the pivotal role of the MGMH, NIH's Grand Challenges in Global Mental Health [21, 22], the United Kingdom's Department for International Development, Grand Challenges Canada, and the Global Alliance for Chronic Disease.

In addition to mhGAP's primary care diagnostic and predominantly pharmacological management, there has been a concerted effort to evaluate and expand psychological interventions globally [32]. These psychological interventions use non-specialists as the cadre of trainees [55, 94], which are typically community health volunteers. In India, there are more than 2 million community health workers (CHWs), including Anganwadi (rural childcare) workers, accredited social health activists (ASHAs), and auxiliary nurse midwives; at a population level, this is 1 CHW per 1000 people [1]. In Ethiopia, there are more than 40,000 health extension workers: 1 per 2500 people. There are more than 3000 in Haiti: 1 per 3000 people; and there are similar ratios in Nigeria, Mozambique, and the Philippines.

Other persons trained to deliver these psychological interventions are teachers, nurses, laypersons in refugee camps, informal or traditional birth attendants, law enforcement officers, religious leaders, and family members. There is an initiative in Uganda to train teachers to address mental health needs of more than 3000 students, and, if successful, to scale the program nationwide [95]. In Liberia, an initiative is underway to train representative officers at every police depot in the country to assure Crisis Intervention Team (CIT) collaborations for law enforcement and mental health clinicians reach the national population of more than four million people [11]. Since in all countries law enforcement is a principal point of contact between the mentally ill and society's institutions, educating police officers about mental illness will likely be critical.

These interventions are designed using core components of psychological treatment classes, such as interpersonal psychotherapy (IPT), cognitive behavioral therapy (CBT), behavioral activation (BA), motivational enhancement, and trauma-focused techniques. Examples of non-specialist psychological treatments include the Thinking Healthy Program, a version of CBT for peripartum women in Pakistan [86], including a peer-delivered version in India and Pakistan [37, 93]; the Healthy Activity Program, a modified version of behavioral activation for depression in India [80]; Counseling for Alcohol Problems, a modified version of motivational enhancement for alcohol use disorder in India [71]; the Friendship Bench in Zimbabwe, which includes individual and group components built on problem-solving [17]; Problem Management Plus (PM+), also a problem-solving approach effective in individual and group formats in Pakistan [84, 85]; cognitive processing therapy for survivors of sexual violence in the Democratic Republic of Congo [7]; and group IPT for adults, adolescents, and specific vulnerable populations in Uganda [14, 15, 70]. For children and adolescents, examples include trauma-focused CBT in Zambia [69], Classroom-Based Interventions in post-conflict settings [45], and group-based psychosocial interventions based on psychosocial support and stress alleviation [74]. There has also been development of a common elements treatment approach (CETA) that is transdiagnostic and includes multiple psychological treatment classes [16, 100]. In addition, a version of guided self-help, Self-Help Plus (SH+), has also been developed [99]. As of 2017, there were 25 RCTs of psychological interventions with a pooled moderate effect size (0.49) for common mental disorders [94].

In 2016, the World Bank held their first meeting dedicated to mental health, *Out of the Shadows: Making Mental Health a Global Priority*, which included dissemination of findings that $1 of economic support for depression and anxiety care yields $4 to $5 return on investment [18]. In 2018, the United Kingdom hosted the first global ministerial mental health summit, bringing together politicians and service users from around the world to encourage global efforts of taking on the burden of mental illness. This also coincided with the release of *The Lancet Commission on*

Global Mental Health and Sustainable Development Goals [78]. In recent years, the Canadian government, UK Department for International Development, and other members of the Global Alliance for Chronic Disease have made significant investments into research to inform mental health services and innovative solutions. LMICs such as Ghana have also begun making great strides in passing mental health services legislation and investigating innovative implementation solutions to contextual challenges [2, 26, 72].

The attention in recent years on LMICs has coincided with a growing recognition that most high-income countries also have large swaths of the population who go without treatment, especially in rural areas and among cultural and ethnic minorities [3, 25, 43, 98]. Global mental health has been amassing evidence in numerous areas, ranging from demonstrating effectiveness for non-specialists delivering psychological treatments to innovations in technology to new approaches for dissemination and implementation [78, 94].

There have been a range of critiques of the current incarnation of global mental health [96]. Patel [77], in a response to these critiques, categorizes them into four categories: psychiatric diagnostic categories are not valid cross-culturally; biomedical interventions have a limited role for socially determined health problems; pharmaceutical companies drive the agenda and practice for the global mental health movement; and global mental health is a form of medical imperialism. At a conceptual level, the critiques of global mental health relate to power, knowledge, and practice: for example, who has the authority to generate knowledge and evidence? What forces endow different systems of knowledge with greater power for dissemination and implementation? Who within healthcare systems and beneficiary communities is culturally authorized to provide feedback and critique in reshaping practice? How is such feedback provided and incorporated into practice, and ultimately? What medical, social, and economic ends are served by cross-cultural, international, and global efforts in psychiatry? These debates are not unique to global *mental* health, as global health struggles with similar challenges regarding power relations in diagnostic labeling, practice, policy, and funding [10, 35].

There are continued efforts to develop a DSM that is more transparent about the cultural assumptions and biases that shape mental health categorization. With the revision of the DSM-5, the goal is to provide more context on the populations from whom diagnostic criteria are developed to help highlight that many of the symptom framings are based on relatively small slices of the human population excluding much of the global diversity. More recent research by biocultural anthropologists, critical cultural neuroscientists, and neuroanthropologists—as well psychiatric geneticists—has demonstrated that the traditional split between pathogenic and pathoplastic is not consistent with research on the origins and mechanisms of mental illness [19, 59]. Instead, processes traditionally labeled as culture and biology are constantly in transaction to shape one another, thus driving emotion, behavior, and cognition. Concepts such as bio-looping illustrate that culturally shaped perception drives biological processes. Kirmayer [48] has framed the relationship as "culture is a product of biology" in that biological processes determine what is perceived, learned, and transmitted from individual or generation to another, and "biology is a product of culture" in that what is referred to as biology is a cultural construct with specific presumptions about what does and does not comprise biology.

Ultimately, it is important to understand the historical legacy of practices and theories that were tied to knowledge and politics at the time. No scientific theory or medical practice is independent of the sociocultural processes when they are developed. Going forward, understanding this history will guide practices to create a more equitable global mental health practice.

References

1. Advancing Partners & Communities. (2019). *Community health systems catalog*. Retrieved from https://www.advancingpartners.org/resources/chsc.
2. Ae-Ngibise, K., Cooper, S., Adiibokah, E., Akpalu, B., Lund, C., Doku, V., & The, M. R. P. C. (2010). 'Whether you like it or not people with mental problems are going to go to them': A qualitative exploration into the widespread use of traditional and faith healers in the provision of mental health care in Ghana. *International Review of Psychiatry, 22*(6), 558–567. https://doi.org/10.3109/09540261.2010.536149.
3. Alonso, J., Liu, Z., Evans-Lacko, S., Sadikova, E., Sampson, N., Chatterji, S., et al. (2018). Treatment gap for anxiety disorders is global: Results of the world mental health surveys in 21 countries. *Depression and Anxiety, 35*(3), 195–208. https://doi.org/10.1002/da.22711.
4. Applbaum, K. (2009). Getting to yes: Corporate power and the creation of a psychopharmaceutical blockbuster. *Culture, Medicine and Psychiatry, 33*(2), 185–215. https://doi.org/10.1007/s11013-009-9129-3.
5. Applbaum, K. (2010). Shadow science: Zyprexa, Eli Lilly and the globalization of pharmaceutical damage control. *BioSocieties, 5*(2), 236–255. https://doi.org/10.1057/biosoc.2010.5.
6. Basaglia, F., Lovell, A., & Scheper-Hughes, N. (1987). *Psychiatry inside out: Selected writings of Franco Basaglia*. New York: Columbia University Press.
7. Bass, J. K., Annan, J., McIvor Murray, S., Kaysen, D., Griffiths, S., Cetinoglu, T., et al. (2013). Controlled trial of psychotherapy for congolese survivors of sexual violence. *The New England Journal of Medicine, 368*(23), 2182–2191.
8. Benedict, R. (1934). *Patterns of culture*. Boston: Houghton Mifflin.
9. Biehl, J. (2004). Life of the mind: The interface of psychopharmaceuticals, domestic economies, and social abandonment. *American Ethnologist, 31*(4), 475–496.
10. Biehl, J., & Petryna, A. (2013). *When people come first: Critical studies in global health*. Princeton: Princeton University Press.
11. Boazak, M., Kohrt, B. A., Gwaikolo, W. S., Yoss, S., Sonkarlay, S., Strode, P., et al. (2019). Law enforcement and clinician partnerships: Training of trainers for CIT teams in Liberia, West Africa. *Psychiatric Services, 70*(8), 740–743. https://doi.org/10.1176/appi.ps.201800510.
12. Bock, P. K. (1999). *Rethinking psychological anthropology: Continuity and change in the study of human action* (2nd ed.). Prospect Heights: Waveland Press.
13. Bock, P. K. (2000). Culture and personality revisited. *The American Behavioral Scientist, 44*(1), 32–40.
14. Bolton, P., Bass, J., Betancourt, T., Speelman, L., Onyango, G., Clougherty, K. F., et al. (2007). Interventions for depression symptoms among adolescent survivors of war and displacement in northern Uganda: A randomized controlled trial. *JAMA, 298*(5), 519–527.
15. Bolton, P., Bass, J., Neugebauer, R., Verdeli, H., Clougherty, K. F., Wickramaratne, P., et al. (2003). Group interpersonal psychotherapy for depression in rural Uganda: A randomized controlled trial. *JAMA, 289*(23), 3117–3124.

16. Bolton, P., Lee, C., Haroz, E. E., Murray, L., Dorsey, S., Robinson, C., et al. (2014). A trans-diagnostic community-based mental health treatment for comorbid disorders: Development and outcomes of a randomized controlled trial among Burmese refugees in Thailand. *PLoS Medicine, 11*(11), e1001757. https://doi.org/10.1371/journal.pmed.1001757.
17. Chibanda, D., Weiss, H. A., Verhey, R., et al. (2016). Effect of a primary care–based psychological intervention on symptoms of common mental disorders in Zimbabwe: A randomized clinical trial. *JAMA, 316*(24), 2618–2626. https://doi.org/10.1001/jama.2016.19102.
18. Chisholm, D., Sweeny, K., Sheehan, P., Rasmussen, B., Smit, F., Cuijpers, P., & Saxena, S. (2016). Scaling-up treatment of depression and anxiety: A global return on investment analysis. *Lancet Psychiatry, 3*(5), 415–424. https://doi.org/10.1016/S2215-0366(16)30024-4.
19. Choudhury, S., & Kirmayer, L. J. (2009). Cultural neuroscience and psychopathology: Prospects for cultural psychiatry. *Progress in Brain Research, 178*, 263–283.
20. Cohen, A. (1992). Prognosis for schizophrenia in the third world: A reevaluation of cross-cultural research. *Culture, Medicine and Psychiatry, 16*(1), 53–75.
21. Collins, P. Y., Insel, T. R., Chockalingam, A., Daar, A., & Maddox, Y. T. (2013). Grand challenges in global mental health: Integration in research, policy, and practice. *PLoS Medicine/Public Libr Sci, 10*(4), e1001434. https://doi.org/10.1371/journal.pmed.1001434.
22. Collins, P. Y., Patel, V., Joestl, S. S., March, D., Insel, T. R., Daar, A. S., et al. (2011). Grand challenges in global mental health. *Nature, 475*(7354), 27–30. https://doi.org/10.1038/475027a.
23. Craig, T. J., Siegel, C., Hopper, K., Lin, S., & Sartorius, N. (1997). Outcome in schizophrenia and related disorders compared between developing and developed countries. A recursive partitioning re-analysis of the WHO DOSMD data [see comment]. *The British Journal of Psychiatry, 170*, 229–233.
24. Csordas, T. J. (1994). *Embodiment and experience: The existential ground of culture and self.* New York: Cambridge University Press.
25. Degenhardt, L., Glantz, M., Evans-Lacko, S., Sadikova, E., Sampson, N., Thornicroft, G., et al. (2017). Estimating treatment coverage for people with substance use disorders: An analysis of data from the World Mental Health Surveys. *World Psychiatry, 16*(3), 299–307. https://doi.org/10.1002/wps.20457.
26. Doku, V. C. K., Wusu-Takyi, A., & Awakame, J. (2012). Implementing the Mental Health Act in Ghana: Any challenges ahead? *Ghana Medical Journal, 46*(4), 241–250.
27. Drew, N., Funk, M., Tang, S., Lamichhane, J., Chavez, E., Katontoka, S., et al. (2011). Human rights violations of people with mental and psychosocial disabilities: An unresolved global crisis. *Lancet, 378*(9803), 1664–1675. https://doi.org/10.1016/S0140-6736(11)61458-X.
28. Ecks, S. (2005). Pharmaceutical citizenship: Antidepressant marketing and the promise of demarginalization in India. *Anthropology & Medicine, 3*(2005), 239–254.
29. Ecks, S., & Basu, S. (2009). The unlicensed lives of antidepressants in India: Generic drugs, unqualified practitioners, and floating prescriptions. *Transcultural Psychiatry, 46*(1), 86–106. https://doi.org/10.1177/1363461509102289.
30. Edgerton, R. B., & Cohen, A. (1994). Culture and schizophrenia: The DOSMD challenge. *The British Journal of Psychiatry, 164*(2), 222–231.
31. Estroff, S. E. (1981). *Making it crazy: An ethnography of psychiatric clients in an American community.* Berkeley: University of California Press.
32. Fairburn, C. G., & Patel, V. (2014). The global dissemination of psychological treatments: A road map for research and practice. *American Journal of Psychiatry, 171*(5), 495–498.
33. Farmer, P. (2003). *Pathologies of power: Health, human rights, and the new war on the poor* (Vol. 4). Berkeley: University of California Press.
34. Farmer, P. (2004). Sidney W. Mintz Lecture for 2001 – an anthropology of structural violence. *Current Anthropology, 45*(3), 305–325.
35. Farmer, P., Kim, J., Kleinman, A., & Basilico, M. (2013). *Reimagining global health. An introduction.* Berkeley: University of California Press.
36. Foucault, M. (1965). *Madness and civilization; a history of insanity in the age of reason.* New York: Pantheon Books.

37. Fuhr, D. C., Weobong, B., Lazarus, A., Vanobberghen, F., Weiss, H. A., Singla, D. R., et al. (2019). Delivering the thinking healthy programme for perinatal depression through peers: An individually randomised controlled trial in India. *Lancet Psychiatry, 6*(2), 115–127. https://doi.org/10.1016/S2215-0366(18)30466-8.

38. Gaines, A. D. (1992). Ethnopsychiatry: The cultural construction of psychiatries. In A. D. Gaines (Ed.), *Ethnopsychiatry: The cultural construction of professional and folk psychiatries* (pp. 3–50). Albany: State University of New York Press.

39. Galtung, J. (1969). Violence, peace, and peace research. *Journal of Peace Research, 6*(3), 167–191.

40. Grinker, R. R. (2008). *Unstrange minds: Remapping the world of autism.* New York: Basic Books.

41. Hallowell, A. I. (1941). The social function of anxiety in a primitive society. In R. Littlewood & S. Dein (Eds.), *Cultural psychiatry and medical anthropology: An introduction and reader (2000)* (pp. 114–128). New Brunswick: The Athlone Press.

42. Harrison, G., Hopper, K., Craig, T., Laska, E., Siegel, C., Wanderling, J., et al. (2001). Recovery from psychotic illness: A 15- and 25-year international follow-up study. *The British Journal of Psychiatry, 178*, 506–517.

43. Hoeft, T. J., Fortney, J. C., Patel, V., & Unützer, J. (2018). Task-sharing approaches to improve mental health care in rural and other low-resource settings: A systematic review. *The Journal of Rural Health, 34*(1), 48–62. https://doi.org/10.1111/jrh.12229.

44. Jilek, W. G. (1995). Emil Kraepelin and comparative sociocultural psychiatry. *European Archives of Psychiatry and Clinical Neuroscience, 245*(4–5), 231–238. https://doi.org/10.1007/BF02191802.

45. Jordans, M. J., Tol, W. A., Susanty, D., Ntamatumba, P., Luitel, N. P., Komproe, I. H., & de Jong, J. T. (2013). Implementation of a mental health care package for children in areas of armed conflict: A case study from Burundi, Indonesia, Nepal, Sri Lanka, and Sudan. *PLoS Medicine/Public Libr Sci, 10*(1), e1001371. https://doi.org/10.1371/journal.pmed.1001371.

46. Kakuma, R., Minas, H., van Ginneken, N., Dal Poz, M. R., Desiraju, K., Morris, J. E., et al. (2011). Human resources for mental health care: Current situation and strategies for action. *Lancet, 378*(9803), 1654–1663.

47. Kirmayer, L. J. (2002). Psychopharmacology in a globalizing world: The use of antidepressants in Japan. *Transcultural Psychiatry, 39*(3), 295–322.

48. Kirmayer, L. J. (2006). Beyond the new cross-cultural psychiatry: Cultural biology, discursive psychology and the ironies of globalization. *Transcultural Psychiatry, 43*(1), 126–144.

49. Kleinman, A. (1988). *Rethinking psychiatry: From cultural category to personal experience.* New York: Free Press, Collier Macmillan.

50. Kleinman, A. (1995). *Writing at the margin: Discourse between anthropology and medicine.* Berkeley: University of California Press.

51. Kleinman, A. (1997). "Everything that really matters" + examining the convergence of medical anthropology and the study of religion: Social suffering, subjectivity, and the remaking of human experience in a disordering world. *Harvard Theological Review, 90*(3), 315–335.

52. Kleinman, A. (2006). *What really matters: Living a moral life amid uncertainty and danger.* New York: Oxford University Press.

53. Kleinman, A., & Good, B. (1985). *Culture and depression: Studies in the anthropology and cross-cultural psychiatry of affect and disorder.* Berkeley: University of California Press.

54. Kleinman, A. M. (1982). Neurasthenia and depression: A study of somatization and culture in China. *Culture, Medicine and Psychiatry, 6*, 117–190.

55. Kohrt, B., Asher, L., Bhardwaj, A., Fazel, M., Jordans, M., Mutamba, B., et al. (2018). The role of communities in mental health care in low- and middle-income countries: A meta-review of components and competencies. *International Journal of Environmental Research and Public Health, 15*(6), 1279.

56. Laing, R. D. (1970). *Self and others* (2nd rev ed.). New York: Pantheon Books.

57. Laing, R. D. (1985). *Wisdom, madness, and folly: The making of a psychiatrist.* New York: McGraw-Hill.

58. Leff, J., Sartorius, N., Jablensky, A., Korten, A., & Ernberg, G. (1992). The international pilot study of schizophrenia: Five-year follow-up findings. *Psychological Medicine, 22*(1), 131–145.
59. Lende, D. H., & Downey, G. (Eds.). (2012). *The encultured brain: An introduction to neuro-anthropology*. Cambridge, MA: MIT Press.
60. LeVine, R. A. (2001). Culture and personality studies, 1918-1960: Myth and history. *Journal of Personality, 69*(6), 803–818.
61. Littlewood, R. (1990). From categories to contexts: A decade of the 'new cross-cultural psychiatry'. *The British Journal of Psychiatry, 159*, 308–327.
62. Littlewood, R. (2002). *Pathologies of the west: An anthropology of mental illness in Europe and America*. Ithaca: Cornell University Press.
63. Littlewood, R., & Dein, S. (2000). Introduction. In R. Littlewood & S. Dein (Eds.), *Cultural psychiatry and medical anthropology: An introduction and reader* (pp. 1–34). New Brunswick: The Athlone Press.
64. Lovell, A., & Scheper-Hughes, N. (1987). Introduction. In A. Lovell & N. Scheper-Hughes (Eds.), *Psychiatry inside out: Selected writings of Franco Basaglia* (pp. 1–50). New York: Columbia University Press.
65. Luhrmann, T. M. (2000). *Of two minds: The growing disorder in American psychiatry* (1st ed.). New York: Knopf; distributed by Random House.
66. Mead, M. (1949). *Male and female: A study of the sexes in a changing world*. New York: W. Morrow.
67. Murphy, H. B., Wittkower, E. D., & Chance, N. A. (1964). Cross-cultural inquiry into the symptomatology of depression. *Transcultural Psychiatric Research Review, 1*, 5–21.
68. Murphy, J. M. (1976). Psychiatric labeling in cross-cultural perspective. *Science, 191*, 1019–1028.
69. Murray, L. K., Skavenski, S., Kane, J. C., Mayeya, J., Dorsey, S., Cohen, J. A., et al. (2015). Effectiveness of trauma-focused cognitive behavioral therapy among trauma-affected children in Lusaka, Zambia: A randomized clinical trial. *JAMA Pediatrics, 169*(8), 761–769.
70. Mutamba, B. B., Kane, J. C., De Jong, J., Okello, J., Musisi, S., & Kohrt, B. A. (2018). Psychological treatments delivered by community health workers in low-resource government health systems: Effectiveness of group interpersonal psychotherapy for caregivers of children affected by Nodding Syndrome in Uganda. *Psychological Medicine, 48*(15), 2573. https://doi.org/10.1017/S0033291718000193.
71. Nadkarni, A., Weobong, B., Weiss, H. A., McCambridge, J., Bhat, B., Katti, B., et al. (2017). Counselling for Alcohol Problems (CAP), a lay counsellor-delivered brief psychological treatment for harmful drinking in men, in primary care in India: A randomised controlled trial. *Lancet, 389*(10065), 186–195. https://doi.org/10.1016/s0140-6736(16)31590-2.
72. Ofori-Atta, A., Read, U., & Lund, C. (2010). A situation analysis of mental health services and legislation in Ghana: Challenges for transformation. *The African Journal of Psychiatry, 13*(2), 99–108.
73. Packard, R. M. (2016). *A history of global health: Interventions into the lives of other peoples*. Baltimore: Johns Hopkins University Press.
74. Panter-Brick, C., Dajani, R., Eggerman, M., Hermosilla, S., Sancilio, A., & Ager, A. (2017). Insecurity, distress and mental health: Experimental and randomized controlled trials of a psychosocial intervention for youth affected by the Syrian crisis. *Journal of Child Psychology and Psychiatry, 59*, 523–541. https://doi.org/10.1111/jcpp.12832.
75. Patel, V., Cohen, A., Thara, R., & Gureje, O. (2006). Is the outcome of schizophrenia really better in developing countries? *Revista Brasileira de Psiquiatria, 28*(2), 149–152.
76. Patel, V., Collins, P. Y., Copeland, J., Kakuma, R., Katontoka, S., Lamichhane, J., et al. (2011). The movement for global mental health. *The British Journal of Psychiatry, 198*, 88–90.
77. Patel, V., Minas, H., Cohen, A., & Prince, M. (2014). *Global mental health: Principles and practice*. Oxford: Oxford University Press.

78. Patel, V., Saxena, S., Lund, C., Thornicroft, G., Baingana, F., Bolton, P., et al. (2018). The Lancet Commission on global mental health and sustainable development. *Lancet, 392*(10157), 1553–1598. https://doi.org/10.1016/S0140-6736(18)31612-X.

79. Patel, V., & Thornicroft, G. (2009). Packages of care for mental, neurological, and substance use disorders in low- and middle-income countries: PLoS Medicine Series. *PLoS Medicine/ Public Libr Sci, 6*(10), e1000160.

80. Patel, V., Weobong, B., Weiss, H. A., Anand, A., Bhat, B., Katti, B., et al. (2017). The Healthy Activity Program (HAP), a lay counsellor-delivered brief psychological treatment for severe depression, in primary care in India: A randomised controlled trial. *Lancet, 389*(10065), 176–185. https://doi.org/10.1016/s0140-6736(16)31589-6.

81. Petryna, A., Lakoff, A., & Kleinman, A. (2006). *Global pharmaceuticals: Ethics, markets, practices*. Durham: Duke University Press.

82. Prince, M., Patel, V., Saxena, S., Maj, M., Maselko, J., Phillips, M. R., & Rahman, A. (2007). No health without mental health. *Lancet, 370*(9590), 859–877.

83. Prince, R. (1985). The concept of culture-bound syndromes: Anorexia nervosa and brain-fag. *Social Science & Medicine, 21*(2), 197–203.

84. Rahman, A., Hamdani, S. U., Awan, N. R., Bryant, R. A., Dawson, K. S., Khan, M. F., et al. (2016). Effect of a multicomponent behavioral intervention in adults impaired by psychological distress in a conflict-affected area of Pakistan a randomized clinical trial. *JAMA, 316*(24), 2609–2617. https://doi.org/10.1001/jama.2016.17165.

85. Rahman, A., Khan, M. N., Hamdani, S. U., Chiumento, A., Akhtar, P., Nazir, H., et al. (2019). Effectiveness of a brief group psychological intervention for women in a post-conflict setting in Pakistan: A single-blind, cluster, randomised controlled trial. *Lancet, 393*(10182), 1733–1744. https://doi.org/10.1016/S0140-6736(18)32343-2.

86. Rahman, A., Malik, A., Sikander, S., Roberts, C., & Creed, F. (2008). Cognitive behaviour therapy-based intervention by community health workers for mothers with depression and their infants in rural Pakistan: A cluster-randomised controlled trial. *Lancet, 372*(9642), 902–909.

87. Rhodes, L. A. (1991). *Emptying beds: The work of an emergency psychiatric unit*. Berkeley: University of California Press.

88. Rivers, W. H. R. (1924). *Medicine, magic, and religion: The Fitz Patrick lectures*. New York: Harcourt, Brace, and Company, Inc..

89. Sartorius, N., Jablensky, A., & Shapiro, R. (1977). Two-year follow-up of the patients included in the WHO International Pilot Study of Schizophrenia. *Psychological Medicine, 7*(3), 529–541.

90. Sartorius, N., Shapiro, R., Kimura, M., & Barrett, K. (1972). WHO international pilot study of schizophrenia. *Psychological Medicine, 2*(4), 422–425.

91. Scheper-Hughes, N. (1979). *Saints, scholars, and schizophrenics: Mental illness in rural Ireland*. Berkeley: University of California Press.

92. Shorter, E. (1997). *A history of psychiatry: From the era of the asylum to the age of Prozac*. New York: Wiley.

93. Sikander, S., Ahmad, I., Atif, N., Zaidi, A., Vanobberghen, F., Weiss, H. A., et al. (2019). Delivering the thinking healthy programme for perinatal depression through volunteer peers: A cluster randomised controlled trial in Pakistan. *Lancet Psychiatry, 6*(2), 128–139. https:// doi.org/10.1016/S2215-0366(18)30467-X.

94. Singla, D. R., Kohrt, B. A., Murray, L. K., Anand, A., Chorpita, B. F., & Patel, V. (2017). Psychological treatments for the world: Lessons from low- and middle-income countries. *Annual Review of Clinical Psychology, 13*(April), 5.1–5.33. https://doi.org/10.1146/ annurev-clinpsy-032816-045217.

95. Ssewamala, F. M., Sensoy Bahar, O., McKay, M. M., Hoagwood, K., Huang, K.-Y., & Pringle, B. (2018). Strengthening mental health and research training in Sub-Saharan Africa (SMART Africa): Uganda study protocol. *Trials, 19*(1), 423. https://doi.org/10.1186/ s13063-018-2751-z.

96. Swartz, L. (2012). An unruly coming of age: The benefits of discomfort for global mental health. *Transcultural Psychiatry, 49*(3–4), 531–538. https://doi.org/10.1177/1363461512454810.
97. Szasz, T. S. (1961). *The myth of mental illness: Foundations of a theory of personal conduct.* New York: Dell.
98. Thornicroft, G., Chatterji, S., Evans-Lacko, S., Gruber, M., Sampson, N., Aguilar-Gaxiola, S., et al. (2017). Undertreatment of people with major depressive disorder in 21 countries. *The British Journal of Psychiatry, 210*(2), 119–124. https://doi.org/10.1192/bjp.bp.116.188078.
99. Tol, W. A., Augustinavicius, J., Carswell, K., Brown, F. L., Adaku, A., Leku, M. R., et al. (2018). Translation, adaptation, and pilot of a guided self-help intervention to reduce psychological distress in South Sudanese refugees in Uganda. *Global Mental Health, 5*, e25. https://doi.org/10.1017/gmh.2018.14.
100. Weiss, W. M., Murray, L. K., Zangana, G. A. S., Mahmooth, Z., Kaysen, D., Dorsey, S., et al. (2015). Community-based mental health treatments for survivors of torture and militant attacks in Southern Iraq: A randomized control trial. *BMC Psychiatry, 15*, 249. https://doi.org/10.1186/s12888-015-0622-7.
101. Wittkower, E. D. (1970). Transcultural psychiatry in the Caribbean: Past, present, and future. *American Journal of Psychiatry, 127*(2), 162–166.
102. World Health Organization. (1981). *World Health Organization: schizophrenia: An international follow-up study.* Chichester: Wiley.
103. World Health Organization. (2001). *The world health report 2001: Mental health: New understanding, new hope.* Geneva: World Health Organization.
104. World Health Organization. (2008). *Task shifting: Rational redistribution of tasks among health workforce teams: Global recommendations and guidelines.* Geneva: World Health Organization.
105. World Health Organization. (2010). *mhGAP intervention guide for mental, neurological and substance-use disorders in non-specialized health settings: Mental health Gap Action Programme (mhGAP).* Geneva: World Health Organization.
106. World Health Organization. (2016). *mhGAP intervention guide for mental, neurological and substance use disorders in non-specialized health settings: Mental health Gap Action Programme (mhGAP) – version 2.0.* Geneva: World Health Organization. http://www.who.int/mental_health/mhgap/mhGAP_intervention_guide_02/en/.
107. Young, A. (1995). *The harmony of illusions: Inventing post-traumatic stress disorder.* Princeton: Princeton University Press.
108. Murthy, R. S., Wig, N. N. (1983). The WHO collaborative study on strategies for extending mental health care, IV: A training approach to enhancing the availability of mental health manpower in a developing country. Am J Psychiatry. *140*(11), 1486–90.
109. Westermeyer, J. (1976). The pro-heroin effects of anti-opium laws in Asia. Archives of General Psychiatry, *33*(9), 1135–1139. https://doi.org/10.1001/archpsyc.1976.01770090125014.
110. Desjarlais, R., Eisenberg, L., Good, B., & Kleinman, A. (1995). World mental health: Problems and priorities in low-income countries. Oxford University Press.
111. Weine S, Kohrt BA, Collins PY, Cooper J, Lewis-Fernandez R, Okpaku S, Wainberg ML. (2020) Justice for George Floyd and a reckoning for global mental health. Global Mental Health. 7:e22. https://doi.org/10.1017/gmh.2020.17.
112. Mead, M. 1935. Sex and temperament in three primitive societies. New York: W. Morrow & Company.

Global Mental Health Law and the Interface with Ethics

3

Maya Prabhu

Introduction

Global mental health processes have, until recently, been somewhat removed from the many disruptive forces in global public health over the past 20 years. Infectious outbreaks like Severe Acute Respiratory Syndrome (SARS) in 2002, the global spread of H5N1 beginning in 2005, and the Ebola crisis of 2014 have all demonstrated the political and economic havoc that cross-border health emergencies can trigger. Numerous new nonstate players have entered the global health arena, including inter-governmental organizations, professional associations, transnational corporations, and initiatives and funders crowding the landscape for global health [6]. The rise of private-sector actors, particularly hybrid partnerships such as the *Global Alliance for Vaccines and Immunization* (GAVI Alliance) and *The Global Fund to Fight AIDS, Tuberculosis, and Malaria* has prompted both excitement and anxiety about corporate influence and norm-setting [7]. Many public health issues have been reframed as health and economic "security challenges" in an age of globalization. These emergent energies and directions have all reconfigured the global health agenda's values and priorities. One important response has been a resurgence of interest in international laws, norms, and policies in order to better govern global health actors, coordinate their efforts, and mediate between their competing visions (Fig. 3.1).[1]

---

[1] For the purposes of this chapter, the authors will use the term "global health law" interchangeably with "international health law" to encompass the range of rules, regulations, and laws implemented by international actors with a primary focus on health. However, there are important distinctions between the use of the term "international," traditionally referring to efforts by state actors versus "global" encompassing a broader set of actors and processes. For more on this distinction and evolution of terms see Ng & Ruger [31].

M. Prabhu (✉)
Yale School of Medicine, New Haven, CT, USA
e-mail: maya.prabhu@yale.edu

© Springer Nature Switzerland AG 2021
A. R. Dyer et al. (eds.), *Global Mental Health Ethics*,
https://doi.org/10.1007/978-3-030-66296-7_3

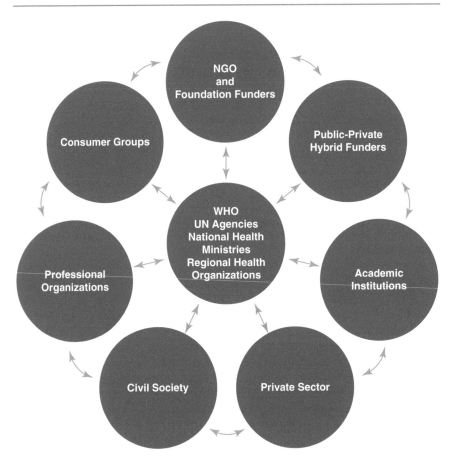

Fig. 3.1 Global Mental Health Actors

Accordingly, the global mental health agenda has acquired a new urgency as has the parallel need to create supportive global mental health laws. In 2007, the World Health Organization launched *mhGAP* (*Mental Health Global Action Program*), its flagship program to scale up mental health treatments in low and middle income countries. This was followed in 2010 by the *World Health Assembly Global Strategy to Reduce the Harmful Use of Alcohol* and the WHO *Mental Health Action Plan 2013–2020* [45, 46]. These paved the way for the United Nations' 2015 Sustainable Development Goals (SDGs) that will shape states' political and social policies until 2030. For the first time, the SDGs recognized that "mental health and substance use ought to be health priorities within the global development agenda" [43] (Fig. 3.2).

The WHO and national governments have identified the development of *mental health laws and legal expertise* as critical to meeting these sustainable development

Mental Health in the Sustainable Development Goals

Target	Indicator
3.4: By 2030, reduce by one third premature mortality from non-communicable diseases through prevention and treatment and promote mental health and well-being	**3.4.2:** Suicide mortality rate
3.5 Strengthen the prevention and treatment of substance abuse, including narcotic drug abuse and harmful use of alcohol	**3.5.1** Coverage of treatment interventions (pharmacological, psychosocial and rehabilitation and aftercare services) for substance use disorders **3.5.2** Harmful use of alcohol, defined according to the national context as alcohol per capita consumption (aged 15 years and older) within a calender year in litres of pure alcohol

Reference: United Nations.

Fig. 3.2 Mental Health in the SDGs

and mental health ambitions [47]. While most clinicians will have had some exposure to domestic health laws and regulations, international laws may remain opaque. Legal tools or "instruments" can take many forms including international agreements and conventions, national and subnational legislation, administrative regulations, fiscal measures, human rights norms, and the judgments of courts and tribunals [22]. Global health law in particular is complex as it is not a single treaty or organized body of laws overseen by a single agency. Yet, knowing when and how to reference international standard-setting instruments can be invaluable for mental health advocates seeking to implement domestic legislation that is important for health.

This chapter will consider some important international legal instruments and processes that could support global mental health goals. In particular, this chapter will examine the WHO's legal capacities and its past and potential contributions to mental health law and practice. In the last two decades, the WHO has embarked on two major international legal endeavors, the *Framework Convention on Tobacco Control (FCTC)* [34] and a revision of the *International Health Regulations (IHR)* [43, 47]. Both were heralded as game-changers for global health and models for future mental-health specific legislation. Taking a wider view of these WHO legal efforts means an opportunity to reflect on some of the gains and limitations of international tools. There have also been many gaps that have been exposed in the ethical underpinnings of the right to health and the global mental health law agenda. This chapter will lay out ideas for expanded ethical inquiry as the field of global mental health law evolves.

The WHO as a Source of Global Health Law

The WHO's Soft Law Functions

As many readers of this textbook are already aware, the international organization charged with directing and coordinating international health work is the WHO, an agency of the United Nations. The WHO's membership consists of 194 countries who convene annually at the World Health Assembly (WHO), the decision-making body of WHO. Health practitioners are likely to be familiar with the WHO's core work with other UN agencies, national health ministries, professional and nongovernmental organizations (NGOs) to define the global health research agenda, provide technical expertise and support capacity-building on the widest range of health issues, including mental health.

The WHO has issued dozens of technical treatment guidelines to ensure optimal health care based on evidence-based literature. Of relevance to mental health practitioners, for example, are *"Guidelines on management of physical health conditions in adults with severe mental disorders"* (2018) and *"Pharmacological treatment of mental disorders in primary health care"* (2010). Most recently, the WHO initiated *"SAFER,"* a technical package to reduce alcohol use including drunk-driving countermeasures, increased access to alcohol screening and treatment, bans and restrictions on alcohol advertising, and increased prices through taxes and pricing policies. What gives WHO guidelines their legitimacy and authority is the organization unparalleled ability to convene subject-matter experts and disseminate health information.

Less well-known is the WHO's role as a creator of international law, both "soft" (nonbinding) and "hard" (binding). The WHO Constitution provides for the adoption of international conventions such as the *Framework Convention on Tobacco Control* (an example of hard law described below) via Article 19, binding regulations such as the *International Health Regulations* via Article 21, and recommendations to member states via Article 23. Two of the better known of the WHO's recommendations are the *International Code of Marketing of Breast-Milk Substitutes* (1981) and the *Global Code of Practice on the Recruitment of Health Personnel* (2010) [20] (Fig. 3.3).

Earlier critiques of the WHO commented on its past indifference to its own binding legal capacities and its preference for addressing health problems with an evidence-driven scientific or technical approach. Fidler described this technocratic stance as consistent with public health and medical professions' preference for education, consensus building, and voluntary compliance with health measures over "coercive" legal obligations. This has resulted in numerous political instruments including World Health Assembly declarations and resolutions, charters, codes of practice and guidance, regulations, "programs of action," and normative statements. Though these are considered soft law, they carry moral weight and member states are expected to comply with them.

Milestones in Global Mental Health Law and Policy

Year	Instrument
1948	Universal Declaration of Human Rights
1950	European Convention for the Protection of Human Rights and Fundamental Freedoms
1966	International Covenant on Civil and Political Rights and the International Covenant on Economic, Social and Cultural Rights
1981	African (Banjul) Chapter on Human and Peoples' Rights
1990	Declaration of Caracas
1991	Principles for the protection of persons with mental illness and the improvement of mental health care, Adopted by General Assembly resolution 46/119 of 17 December 1991
1993	UN Principles for the Protection od Persons with Mental Illness
1996	Declaration of Madrid
1996	WHO Mental Health Care Law: Ten Basic Principles
1996	WHO Guidelines for the Promotion of Human Rights of Persons with Mental Disorders
1999	Inter-American Convention on the Elimination of all Forms of Discrimination against Persons with Disabilities
2005	WHO Resource Book on Mental Health, Human Rights and Legislation
2007	WHO MhGAP (Mental Health Global Action Program)
2010	WHA Global Strategy to Reduce the Harmful use of Alcohol
2013	WHO Mental Health Action Plan 2013-2020
2015	UN Sustainable Development Goals

References Multiple Sources.

Fig. 3.3 WHO Legal Authority

The WHO and the Right to Health

An essential aspect of the WHO's issuances is that they are consistent with a "right to health" approach. The right to health was first articulated in the Preamble to the 1946 WHO Constitution which asserted that "the enjoyment of the highest attainable standard of health is one of the fundamental rights of every human being without distinction of race, religion, political belief, economic or social condition" [26]. The right to health was further elaborated in the *1948 Universal Declaration of Human Rights* and the *1966 International Covenant on Economic, Social, and Cultural Rights* [25] which identified core obligations such as the right of access to health facilities, basic shelter, housing and sanitation, essential drugs, a national public health strategy, and plan of action which addresses the health concerns of all populations. These documents underscore that the realization of the right to health is closely aligned with the achievement of basic civil, political, economic, social, and cultural rights. Moreover, state obligations apply to mental health just as much as to physical health.

There is an animated debate about whether human rights law can be considered binding on sovereign nations. The WHO's stance has been that international human rights instruments are generally accepted as "legitimate norms" which create obligations on the part of states. All states in the world have signed at least one international instrument that recognizes the right to health [48] and the right to health, or the aspiration to protect the right to public health, is enshrined in a quarter (25%) of WHO member state constitutions [25]. The WHO's work, therefore, can be seen not only as embracing the right to health, but also as helping to operationalize a rights-based approach to health. In other words, the WHO not only promotes the right to health but also seeks to provide guidance about how to translate it into specific outcomes.

The WHO and Mental Health

There are many examples of WHO guidance on mental health policies that fully incorporate the right to health. In 1993, the UN General Assembly adopted the *Principles for the Protection of Persons with Mental Illness and of the Improvement of Mental Health Care (MI Principles)* [40]. The *MI Principles* were considered, for their time, the most wide-ranging standards for persons with mental disabilities. They established minimum standards of practice in the mental health field requiring a more humane, less restrictive, and more individualized treatment approach. It was against this backdrop that the WHO followed with *Mental Health Care Law: Ten Basic Principles (Ten Principles)* based on its analysis of mental health legislation in 45 countries around the world and the United Nations' *MI Principles* [46]. These *Ten Principles* emphasized that mental health care should be provided in the least restrictive fashion possible: where decisions affect a person's liberty, there must be automatic periodic review. Any mental health clinician who has had to admit patients to a hospital and inform them of their rights to a legal advisor and review of their admission is operating under mental health laws informed by these UN and WHO principles. Alongside the *Ten Principles,* the WHO developed *Guidelines for the Promotion of Human Rights of Persons with Mental Disorders*, a tool to help countries apply *MI Principles* and evaluate human rights conditions in institutions [45]. In 2009, the WHO issued "Improving Health Systems and Services for Mental Health" which detailed essential steps for governments to integrate mental health into its health systems including mental health legislation as a complement to mental health policy [48] (Fig. 3.4).

The embrace of a human rights perspective on mental health law and policy culminated in 2013 with the World Health Assembly's adoption of the *Comprehensive Mental Health Action Plan 2013–2020*. This action plan establishes benchmarks to improve mental health leadership, prevent mental illness, integrate care in community settings, and strengthen research. Throughout the plan are calls for robust mental health laws to "promote human rights and the development of accessible health and social services in the community." Of specific interest is the *Plan's* call for mental health legislation that is compatible with the 2006 *Convention on the Rights of Persons with Disabilities (CRPD)* [42]. The *CRPD* is not a WHO treaty but is the first international human rights instrument specifically designed to protect persons

MENTAL HEALTH CARE LAW: TEN BASIC PRINCIPLES

1. Promotion of Mental Health and Prevention of Mental Disorders

2. Access to Basic Mental Health Care

3. Mental Health Assessments in Accordance with internationally Accepted Principles

4. Provision of the Least Restrictive Type of Mental Health Care

5. Self-Determination

6. Right to be Assisted in the Exercise of Self-Determination

7. Availability of Review Procedure

8. Automatic Periodical Review Mechanism

9. Qualified Decision-Maker

10. Respect of the Rule of Law

Reference: WHO (1996b),

Fig. 3.4 Ten Mental Health Principles

WHO LEGAL AUTHORITY

Legal Tool	Authority	Examples	Force
Conventions	Granted by Art, 19, WHO Constitution	-Framework Convention on Tobacco Control	"Binding"hard law
Regulations	Granted by Art, 21, WHO Constitution	-International Health Regulations -Nomenclature Regulations	"Binding"hard law
Recommendations	Granted Art, 23, WHO Constitution	-Pandemic Influenza Preparedness Framework -Global Code of Practice on International Recruitment of Health Personnel	"Nonbinding" but persuasive

Fig. 3.5 Milestones in Global Mental Health Law and Policy

with disabilities, including persons diagnosed with mental illness. It is legally binding, with countries committed to harmonizing their domestic laws and practices in order to comply with it. Though the *CRPD* has generated controversy in a number of areas relevant to patients with psychiatric illness (which will be discussed below), it is incontrovertible that the *Convention* has generated paradigm-shifting discussions about how to include persons with disabilities and mental illness fully into community life (Fig. 3.5).

Binding Hard Law

The WHO also creates "hard" or binding law in two ways: by approving regulations in specifically delineated subject areas covered by Article 19 of its Constitution, or by approving conventions under Article 21. Thus far, the WHO's work in both of these areas has been unrelated to mental health. The only sets of regulations that have been adopted are related to Nomenclature (standardizing names) and the "*International Health Regulations*" (*IHR*).

The original *International Health Regulations* of 1969 was the WHO's first binding instrument, designed to monitor six specific infectious diseases (cholera, plague, yellow fever, smallpox, relapsing fever, and typhus). When the *IHR* were revised in 2005, the number of "critical health events" that could trigger a "public health emergency of international concern" was expanded to include many more infectious diseases as well as biological, chemical, or radiological incidents. The *IHR* restricts the measures countries may take to address those public health emergencies to those that are supported by scientific evidence and are commensurate with the risks involved. The IHR is also anchored in the "full respect for the dignity, human rights and fundamental freedoms of persons" [43].

The *Framework Convention on Tobacco Control* however, is more instructive for potential global mental health law. The *FCTC* addresses the management of tobacco on both of the supply and demand sides, regulating tobacco product contents, advertising, pricing, taxation, consumer education efforts, and calling for legislation against smuggling. It is considered the first "evidence-based treaty" and a global health law success story with more than 168 signatories. Although the FCTC is an extremely technically precise document, it is also steeped in concerns about the right to health. Articles that address exposure to tobacco smoke are related to the right to safe working conditions and a healthy environment; articles that counter the employment of children in the tobacco industry are intended to realize the rights of children to an adequate standard of living and barriers to education. Conventions modeled on the *FCTC* have been proposed for health concerns ranging from antimicrobial resistance, nutrition, obesity, elder care, corruption in health care settings, to counterfeit medicines.

The revised *IHR* and the *FCTC* stoked excitement about a new era for WHO activism and country commitment to binding treaties for health. Most important, it has been argued that such international conventions establish "norms" or behavioral expectations in support of domestic antismoking efforts. One review of 96 legal challenges to tobacco control measures found that the *FCTC* "made a substantial contribution to courts' reasoning" and "strengthened governments' arguments in defending litigation" [48,. For example, in 2012, the South African Appeals Court upheld an advertising ban on tobacco products after a challenge that the ban imposed unreasonable limits against commercial speech (*British American Tobacco South*

Africa Ltd v *Minister of Health*). The Court concluded that South African courts are obliged to "have regard to international law" even when interpreting domestic rights. The court specifically affirmed South Africa's "clear obligations" to the *FCTC*, underscoring that *FCTC* practices were reflected "in many other open and democratic societies." In the case of *Philip Morris v. Uruguay* [34], an investment tribunal upheld Uruguay's graphic health messages against smoking as part of good-faith efforts to protect public health.

The *FCTC* has been cited as a model for the regulation of other "unhealthy products," such as sugar and trans fats, but particularly alcohol [26]. As with tobacco, the global mental and physical health burden of alcohol is high, and the cross-border nature of the alcohol industry, including its illicit trade, is a challenge for national governments. Advocates for a convention for alcohol hope that it can slow the specific expansion of alcohol markets to young people, support national regulations, and reduce harmful consumption [22].

Limits to a Framework Convention Approach

There are reasons to be cautious about the capacity of international treaties to change health outcomes. First, it is self-evident that the negotiation of such international frameworks requires significant investments of time and resources. The *FCTC* required 8 years from initiation to adoption by the World Health Assembly, the revised *IHR*, 10 years. In the process of negotiation, the compromises needed to build international support may well have weakened the instruments. The revised *IHR*, for example, did not create any new enforcement mechanism for addressing compliance failure (as was dramatically illustrated when China and Indonesia declined to provide the WHO access to Avian Flu samples). Similarly, the *FCTC* did not include a mechanism to settle disputes, nor did it make provisions for financial assistance to developing countries to implement it. This allowed for wider support for and ratification of the *FCTC,* but may have compromised its effectiveness.

Additionally, some critics have raised ethical concerns that international frameworks assert the priorities and means of powerful states based on their own needs, obligating developing countries to subordinate their local agendas [19]. Lastly, it would appear that some measures supported by international frameworks may be more feasible than others for developing countries. Assessments of the *FCTC's* effectiveness showed the most progress in mandates such as smoke-free laws, health warnings, and media campaigns, but less progress in domains that might require robust litigation such as the "implementation of measures to counter industry interference, regulate tobacco product contents, promote alternative livelihoods, and protect the environment and health of tobacco workers" [8]. Litigation, a favored tool of developed country NGOS and plaintiffs, is particularly cost-ineffective in the legal systems of already overburdened developing countries.

Overall, it would appear that, as with all global health goals, a multifactorial approach must involve clear targets, support for local implementation, monitoring, and a sustained effort. "[U]nder the right circumstances, international law can contribute to the success of [public health] strategies but cannot substitute for them" [4].

Lack of a Normative Framework for Global Health Law

There remains a broader question about the moral underpinnings of global health law. What is the normative framework for determining global health policy, and which values ought to be prioritized in legal tools when there are competing concerns? Many writers have been struck by the lack of a fully conceived normative vision for global health law and have interrogated competing ethical foundations [5]. Others have wondered whether global *mental* health laws have distinct ethical considerations given the unique vulnerability of persons with serious mental illnesses.

The lack of clear values undergirding global health law may be an artifact of their original iterations. The earliest international health laws were bilateral or multilateral agreements between states designed to limit the spread of infectious diseases, transboundary pollutants, alcohol, and opium. They were intended to avoid affecting trade and national security. Pragmatism and rational self-interest were the primary motivations.

As global health has emerged as a field, Gostin and Powers are among those who have asserted that the moral foundation of global health law ought to be social justice (2006). Social justice can be understood as "fair and equal distribution across racial, gender, and economic differences" with particular attention called to the most impoverished populations. In this conception, global health is a shared responsibility or moral imperative with shared risks and obligations. Jennifer Shah Ruger [29] is among a group of scholars who emphasize "equity" as the basis for law with individuals as the "moral unit" for health outcomes. Global mental health equity therefore is the global equal realization of an individual's full potential. In both conceptions, states continue to have the most pressing obligations but require support from global actors and institutions.

In the absence of a unifying moral framework for global health laws, multiple alternate framing devices have been put forward. These justify financing and laws for global health goals along the lines of national security, human security, economic development, and health as a global public good. The logic of "securitization" paradigms is strongest for infectious pathogens but risks "global health fatigue" with never-ending declarations of "health crises" that fail to address the health infrastructure and socio-economic factors that place some populations and countries at higher risk for disease [30, 38]. The Ebola crisis in Guinea, Liberia, and Sierra Leone in 2014–15 exemplifies this bind, yielding $4.5 billion in funds from the United States alone but highlighting chronically underfunded health infrastructures [44].

For noncommunicable diseases like mental illness, human rights language and approaches have tended to fill the "moral gap." In these formulations, the core concept of the right to health defines state responsibilities for health and determinants of health. Rights language thus frames health "not as an externality, investment, or issue of compassion but as a legal entitlement and fundamental matter of social justice" [26].

Critiques of a Human Rights Approach

Human rights approaches can nonetheless be criticized on a variety of grounds. Human rights health obligations can be difficult to enforce within states even when human rights failures are well-documented. Highly visible vulnerable populations such as refugees and asylum seekers are not accorded minimal mental health access in many countries. There has been along and sad history of the "misuse and abuse" of mental health systems: diagnoses and interventions under the former Soviet Union and apartheid South Africa, and the treatment of political detainees at Guantanamo [4, 24, 30]. The right to health can feel like a hollow aspiration when deliberate attacks on health care providers in war zones seem to occur with frequency and impunity. This has led many to wonder whether the "generic recognition" of the right to health is simply an insufficient basis for better health outcomes. To be fair, this may not be a problem only for human rights theory; it may apply to any ethics framework that is not adequately operationalized.

Second, a human rights perspective, in the absence of ethical guidance, may not resolve situations where different rights themselves are in conflict. For example, several instances of competing rights can be found within the *Disabilities Convention*. In the first instance, the *Convention* explicitly prohibits using the criterion of disability for detention and treatment of a nonconsenting patient (including the mentally ill) [10]. The expert Committee that interprets the *Convention* opined that such a ban on involuntary hospitalization of persons extended to hospitalizations based on risk or dangerousness, regardless of what due process safeguards are in place. Especially where the risk might be to other people, this stance does not appear to strike a fair balance between the rights of the individual and legitimate concerns of society.

In a second instance, the *Convention* appears to require the elimination of all substitute decision-makers (for example, a health care proxy) in lieu of "supported decision-making." This is based on the premise that the concept of incapacity is incompatible with respecting the autonomy and preferences of persons with disabilities [14]. For clinicians who care for persons with conditions that impair decision-making capacities (such as dementia, schizophrenia, delirium), this position undermines the current health and safety of some patients as well as less obvious future interests. Appelbaum [1] envisions the following: "The decisions of all patients able to say "no," for example, to life-saving treatment for pneumonia— although demented, delirious, or psychotic—would have to be respected...Nor could [treaters] step in to stop persons in the manic phase of bipolar disorder from dissipating the savings accumulated over a lifetime, rendering themselves and their families penurious." To many observers, this undermines other *CRPD* goals such as the humane treatment of the disabled [2, 37].

In a third example, the United Nations High Commissioner has indicated that the *Convention* required replacing criminal defenses that are "based on mental or intellectual disability" with "disability neutral" doctrines. Numerous scholars have interpreted this as requiring the elimination of "not criminally responsible" or "diminished responsibility" defenses for those with mental illness [2, 9, 24]. The rationale is that withholding criminal responsibility on the basis of mental incapacity is itself "a particular kind of social exclusion, or withdrawal of the recognition that we normally extend to others." But the removal of such defenses would inevitably "lead to the conviction and imprisonment of defendants with severe mental illnesses who would not previously have been held responsible for their actions…." [1]. It is difficult to conceive of a more severe deprivation of liberty and social exclusion than extended incarceration.

A final appraisal comes from transcultural psychiatrists. The global mental health project has been critiqued for failing to adequately consider local and culturally specific understandings of health, wellness, distress, and personhood against a deeply biological Western bias. By extension, global mental health law is critiqued for its emphasis on rights-based legal instruments (such as those discussed in this chapter) from international agencies still dominated by the Global North. This is ironic because the right to health is intended to be implemented in a culturally respectful manner as well as a manner that protects against cultural approaches that are harmful to health. While there are many interpretations of the right to health and culture by UN committees working in reproductive health, much work still needs to be done to elaborate the cultural dimensions of the right to mental health [13].

Areas for Future Ethical Inquiry

The field of global mental health law is still nascent. Consequently, there are potentially limitless areas for ethical inquiry. The *Convention on the Rights of Persons for Disability* which calls for new norms of autonomy and capacity will require ongoing consideration about its implementation in clinical settings where the immediate- and long-term interests of the patient may diverge. The incorporation of cultural and local communities in the drafting of global health care laws and policies will assist in determining what is "culturally appropriate" mental health care. The right to health may be applied universally but not implemented uniformly. Finally, global mental health law will benefit from elaboration of its normative underpinnings beyond what is fiscally and politically expedient.

There is an additional important area: Many critics of global mental health argue that "the scaling up of services" from developed countries to under-resourced countries will inevitably favor medication as the primary treatment at the expense of the structural and social determinants of mental health. This concern about the pharmaceutical industry agenda is heightened by the severe shortage of a skilled mental health labor force in many parts of the world. The concern about pharmaceutical industry influence is not hypothetical: researchers advising the WHO on the A/H1N1 "Swine flu" influenza pandemic in 2011 were found to have close ties to the pharmaceutical industry [9]. The "swine flu scandal" resulted in the creation of the Framework of Engagement with NonState Actors (FENSA) which was approved by the WHO in 2016. It established careful rules of collaboration between the WHO and private sector entities (and other actors). Going forward, it will be crucial to monitor FENSA's monitoring of undue industry influence.

Conclusions

This chapter provides a primer on some key international health law instruments that might support future global mental health policy. What the community hopes is clear, however, is that while global health law approaches – both hard and soft – are invaluable, they alone are insufficient. Rather, in a rapidly changing health land-scape, multiple actors, institutions, and tools must advance mental health goals in a multi-sector approach. In this sense, global public health best practices remain as they always were – a full-scale effort by all of civil society to move the right to health from aspiration to implementation.

References

1. Appelbaum, P. S. (2016). Protecting the rights of persons with disabilities: An international convention and its problems. *Psychiatric Services, 67*(4), 366–368. https://doi.org/10.1176/appi.ps.201600050.
2. Bartlett, P. (2012). The United Nations convention on the rights of persons with disabilities and mental health law. *Modern Law Review, 75*(5), 752–778. Retrieved January 2, 2020 from www.jstor.org/stable/41682870.
3. Bollyky, T., & Fidler, D. *Has a global tobacco treaty made a difference?* The Atlantic 2015. Retrieved from https://www.theatlantic.com. British American Tobacco South Africa (Pty) Ltd v Minister of Health (463/2011) [2012] ZASCA 107.
4. Bonnie, Richard J. (2002). Political Abuse of Psychiatry in the Soviet Union and in China: Complexities and Controversies. J Am Acad Psychiatry Law. 30(1), 136–44.
5. Brown, G. W. (2012). Distributing who gets what and why: Four normative approaches to global health. *Global Policy, 3*(3), 292–302. https://doi.org/10.1111/j.1758-5899.2012.00180.x.
6. Chan, M. *Introductory remarks on programmes and priority setting at the Executive Board special session on WHO reform.* WHO 2011. Retrieved January 2, 2020 from http://www9.who.int/dg/speeches/2011/reform_priorities_01_11/en/
7. Civil Society Statement. *On the World Health Organization's proposed Framework of Engagement with Non-State Actors (FENSA) 2016.* Retrieved on January 2, 2020 from: http://www.babymilkaction.org/wp-content/uploads/2016/05/Civil-Society-Statement-64.pdf
8. Chung-Hall, J., Craig, L., Gravely, S., et al. (2019). Impact of the WHO FCTC over the first decade: A global evidence review prepared for the Impact Assessment Expert Group. *Tobacco Control, 28*, s119–s128.
9. Cohen, D., & Carter, P. (2010). WHO and the pandemic flu "conspiracies". *BMJ, 340*, c2912.
10. Craigie, J. (2015). Against a singular understanding of legal capacity: Criminal responsibility and the convention on the rights of persons with disabilities. *International Journal of Law and Psychiatry, 40*, 6–14. Available at SSRN: https://ssrn.com/abstract=3015824.
11. Cronin, T., Gouda, P., McDonald, C., & Hallahan, B. (2017). A comparison of mental health legislation in five developed countries: A narrative review. *Irish Journal of Psychological Medicine, 34*(4), 261–269. https://doi.org/10.1017/ipm.2017.48.
12. Donders, Y. M. (2015). Exploring the cultural dimensions of the right to the highest attainable standard of health. *PER: Potchefstroomse Elektroniese Regsblad, 18*(2), 180–222. https://doi.org/10.4314/PELJ.V18I2.05.

13. Dufour, M., Hastings, T., & O'Reilly, R. (2018). Canada should retain its reservation on the United Nation's convention on the rights of persons with disabilities. *Canadian Journal of Psychiatry, 63*(12), 809–812. https://doi.org/10.1177/0706743718784939.
14. Fidler, D. (1998). The future of the World Health Organization: What role for international law? *Vanderbilt Journal of Transnational Law, 5*(31), 1079–1126. Available at https://www. repository.law.indiana.edu/cgi/viewcontent.cgi?article=1699&context=facpub.
15. Gostin, L. O, Powers M. (2006). What does social justice require for the public's health? Public health ethics and policy imperatives. Health Aff (Millwood). 25(4):1053–60. https:// doi.org/10.1377/hlthaff.25.4.1053.
16. Gostin, L. O., Sridhar, D., & Hougendobler, D. (2015). The normative authority of the World Health Organization. Public Health, 129(7), 854–863. https://doi.org/10.1016/j.puhe. 2015.05.002. https://scholarship.law.georgetown.edu/facpub/1498.
17. Gostin, L. O. (2015). The future of the World Health Organization: Lessons learned from Ebola. *The Milbank Quarterly, 93*(3), 475–479. https://doi.org/10.1111/1468-0009.12134.
18. Haysom, N., Strous, M., & Vogelman, L. (1990). The Mad Mrs Rochester Revisited: The Involuntary Confinement of the Mentally Ill in South Africa. *South African Journal on Human Rights, 6*(3), 341–362. https://doi.org/10.1080/02587203.1990.11827818.
19. Hoffman, S., Røttingen, J.A. (2012). Alcohol control: Be sparing with international laws. Nature. 483. 275. 10.1038/483275e.
20. Heymann, J., Cassola, A., Raub, A., & Mishra, L. (2013). Constitutional rights to health, public health and medical care: The status of health protections in 191 countries. *Global Public Health, 8*(6), 639–653. https://doi.org/10.1080/17441692.2013.810765.
21. Lien, G., & DeLand, K. (2011). Translating the WHO Framework Convention on Tobacco Control (FCTC): Can we use tobacco control as a model for other non-communicable disease control? *Public Health, 125*(12), 847–853. https://doi.org/10.1016/j.puhe.2011.09.022.
22. Sridhar, D. (2012). Regulate alcohol for global health. Nature. 482, 302. https://doi. org/10.1038/482302a.
23. Magnusson, R. S., McGrady, B., Gostin, L., Patterson, D., & Abou Taleb, H. (2019). Legal capacities required for prevention and control of noncommunicable diseases. *Bulletin of the World Health Organization, 97*(2), 108–117. https://doi.org/10.2471/BLT.18.213777.
24. Miles, S. (2007). Medical ethics and the interrogation of Guantanamo 063. *The American Journal of Bioethics, 7*(4), 5–11. https://doi.org/10.1080/15265160701263535.
25. Ng, N. Y., & Ruger, J. P. (2011). Global health governance at a crossroads. *Global Health Gov, 3*(2), 1–37.
26. Ooms G, Hammonds R. (2010). Taking up Daniels' challenge: The case for global health justice. Health Hum Rights. 12(1):29–46.
27. Philip Morris Brands SARL v Oriental Republic of Uruguay (Award), ICSID Case No. ARB/10/7 (8 Jul 2016).
28. Ruger, J. P. (2008). Normative foundations of global health law. *Georgetown Law of Journal, 96*(2), 423–443. Available at https://www.law.georgetown.edu/georgetown-law-journal/.
29. Ruger J. P. (2008). Normative Foundations of Global Health Law. The Georgetown law journal. *96*(2), 423–443.
30. Scholten, M., & Gather, J. (2018). Adverse consequences of article 12 of the UN Convention on the Rights of Persons with Disabilities for persons with mental disabilities and an alternative way forward. *Journal of Medical Ethics, 44*(4), 226–233. https://doi.org/10.1136/ medethics-2017-104414.
31. Slobogin, C. (2015). Eliminating mental disability as a legal criterion in deprivation of liberty cases: The impact of the Convention on the Rights of Persons with Disability on the insanity defense, civil commitment, and competency law. *International Journal of Law and Psychiatry, 40*, 36–42. Available at https://www.journals.elsevier.com/ international-journal-of-law-and-psychiatry.
32. United Nations. *Universal declaration of human rights, G.A. Res. 217A (III), U.N. Doc A/810 at 71 (1948) 1948.* Retrieved on January 2, 2020 from https://www.un.org/en/ universal-declaration-human-rights/

33. United Nations. *Constitution of the world health organization 1946*. Retrieved on January 2, 2020 from https://www.who.int/governance/eb/who_constitution_en.pdf
34. UN General Assembly. *Principles for the protection of persons with mental illness and the improvement of mental health care 1993*. Retrieved on January 2, 2020 from https://www.who.int/mental_health/policy/en/UN_Resolution_on_protection_of_persons_with_mental_illness.pdf
35. UN General Assembly. *Convention on the rights of persons with disabilities, A/RES/61/106, Annex I2006*. Retrieved on January 2, 2020 from https://www.refworld.org/docid/4680cd212.html
36. UN General Assembly. *Transforming our world: The 2030 agenda for sustainable development, 21 October 2015, A/RES/70/12015*. Retrieved on January 2, 2020 from https://sustainabledevelopment.un.org/index.php?page=view&type=111&nr=8496&menu=35
37. Wenham, C. (2019). The oversecuritization of global health: Changing the terms of debate. *International Affairs, 95*(5), 1093–1110. https://doi.org/10.1093/ia/iiz170.
38. WHO. *Guidelines for the promotion of human rights of persons with mental disorders 1996*. Retrieved on January 2, 2020 from https://apps.who.int/iris/handle/10665/41880
39. WHO. *Mental health care law: Ten basic principles: With annotations suggesting selected actions to promote their implementation*. World Health Organization 1996. Retrieved on January 2, 2020 from https://apps.who.int/iris/handle/10665/63624
40. WHO. *WHO framework convention on tobacco control 2003*. Retrieved on January 2, 2020 from https://treaties.un.org/doc/Treaties/2003/05/20030506%2002-12%20PM/Ch_IX_04p.pdf
41. WHO. *International health regulations 2005*. Retrieved on January 2, 2020 from https://www.who.int/ihr/publications/9789241596664/en/
42. WHO (2005). International Health Regulations. 2nd edition. Geneva, Switzerland: World Health Organization; 2008. Retrieved on March 1, 2021. Available at: http://whqlibdoc.who.int/publications/2008/9789241580410_eng.pdf.
43. WHO. (July 4, 2006). *Improving health systems and services for mental health*. World Health Organization 2009. Retrieved on January 2, 2020 from https://apps.who.int/iris/handle/10665/44219. Ximenes Lopes v. Brazil, Inter-Am. Ct. H.R. (ser. C) No. 149.
44. WHO. *The right to health*. Fact Sheet No. 31, 2008. Retrieved on January 2, 2020 available at: https://www.ohchr.org/Documents/Publications/Factsheet31.pdf
45. WHO (2010). Global Strategy to Reduce the Harmful Use of Alcohol. Retrieved on January 31, 2020. Available at: https://www.who.int/substance_abuse/msbalcstragegy.pdf.
46. WHO (2013). Mental health action plan 2013–2020. Retrieved on March 1, 2021. Available at: https://www.who.int/publications/i/item/9789241506021.
47. WHO (2017). Mental Health Atlas. Retrieved on January 31, 2020. Available at . https://www.who.int/mental_health/evidence/atlas/mental_health_atlas_2017/en/.
48. Zhou S. Y., Liberman J. D., Ricafort, E. (2019) The impact of the WHO Framework Convention on Tobacco Control in defending legal challenges to tobacco control measures. Tobacco Control. s113–s118.

Ethical Considerations in Global Mental Health Research

4

Sana Loue

Background

Significant global mental health inequities exist with respect to access to care, service utilization, and mental health outcomes across geographical regions, socioeconomic status, race, ethnicity, sex, and sexual orientation [160, 162]. Estimates indicate that four out of every five people with serious mental disorders living in low- and middle-income countries are unable to obtain needed mental health services [160]. Poverty, in particular, has been identified as a determinant of poor mental health but is also a consequence due to the impact of mental illness on individuals' ability to function [39, 74, 111]. Stigmatization of and discrimination against both the sufferer and his or her family members may exacerbate the difficulties of coping with a mental illness [121, 138].

Access to needed, appropriate mental health treatment may be particularly problematic for those living in low-income countries. The median mental health expenditure per capita in low-income countries is only $0.20, compared to $44.84 in high-income countries [160]. The limited availability of psychiatric and other mental health care due to scarce resources and a limited infrastructure [160, 161] may be compounded by the reluctance of medical professionals to enter the field of psychiatry [122, 154], physicians' own beliefs in supernatural causes of mental illness [10], and their migration to either more developed urban centers or more developed nations [44, 132]. Data indicate that there is a median rate of 0.05 psychiatrists per 100,000 persons in low-income countries, compared to 8.59 in high-income countries [160]. Unsurprisingly, difficulties in accessing adequate mental health care may lead patients and/or their concerned family members to rely on untrained faith and traditional healers [137]. However, in their efforts to ameliorate illness

S. Loue (✉)
Case Western Reserve University, Department of Bioethics, Cleveland, OH, USA
e-mail: sxl54@case.edu

© Springer Nature Switzerland AG 2021
A. R. Dyer et al. (eds.), *Global Mental Health Ethics*,
https://doi.org/10.1007/978-3-030-66296-7_4

symptoms or cure the disease, healers' lack of mental health knowledge and their own beliefs related to the causes of mental illness may lead to the use of abusive practices [7].

These data suggest that there is a critical need to engage in global mental health research to identify both efficacious, affordable treatments and interventions and delivery mechanisms that will optimize access for those in need of such services. All such research, however, must be both scientifically and ethically sound. As indicated in the *International Guidelines for Health-Related Research Involving Humans* [37, p. 1].

Although scientific and social value are the fundamental justification for undertaking research, researchers, sponsors, research ethics committees, and health authorities have a moral obligation to ensure that all research is carried out in ways that uphold human rights and respect, protect, and are fair to study participants and the communities in which the research is conducted. Scientific and social value cannot legitimate subjecting study participants or their communities to mistreatment or injustice.

Governing Principles

Although there exist numerous conceptual frameworks for bioethical analysis, e.g., feminist ethics [127, 133, 134], the ethic of care [54], deontology, [12, 70] virtue ethics [85], utilitarianism [24, 103], casuistry [69], and communitarianism [49], international guidelines and the regulatory provisions of the United States and other countries have adopted to greater or lesser degree the principlist model of bioethics. The three principles of respect for persons, beneficence, and justice derive from the provisions of the Nuremberg Code (1949) and the *Belmont Report* [113] and are reflected in various international documents [37, 163]. The principle of nonmaleficence, the corollary to beneficence, has also been noted in the extant literature. More recently, it has been suggested that the concept of vulnerability, discussed in greater detail below, similarly warrants recognition as a guiding principle of research ethics. As will be seen below, it is not possible to maximize the application of each of these principles simultaneously.

Respect for Persons

The principle of respect for persons encompasses the concept of individual autonomy and serves as the basis for the requirement of voluntary informed consent, discussed in detail below. The *Belmont Report* [113] defines an autonomous individual as one who "is capable of deliberation about personal goals and of acting under the direction of such deliberation."

Although international guidelines and national regulations emphasize the importance and necessity of individual informed consent (and assent where indicated), the concept of the individual as an autonomous decision-maker is far from universal. As an example, although males in Uganda are legally able to make their own decisions once they have reached the age of 18 years, it is customary to seek their fathers' consent prior to entering into any obligation [88]. Additionally, women may seek their husbands' consent prior to enrolling in a research study. Kass and Hyder [71] found from their survey of 540 investigators from developing countries that almost one-fifth sought consent from a family member other than the prospective research participant.

Respect for persons also encompasses the requirement that persons with diminished autonomy be provided with additional protections. Diminished autonomy may be due to a variety of factors, including age, as is the case with young children; to mental health status; to confinement in an institutional environment such as a prison or detention facility; or to marginalization or oppression, among others. Although the requirement of special protections is often framed in terms of diminished autonomy, vulnerability in research may arise from a plethora of circumstances which call for consideration of additional protections. These circumstances are addressed more fully below in the context of vulnerability in research.

Beneficence and Nonmaleficence

The principle of beneficence refers to the ethical obligation to maximize possible benefits, while nonmaleficence refers to the obligation to do no harm and to minimize possible harms [113]. The conduct of mental health research frequently requires an evaluation of study aims and protocol against these principles.

As an example, research designed to assess the prevalence of mental disorders or the need for mental health services among internally displaced persons and refugees may inadvertently lead to the retraumatization of individuals who have escaped from traumatic or abusive situations [135]. The discontinuation of antipsychotic medication in a well-intentioned study designed to assess the efficacy of a new medication may lead to a relapse in symptoms [47]. It is not farfetched to suggest that, depending upon the duration of response time to the reintroduction of antipsychotic treatment, an individual experiencing a severe relapse in symptoms may also face adverse social consequences. Consideration of beneficence and nonmaleficence in such situations requires that the investigators and sponsors of the specific research study anticipate how benefits may be maximized and harms may be minimized [113].

The consideration of potential harms should extend beyond a focus on only physical or psychological events to include potential social and emotional harms as well. Depending upon the context in which the study is conducted, a failure to maintain the confidentiality of the information provided by the participant could lead to his or her loss of employment or housing, ostracism from family or friends, or abuse. Family members may suffer similar consequences due to their association with the research participant.

Justice

The principle of justice refers to the fair distribution of the benefits and burdens of research [113]. Historically, the populations that have suffered the burdens of research—institutionalized persons [22], prisoners [61], minorities [26], children [158], and patients [158], for example—often lacked access to any resulting benefits. Indeed, in some cases, such as the Tuskegee syphilis study [149], the irradiation experiments at the University of Cincinnati [158], and the Willowbrook hepatitis experiments [79], as well as others, it is doubtful that the experiment produced any benefit and reflected, instead, the exploitation of easily accessed populations.

Exactly what constitutes such a fair distribution of benefit and burdens has been subject to various interpretations. These include distribution (1) of an equal share to each person; (2) to each person according to his or her own need; (3) to each person based on his or her individual effort; (4) to each person according to societal contribution; and (5) to each person according to merit [113].

Vulnerability

The concept of vulnerability has been recognized as foundational to the conduct of ethical research [87] and as "the single most important idea that will shape … the … development of bioethics" [128, p. 380]. The delineation of participants who may be "vulnerable," variously conceived of as an element of respect for persons [36] or as a component of the principle of justice [34], has been reflected in various national and international research guidelines and regulations as referring to specified groups or categories of individuals, such as children, prisoners, pregnant women, fetuses, and those with mental illnesses or intellectual impairments. More recently, however, it has been recognized that the classification of entire groups of individuals, such as mental health service users, as vulnerable in research leads to stereotyping and to their disempowerment and stigmatization and may often foreclose their ability to participate in even low-risk noninterventional research [13, 80, 146]. The categorical approach exemplifies the challenges associated with efforts to maximize the ethical principle simultaneously. An emphasis on beneficence and nonmaleficence in an effort to protect individuals with mental illness leads to a diminution of their autonomous decision-making.

While it is beyond the scope of this chapter to provide a review of the discourse surrounding vulnerability, several points may be key to the conduct of global mental health research. First, individuals may be vulnerable due to the condition of being human and their particular situations, but this may or may not translate to vulnerability *in the context of research*. Vulnerability in research suggests that there is an "increased potential that one's interests cannot be protected" [9, p. 25]. Additionally, "[i]ndividuals or groups may experience vulnerability to different degrees and at different times, depending on their circumstances" [30]. As an example, an individual whose schizophrenia symptoms are intermittently controlled with their medication regimen may demonstrate sufficient capacity and understanding to participate in a study involving semi-structured interviews, but may or may not have the cognitive wherewithal at a specific time to weigh the risks and benefits associated with a placebo-controlled randomized trial of a new medication.

Second, vulnerability in research may be attributable to external or contextual factors as well as to internal or individual factors [166, 167]. Kipnis [78] has suggested that vulnerability may be characterized as follows, which reflect both contextual and individual factors:

- Incapacitational: vulnerability due to a lack of decisional capacity
- Juridic: vulnerability arising due to the authority of another who has an interest in the individual's participation in research
- Deferential: vulnerability arising due to an informal hierarchical relationship such that the individual masks his or her unwillingness to participate in research
- Social: vulnerability of an individual due to the devaluation of the rights or interests of the group of which the individual is a member, resulting from stigma or discrimination
- Situational: vulnerability arising from medical exigency
- Medical: vulnerability due to suffering resulting from a condition for which there is no remedy
- Allocational: vulnerability due to the receipt of goods and services through research participation that would otherwise be unavailable

Although Kipnis focused specifically on vulnerability in pediatric research, these categories are relevant and applicable to adults as well. Consideration of these various dimensions of vulnerability is particularly important in the context of global mental health research in view of the relative lack of mental health services and treatments available in low-income countries and the oppression of minority groups in various locales throughout the world.

Third, vulnerability in research has traditionally been addressed by considering an alternative population for participation in research; requiring additional justifications for the enrollment of vulnerable persons; requiring special protections such as stricter consent requirements or limiting the risks of exposure; or requiring that the research be responsive to the needs of the vulnerable persons [34, 35]. Such protections, however, inure to the individual and rest on the assumption that vulnerability is necessarily attributable to a characteristic of the individual. However, as Luna [90] has noted, individuals may be autonomous and able to assess the risks and benefits of potential research participation, but may be disempowered and marginalized in their society due to oppression, poverty, or other contextual factors. Indeed, the vulnerability of persons everywhere has increased as the result of increasing state emphasis on enterprise and profitability rather than public welfare [168]. ten Have [148] has observed that the usual remedies to vulnerability are inadequate in such circumstances. Rather, vulnerability resulting from systemic forces must be addressed at a systemic or institutional level, which may not be reasonably effectuated by either researchers or bioethicists.

A lack of understanding of systemic forces that create participant vulnerability may inadvertently exacerbate that vulnerability. As an example, Alenichev and Nguyen [11] examined participants' understandings of their experiences in a phase II double-blinded placebo-controlled trial of an Ebola vaccine in West Africa. The locale in which the study was conducted was characterized by high rates of poverty and unemployment. The researchers found that the participants viewed the trial as providing access to medical and socioeconomic benefits and association with more powerful others that would have otherwise been unattainable. They observed, additionally, that the vaccine trial utilized recruitment and retention practices that were similar to those that had been utilized by reintegration programs directed at the rehabilitation of returning soldiers. As a result, research participants perceived "graduation" from the vaccine trial as conferring an advantage in entering the workforce. Following the conclusion of the trial, however, many remained unemployed and additionally faced stigma due to their trial participation. The researchers concluded that the original study team's lack of an adequate contextual understanding had inadvertently led to an exacerbation of participants' vulnerability.

The International Ethics Framework for Conducting Research with Human Participants

Various international organizations have promulgated guidelines for the ethical conduct of research involving human participants. While many of these documents are not legally binding, many countries have integrated their precepts into their national laws. US federal regulations, for example, have operationalized the principles embedded in the Nuremberg Code, discussed below, and the *Belmont Report*, discussed earlier. Additionally, because the principles enunciated in some of these documents are so foundational to the conduct of research with humans and have been adopted by so many countries, their principles may be considered to be "norms of customary international law" [4].

The Nuremberg Code

Nazi physicians forced prisoners to undergo various medical experiments, which included subjection to extremes of temperatures, deliberate infection with bacteria, bone and limb transplants, forced ingestion of seawater, and mustard gas-induced burns [126, 169]. The prisoners were not provided with an opportunity to consent or to decline participation, nor were they advised of any potential risks or benefits that they might experience as a result. The physicians carrying out the experiments made no attempt to minimize harm or to maximize benefit.

The horrors of these experiments prompted the development of the Nuremberg Code (1949), a statement of basic principles that are deemed to be universally applicable to research conducted with human beings. The Nuremberg Code specifies that:

- Voluntary consent of the participant is essential.
- The results of the experiment must be beneficial to society.
- Animal experiments and knowledge of the natural history of the disease are pre-requisites to experimentation with humans.
- Unnecessary suffering and injury during the experiment are to be avoided.
- An experiment should not be conducted if it is believed that death or disabling injury will occur.
- The degree of risk should not exceed the humanitarian importance of the problem under investigation.
- Facilities used must be adequate to protect the participant against injury or death.
- The persons conducting the experiment must be scientifically qualified.
- The participant has the right to withdraw at any time.
- The scientist must be prepared to end the experiment if there is probable cause that it will likely lead to injury, disability, or death of the participant [15].

The frequent characterization of the Nuremberg Code as reflective of a universal approach has been challenged due to its emphasis on individual consent. However, concepts of personhood differ greatly across societies [88]. Additionally, accusations of "ethical imperialism" have been launched against what is perceived to be the imposition of Western ethics on non-Western contexts [129]. Accordingly, although many non-Western countries recognize the principles reflected in the Nuremberg Code, they have also engaged in efforts to develop ethical guidelines and principles that are responsive to the local contexts [119].

The Declaration of Helsinki

The Declaration of Helsinki, initially adopted by the World Medical Association in 1964 and now in its seventh version, is a set of ethical principles to guide the conduct of research involving humans. The Declaration developed the principles first enunciated in the Nuremberg Code. Unlike the Nuremberg Code, the Helsinki Declaration permits a surrogate to provide consent to participate in research on behalf of an individual who is unable either legally or physically to do so himself or herself. Later revisions of the document emphasized the requirement of voluntary informed consent to participate in research [32]. The fifth revision of the Declaration eliminated the original Declaration's distinction between therapeutic and nontherapeutic research in favor of an emphasis on more general research principles and, additionally, introduced provisions relating to social justice, disclosure of conflict of interest, and publication bias.

Of note, the US Food and Drug Administration rejected the 2000 and subsequent revisions of the Declaration [159]. Neither the FDA nor the NIH training in human subject research participant protection refers to the Declaration of Helsinki, raising concerns that the protections for research participants outside the United States are now weakened.

The International Covenant on Civil and Political Rights

The International Covenant on Civil and Political Rights (ICCPR) was drafted by an international committee following the Second World War. Although it was entered into force in 1976, the United States did not ratify it until 1992. It has been signed by 74 countries [151].

Article 7 of the ICCPR links nonconsensual experimentation to torture and inhuman or degrading treatment:

No one shall be subjected to torture or to cruel, inhuman, or degrading treatment or punishment. In particular, no one shall be subjected without his free consent to medical or scientific experimentation.

General Comment 20, adopted by the Human Rights Committee in 1992, provided additional guidance as to the application of this clause:

Article 7 expressly prohibits medical or scientific experimentation without the free consent of the individual concerned … The Committee also observes that special protection in regard to such experiments is necessary in the case of persons not capable of giving valid consent and in particular those under any form of detention or imprisonment.

In contrast to the Nuremberg Code and the Helsinki Declaration, the ICCPR is binding on those countries that have ratified it; the countries agree to enforce it through their own legal systems [170]. However, there is no international mechanism for its enforcement [171]. The treaty is non-self-executing in the United States, meaning that a private right of action for its violation does not exist [172].

Guidelines of the Council for International Organizations of Medical Sciences

Additional international documents provide further guidance on the conduct of research with human beings. Earlier compilations of the Council for International Organizations of Medical Sciences (CIOMS) include guidelines for epidemiological research (1991) and for biomedical research (1993, 2002), which set forth numerous broadly stated guidelines accompanied by relevant commentary. These documents reflect the potential for heterogeneity across cultures in addressing ethical issues in research. Most recently, CIOMS has issued the *International Ethical Guidelines for Health-Related Research Involving Humans* (2016).

Additional Guidance

Many countries that engage in, sponsor, or permit research involving human participants have established their own ethical guidelines. Researchers should familiarize themselves with both these country-specific ethical standards and any governing laws or regulations pertaining to research in the specific venue.

Provisions must be made to adhere to these laws and guidelines in addition to those of the investigator's own country.

Launching the Study

Informed Consent Processes

Informed consent to participate is a prerequisite to the enrollment of a research participant in any study. In situations in which the prospective participant is unable to provide his or her informed consent, assent may be required in addition to the informed consent of a legally authorized representative of the individual, e.g., a parent or guardian. Valid informed consent comprises four elements: information, understanding, capacity to make a decision, and voluntariness. The absence of adequate provisions for informed consent and protection of the research participants may have dire consequences for the participants, the researcher, and/or the researcher's institution. I have seen situations in which a research team's inadequate protections of participant identity and confidentiality have led to a participant's loss of housing and the somewhat careless disclosure of a participant's health condition to his or her stigmatization and ostracism from neighbors. As another example, the suicide of Tony Lamadrid, participant in a NIMH-funded double-blinded antipsychotic drug crossover and removal study conducted at the University of California, Los Angeles, triggered a lawsuit against the institution and a federal investigation of the drug trial and the university's consent review process [59, 63]. The investigation concluded that the researchers and UCLA had failed to adequately protect participants in the informed consent process and required that the university modify its review system.

Information and Understanding Exactly what or how much information is to be provided to prospective participants to enable them to decide whether or not to participate has been a subject of debate. Current federal regulations, discussed in greater detail below, require that the information be such that a reasonable person would want in order to decide whether to enroll in or to decline participation in a given study.

The provision of information is, however, inadequate if prospective participants are unable to understand it. Written informed consent may present a challenge in any setting due to the length of the document, the use of technical language, and the readability level of the form. In the United States, for example, it has been estimated that one out of every five individuals is functionally illiterate and lacks the reading and writing skills necessary to conduct daily activities [41]. The lower the reading level of the document, the more likely it is that the prospective research volunteer will be able to understand the information presented [89, 164].

Other factors may also affect comprehension. Research has indicated that understanding may be enhanced if the information is presented by nonmedical personnel

[23, 173]. Providing the individual with additional time to digest the information prior to consenting has also been found to increase understanding ([174, 175] Byrne, Rice, & Cuschieri 1993; Moorow, Gootnick, & Schmale 1978), an approach that has been recommended in Uganda [88]. Varying the size of the type or spacing or information [141], using a multicomponent approach to providing information [40], and using graphics [124] have also been found to be helpful. The use of a video to explain the research study may aid increasing the comprehension of potential volunteers in psychiatric research [23].

The provision of information in the global setting may present numerous additional challenges. First, differences in language may make it difficult to communicate concepts that are often seen as foundational. Researchers conducting investigations at various sites in Africa, for example, have noted that there is no equivalent to the terms "research" or "candidate gene" in many African languages [71, 92, 94, 108]. Discussions between researchers and bioethicists harkening from diverse disciplinary and cultural backgrounds may also present challenges due to differing understandings of seemingly similar terms, leading to difficulties in their efforts to reach consensus regarding acceptable practices [95].

Second, cultural, social, and regulatory factors often impact understandings of risk and benefit and of what must be communicated as a risk or benefit. As an example, assume that participants in a clinical trial to assess the equivalence of a new pharmaceutical treatment for bipolar disorder will be required to undergo periodic blood draws to monitor various values, including medication level. Many Western industrialized countries would characterize the blood draw as a procedure involving minimal risk. However, in a specific context, the blood draw may constitute a greater than minimal risk due to beliefs about the power of blood and its use in sorcery and witchcraft [94, 139, 142].

The complexities surrounding the provision of information may impact prospective participants' understanding of what will be expected of them and of the risks and benefits associated with the research [93]. Various strategies have been suggested to increase participant understanding, including engaging with the study community in town halls or forums about the research prior to initiating recruitment efforts [52, 125, 155], consultation with local representatives and cultural representatives regarding the most effective means of communicating and obtaining informed consent [165], and the use of pictorial displays [93]. And, because of the potential for misunderstandings and confusion, many researchers in developing countries have suggested that a mechanism to evaluate prospective participants' level of comprehension be incorporated into the informed consent process [65].

The concept of therapeutic misconception refers to a research participant's mistaken belief that, while a participant in a research study, decisions made regarding her care are for her medical benefit [20, 21], a perspective that essentially conflates the role of research participant with that of medical patient [99]. Whereas the aim of clinical care is to provide the best medical care for the individual patient, clinical research seeks to answer a specific scientific question and to generate generalizable knowledge that will benefit future patients [176]. Accordingly, the treating clinician has a duty of beneficence to his or her patient;

the clinical researcher has an obligation to protect the participant from exploitation and unnecessary harm and to ensure the scientific validity of the research [176]. Researchers and clinicians have been found to share the same misunderstanding [68, 143–145]. Participants' confusion may be exacerbated in situations in which recruitment tools and/or informed consent forms use therapeutic terms to describe the research [38, 58, 77].

Therapeutic misconception does not primarily reflect either inadequate disclosure by the research team or a participant's lack of capacity, but rather stems from divergent cognitive frames [83]. It has been suggested that the concept of therapeutic misconception derives from the absence of "rational congruence" between a participant's understanding of the research and that of the researcher [96, p. 159].

The therapeutic misconception raises ethical issues because this misunderstanding may lead a participant to under- or overestimate the risks and/or the benefits associated with the research, i.e., therapeutic misestimation [62], or to believe that he or she is more likely to benefit than is statistically predicted, i.e., therapeutic optimism. A participant's consent may not be truly informed if he or she fails to understand the differing intentions underlying medical care and research and the difference in roles between research staff and clinical care providers [29]. A number of researchers have suggested that optimism should not be ethically problematic [62] and that compelling evidence should be required to override an individual's agreement to participate in research, notwithstanding participant judgments about potential benefits and harms [98]. Nevertheless, in some cases, the misunderstanding may so distort the consent process as to necessitate reliance on consent monitors and scripts [96] or, ultimately, the exclusion of an individual from study participation [98].

Researchers conducting a systematic review of psychiatry research through 2015 identified various factors associated with the presence of therapeutic misconception: lower education, increased age, poor insight, cognitive deficits, increased illness symptoms, poorer self-rated quality of health, and decreased levels of independence [150]. Studies conducted in various international settings suggest that this erroneous belief has underlain individuals' agreement to participate in the investigations. Molyneux, Peshu, and Marsh [108] found that parents in a coastal Kenyan town agreed to their children's participation in a study based on the mistaken belief that the children would benefit medically. Kass et al. [72] reported that almost all of the individuals interviewed regarding their participation in international health studies indicated that they had agreed to do so because they expected assistance or treatment for their medical problem. In a recent pediatric preventive malaria trial conducted in rural Tanzania, researchers found that parents who declined to have their children participate in the trial were more likely to have understood the experimental nature of the trial and less likely to confuse the research with the provision of clinical care, that is, less likely to hold a therapeutic misconception [112].

A recent randomized intervention trial conducted to test the efficacy of an informed consent intervention found that, in comparison with a traditional informed consent procedure, scientific reframing reduced therapeutic misconception among patients considering enrollment in hypothetical clinical trials [33]. The study sample included 154 participants having a diagnosis of major depression diabetes mellitus, hypertension, coronary artery disease, head/neck cancer, or breast cancer. The 12-minute scientific reframing video, delivered to those randomized to the experimental arm prior to the informed consent process, included segments focused on the purpose of the research and the concept of clinical equipoise, a description of randomization, limitations on dosage and adjunctive medications and the importance of the limitations to the study, subject and physician blinding and the reasons therefore, and the use of these strategies to improve the study design and assure study validity rather than improving the care of the research participants. The vast majority of the participants were white, slightly more than one-half were female, and all of those who completed the study were English-speaking.

However, the effectiveness of such an approach in reducing therapeutic misconception among a more diverse population is uncertain. Burke [29] found in her research relating to cancer clinical trial recruitment in a safety net setting that discussions to introduce the possibility of participation in research prior to the initiation of the informed consent process may be critical in recruiting participants who are underserved, vulnerable, and unfamiliar with research and its relationship to medical care [29]. Interviews conducted with patients invited to participate in a clinical trial revealed that many did not remember having been invited to participate in research. Instead, the patients' focus remained on navigating their unstable living situations rather than assessing the risks and benefits of research versus treatment. Importantly, class, inequality, and dependence influenced the ethical engagements that occurred between the clinician-investigators and prospective participants. Burke concluded that the continuing relevance of the usual remedial approach to therapeutic misconception—increasing research literacy—is questionable and may have to give way to an increased emphasis on patient advocacy and social justice.

Capacity Questions have been raised regarding the capacity of individuals with mental illness to participate in research. (Here, it is important to distinguish between the concept of capacity, which refers to an individual's mental ability to make an informed choice, and the concept of incompetence, which refers to a judicial determination that a specific individual lacks the ability to make decisions and care for himself or herself.) The findings from various studies suggest that many individuals who have been diagnosed with a mental illness have adequate capacity to provide informed consent [19, 76, 110].

Although objective measures of capacity to participate in research have been developed, such as the MacArthur Competence Assessment Tool-Clinical Research (MacCAT-CR) [56, 57], their adequacy in the context of longitudinal and qualitative research has been questioned [146]. The MacCAT-CR utilizes a semi-structured interview format, requiring prospective participants to respond to questions relating to their understanding of the research, the effects of participation on their own lives, their reasoning about participation, and their ability to communicate a decision. However, participants' decision-making capacity and understanding may shift during the course of a study. Repeated administration of the same measure may lessen a participant's trust in the research and lead to reduced participation or withdrawal [146]. Additionally, in the context of global mental health research, a chosen measure to assess capacity may not have been translated into the local language and/or validated for the population in which it is to be used.

Voluntariness he extent to which participation in research is voluntary may be impacted by numerous factors depending upon the specific setting. These may include socioeconomic status, caste, tribe, sex, age, level of education, and access to care or other treatment options. Power inequities associated with any of these variables may compel individuals to feel that they must consent to participate in a particular study [93]. Importantly, at least one court in the United States has affirmed that the prohibition against nonconsensual human medical experimentation is a universally accepted "norm of customary international law" [4].

Ethical Considerations in Study Design and Procedures

Study design may be one of the most complex and controversial issues in mental health research. These debates may be even more contentious in the global health context due to health disparities, power differentials, and lack of access to adequate mental health care [140]. Foremost among these issues is the conduct of placebo-controlled trials to test new interventions for the treatment of mental illness or to enhance mental health. Indeed, clinical trials may "constitute a fragile and sporadic therapeutic niche" in countries that lack adequate mental health services [100, 101].

It appears that there exists general agreement that the use of a placebo in a clinical trial is ethical when there is no existing treatment for the disorder under examination and the trial is to involve the testing of a new class of drugs [31] or when the investigational treatment is to be tested in volunteers for whom standard treatments have proven to be ineffective [104]. The use of placebo in other circumstances, however, has prompted vigorous disagreement, particularly in the context of psychiatric research [25] and, more especially, in the context of clinical trials for treatments targeting depression and schizophrenia [131, 157].

Those who argue in support of placebo-controlled trials point to the methodologic advantages. It has been asserted that placebo-controlled trials are necessary in order to effectively distinguish between medications that are efficacious and those that are not, thereby reducing the likelihood that ineffective drugs will be approved [147]; that placebo-controlled trials reflect enhanced efficiency because smaller sample sizes are needed, leading to potential risk exposure for fewer individuals [25, 105]; and that the risks posed to a few people are justified by the potential benefits to be gained from the new knowledge [82, 104]. Placebo-controlled trials have also received support for use in situations in which the standard treatment would not be accessible outside of the trial context for the majority of the population due to its cost [81]. Placebo-controlled studies have also been justified as providing insights into the potential harms that may be associated with noncompliance among those who decline treatment due to intolerable side effects or because they are too ill to follow a medication regimen [130].

Additionally, those who favor placebo-controlled trials for the testing of new treatments dispute the characterization of a placebo as no-treatment, pointing to findings from psychiatric research that appear to demonstrate a high rate of placebo response among individuals diagnosed with panic disorder, depression, and schizophrenia [6, 27, 60, 73, 75]. The placebo itself does not have a pharmacological effect that causes this response; rather, it is the response of the brain to the perception of treatment that triggers the response [14]. But, the higher the placebo response, the more difficult it may be to determine whether a particular treatment is efficacious for the disorder under study. Research indicates that the placebo effect may be impacted by participants' previous involvement in research, the duration of their illness, and various study site characteristics [84].

Supporters of placebo-controlled trials in mental health research have further argued that mechanisms can be implemented to reduce the possibility of participant harm including minimization of the duration of placebo exposure and exclusion of individuals at risk of suicidal behavior, those with psychosis, and those in need of immediate treatment [31]. Additional suggestions from those supportive of placebo-controlled trials in psychiatric research include the provision of treatment optimization to volunteers following the completion of the trial [104] and the use of an add-on design as an alternative, in which patients would be randomized to the standard treatment plus placebo or the standard treatment plus the agent under study [31]. At least one writer has suggested that a distinction be drawn between volunteers' risks that are of "moral concern" but are "tolerated ethically," such as psychic distress, and those that cannot be tolerated ethically, such as severe distress [104, p. 712]. Indeed, some have contended that in the context of clinical trials of treatments for major depressive disorder and anxiety, the "moral worries" regarding harms arising from placebo-controlled trials "are exaggerated relative to the likelihood that such harms might materialize …" [42, p. 388].

Those who oppose placebo-controlled trials maintain that there is no ethical justification for the exposure of trial participants to additional risk or discomfort if a proven treatment exists for the condition under study [53]. It has been suggested that reliance on a placebo when an effective treatment could be used as a control breaches the ethical requirement of clinical equipoise because the placebo is inferior to the standard treatment [102]. Placebo-controlled trials of maintenance treatments, in which participants are randomized to a placebo arm and to a continued treatment arm, are thought to be particularly problematic ethically because of the risk of worsening symptoms or relapse [48, 104, 109]. Several studies have demonstrated that longer duration of untreated psychosis and a greater number of psychotic episodes are associated with disease progression and greater morbidity [46, 55, 123]. Of note, clinicians' withdrawal of medications in the context of clinical trials directly contravenes clinical efforts to encourage patient adherence to the prescribed medical regimen [45, 48].

Emanuel and Miller [43] have attempted to identify a middle ground between these two positions. They suggest that a placebo-controlled trial may be justified ethically if three criteria are met: (1) there is a high response rate to placebo; (2) the disorder under investigation is characterized by frequent spontaneous remissions or a waxing and waning course; and (3) available treatment is only partly effective or is associated with serious side effects [43].

The current iteration of the Declaration of Helsinki [163] specifies in Principle 33 the conditions under which a placebo-controlled trial will be considered to be ethically acceptable:

> The benefits, risks, burdens, and effectiveness of a new intervention must be tested against those of the best proven intervention(s)

Except in the following circumstances: .

- Where no proven intervention exists, the use of placebo, or no intervention, is acceptable; or
- Where for compelling and scientifically sound methodological reasons, the use of any intervention less effective than the best proven one, the use of placebo, or no intervention is necessary to determine the efficacy or safety of an intervention
- and the patients who receive any intervention less effective than the best proven one, placebo, or no intervention will not be subject to additional risks of serious or irreversible harm as a result of not receiving the best proven intervention.

Extreme care must be taken to avoid abuse of this option.

The guidelines of the International Conference on Harmonisation [66] pertaining to the selection of a control group similarly consider the use of placebo to be inappropriate if a treatment known to prevent serious harm in the study population is in existence.

Findings from a survey of national drug regulatory authorities in 93 countries with respect to placebo-controlled trials indicated that 20 of the 30 responding regulatory bodies indicated that their institutions were bound by the Helsinki Declaration provisions relating to placebo-controlled trials, whereas 10, including the United States, indicated that their respective countries are guided by other ethical principles [136]. None of the 30 authorities unequivocally required placebo-controlled trials for drug approval; nine indicated that use of standard treatment was required for a clinical trial to proceed. The United States indicated that several control options are often available and the selection would depend on what is appropriate.

The ideal clinical trial participant is believed to be one who is an autonomous rational volunteer who is active in the consumption of information about his or her health, has options for care outside clinical research, and is able to differentiate and choose among the options given his or her personal health needs [97, p. 1794].

For many reasons, this image of the ideal research volunteer may be inapropos, particularly in the context of global mental health research.

Not surprisingly, comprehension of concepts integral to clinical trial design may be compromised in many global settings due to difficulties surrounding the translation of scientific concepts generally, the absence of equivalent terms in some languages, and low levels of literacy [5, 155]. Kass and Hyder [71] reported from their survey of researchers working in international settings that only 57% of the 302 researchers surveyed believed that their participants understood the meaning of placebo. Burgess et al. [28] found in their assessment of trial participants' understanding of concepts that only 13%, 20%, and 20% understood the concept of randomization, placebo, and blinding, respectively. A recent meta-analysis of informed consent comprehension in African research settings reported that only 47% of 1633 participants in 4 studies comprehended the meaning of randomization, 30% of 753 participants in 5 studies understood the concept of therapeutic misconception, and 48% of 3946 participants in 6 studies understood placebo [8].

Trials designed to assess interventions other than medications may be equally controversial. The Bucharest Early Intervention Project serves as an example of the contextual and ethical issues that must be considered in conducting global mental health research.

The study was a 4-year longitudinal randomized controlled trial of foster care as an intervention for children in institutions in Bucharest, Romania, that was conducted between 2000 and 2005. The investigation sought to identify brain changes during the first years of life that influence specific behavioral outcomes in children raised in orphanages; to assess the impact of the child's experiences on brain development; to determine the extent to which placement in a more favorable environment might remediate abnormalities; and to identify a specific period, if one exists, during which an intervention would be most effective [16, 17]. The study was approved by regulatory authorities in both the United States and Romania, and informed consent was obtained from parents and institutional caregivers prior to commencing the study.

At the time of the study, there were approximately 136,000 children living in institutions in Romania [86]. The children had little exercise, often received inadequate nutrition, had little personal interaction, and had minimal to no educational and recreational opportunities ([177, 178], Beri et al. 2002). Active children were controlled with the use of restraints and/or tranquilizers (Taneja, Sriram, Beri et al. 2002). Hygiene was inadequate, resulting in the transmission of HIV, hepatitis, and/ or parasitic infections [179, 180].

The study enrolled a total of 136 institutionalized children between the ages of 5 and 31 months who were randomized to remain in institutional care or to be placed in foster care. The children were to be compared to 72 never-institutionalized children who were matched by age and sex. Periodic assessments of the children focused on language development, social communication, social interaction, attachment, temperament, and discrimination of facial emotion.

Ethical concerns related to the study were raised at least by 2002. The European deputy to the European Parliament voiced objections about the lack of direct benefit to many of the child participants, the transport of all data and videotapes to the United States in contravention of the European Union's rules on data protection, and the researchers' conduct of the study in Romania, rather than the United States, made possible by exploiting Romania's then-lax government regulations related to research [67]. Multiple scholars continued to raise concerns related to the lack of direct benefit to the participants, the selection of Romania as the site of the study, the absence of clinical equipoise in view of existing literature that clearly documented the adverse effects on children of institutional settings, and the investigators' failure to provide at the conclusion of the study for the placement in foster care of children remaining in institutions if the intervention had been found to be beneficial [18, 50, 51, 86, 156]. Two of these commentaries explicitly compared the investigators' observation of the institutionalized children's progressive cognitive decline to the US-based Tuskegee study, in which investigators observed and assessed the effects of the natural progression of syphilis in black men, despite the availability of a known remedy [51, 86].

The investigators of the Bucharest Early Intervention Project and their consulting bioethicist have variously responded to these critiques by asserting that the institutionalized children experienced minimal risk as a result of their study participation because the continuing institutionalization represented a continuation of their then-life experience; that the policy debate surrounding foster care versus institutional care had not yet been settled in Romania; that the study protocol had been reviewed by more than one ethics review committee; that institutional caregivers or foster parents had assented to the children's participation; and that clinical research is designed to answer scientific questions, not to benefit individuals [106, 107, 181]. When asked by a journalist how he avoided being upset by the conditions in which the children lived, Charles Nelson, one of the investigators, indicated that he detached and went about his work as a scientist [64]. One scholar critical of the research, however, lamented that "the BIEP investigators had lost control of their study [to the Romanian government's agenda] and its moral compass, all with grave consequences" [50].

Research Monitoring and Compliance

The US Regulatory Framework and Compliance

The principles enunciated in the *Belmont Report* [113] are reflected in the US regulatory framework governing research involving human participants. The US Department of Health and Human Services (DHHS) and the US Food and Drug Administration (FDA) relied on the report in 1981 as the basis for the revision of their then-existing regulations.

In 1991, 15 different federal departments and agencies codified in their regulations the Federal Policy for the Protection of Human Subjects, known as the "Common Rule." The Common Rule was revised in 2017 and amended in January 2018; these most recent revisions became effective on January 21, 2019. Twenty different federal agencies are either signatories to the revised Common Rule or have indicated their intent to become an official signatory. These include many agencies from which global mental health researchers may be seeking research funds, such as the Agency for International Development, the Department of Defense, the Department of Veterans Affairs, the Department of Health and Human Services, and the National Science Foundation [152].

The revised Common Rule now specifies that the information provided to each participant must be such that a reasonable person would want in order to decide whether or not to participate. Minimally, this must include the following:

1. A statement that the study involves research, an explanation of the purposes of the research and the expected duration of the subject's participation, a description of the procedures to be followed, and identification of any procedures that are experimental
2. A description of any reasonably foreseeable risks or discomforts to the subject
3. A description of any benefits to the subject or to others that may reasonably be expected from the research
4. A disclosure of appropriate alternative procedures or courses of treatment, if any, that might be advantageous to the subject
5. A statement describing the extent, if any, to which confidentiality of records identifying the subject will be maintained
6. For research involving more than minimal risk, an explanation as to whether any compensation and an explanation as to whether any medical treatments are available if injury occurs and, if so, what they consist of, or where further information may be obtained
7. An explanation of whom to contact for answers to pertinent questions about the research and research subjects' rights and whom to contact in the event of a research-related injury to the subject
8. A statement that participation is voluntary, refusal to participate will involve no penalty or loss of benefits to which the subject is otherwise entitled, and the subject may discontinue participation at any time without penalty or loss of benefits to which the subject is otherwise entitled
9. One of the following statements about any research that involves the collection of identifiable private information or identifiable biospecimens:
   (i) A statement that identifiers might be removed from the identifiable private information or identifiable biospecimens and that, after such removal, the information or biospecimens could be used for future research studies or distributed to another investigator for future research studies without additional informed consent from the subject or the legally authorized representative, if this might be a possibility
   (ii) A statement that the subject's information or biospecimens collected as part of the research, even if identifiers are removed, will not be used or distributed for future research studies [1]

Additional information may be required depending upon the nature of the study.

The revised Common Rule made numerous additional changes with respect to activities classified as human research, the informed consent process, consent documentation, criteria for granting a waiver of consent and documentation of the waiver, exempt categories, review by institutional review boards (IRB), and continuing review. Table 4.1 summarizes these revisions below. However, researchers are urged to consult the regulations and the research office of their respective institutions for more detailed guidance.

Table 4.1 Summary of changes to Common Rule

Domain	Revisions

Definition of research	Four types of activities now identified as not constituting research:
	    Specified scholarly and journalistic activities
	    Specified public health surveillance activities
	    Collection and analysis of specimens, records, or information collected by or for a criminal justice agency for certain criminal justice or investigative purposes
	    Specified authorized operational activities for national security purposes

Informed consent	Prospective participants must be provided with the information that a reasonable person would want to have in order to make an informed decision
	The information must be presented in a manner that enhances understanding of why someone might or might not want to participate in the research
	The informed consent form should be designed in such a way as to help people process complicated information
	The beginning of the form must display the study's purpose, risks, benefits, and alternatives
	The informed consent form must indicate whether participants' information or biospecimens might or will not be stripped of identifiers and used for future research
	For any clinical trial conducted or supported by a department that is a signatory to the Common Rule, one consent form must be posted on a publicly available federal website following the close of recruitment and no later than 60 days after the last study visit. The consent form must have been used to enroll study participants
	If relevant to the study, the informed consent form must also contain:
	    Information about possible commercial profit
	    Information about whether the research participants will be provided with any clinically relevant research results
	    Information about whether activities will or might include whole genome sequencing

Waiver of informed consent and documentation	A signed informed consent form may not be necessary if the participants are members of a distinct cultural group or community in which signing the form is not the norm, and the research involves no more than minimal risk, and there is an alternative method available for the documentation of consent

(continued)

Table 4.1 (continued)

Domain	Revisions

Exempt categories	*Exemption 1*, educational practices: The research must not be likely to adversely impact the student's opportunity to learn required content or the assessment of educators that provide the instruction
	Exemption 2, educational tests, surveys, observation of public behavior:
	  Expanded to include collection of sensitive and identifiable data
	  Not applicable to research involving interventions, collection of biospecimens, linking to personally identifiable information, or research with children, except for some educational tests and some public observation
	  Disclosure of participants' responses outside the research would not damage their educational advancement
	  Limited IRB review may be permissible
	Exemption 3 (new category), benign behavioral interventions:
	  Includes data collected through interaction, e.g., interview, recording, survey
	  Does not include research with children, deception in the absence of prior agreement, physiological data collection methods
	Exemption 4, research on existing data: expanded to permit both prospective and retrospective reviews, maintenance of all identifiers if all data are protected health information and specified research conducted by or for a federal department or agency or using government-collected or – generated information for non-research activities
	Exemption 5, public benefit service: now requires that the project be posted on a federal website
	Exemption 7, permits storage and maintenance of data and/or specimens in a repository, with identifiers, for secondary research collected under broad consent and with an approved IRB protocol
	Exemption 8 (new category): permits secondary research of identifiable data or biospecimens collected under an approved IRB protocol with broad consent:

IRB review and continuing review	Some minimal risk studies will no longer be subject to annual review. Extended approval is not permissible for studies involving FDA-regulated components or oversight, prisoners, or stem cells or SCRO protocols Limited IRB review is available for specified exemptions. In such cases, the IRB must assure that adequate provisions have been made to protect participants' privacy and the confidentiality of the data Most federally funded collaborative US-based research projects will be required to utilize one IRB

Sources: 82 Fed. Reg. 7149-7272 [2]; 83 Fed. Reg. 28497-28520; [3, 153]

Monitoring Mechanisms

One of the primary concerns in conducting research is that of participant safety. As noted earlier, the ethical principles of beneficence and nonmaleficence call upon the investigator to make efforts to maximize benefit and to avoid all unnecessary harm. Accordingly, efforts must be made to oversee the study and assure participant safety during the course of the research. These concerns are reflected in federal policy; the National Institutes of Health requires that all clinical trials have appropriate oversight and monitoring to protect the health, rights, and safety of the participants [115,

116]. The policy encompasses all types of clinical trials, including physiologic, toxicity, and dose-finding studies (phase I); efficacy studies (phase II); and efficacy, effectiveness, and comparative trials (phase III). The form that the monitoring is to take should be appropriate to the level of risk involved.

The investigator of a study is in all situations tasked with the responsibility of overseeing and assuring participant during the course of the research. The investigator may wish to and, in some cases, be required to develop a data safety monitoring plan (DSMP). The National Institute of Mental Health (NIMH), for example, requires that investigators applying to the NIMH for funding include in the Human Subjects section of their proposal a DSMP [117]. NIMH advises the investigative team to consider in the development of the DSMP "the protocol, phase, intervention(s), target population, subject safety and privacy, risks and benefits involved in the study, data integrity and confidentiality, study coordination, and how the team addresses each of these elements" [117]. The DSMP must address the roles and qualifications of the individuals responsible for monitoring the trial; issues related to trial safety including, but not limited to, potential risks and measures in place to mitigate them, consent and assent procedures, stopping rules, procedures for the management of incidental findings, the disclosure and management of conflicts of interest, and data security; a description of reportable events and how they are to be handled; and issues related to data management, analysis, and quality assurance [117].

However, this responsibility is not left to the investigator alone. The sponsor (funder) of the study also bears responsibility for oversight. This suggests that, minimally, the sponsor of research should not fund studies that are characterized by inadequate protections of the research participants or that anticipate severe injury or death due to participation.

Institutional review boards (IRBs) are administrative bodies that are charged with the responsibility of following ethical standards for the conduct of studies and ensuring that the identity, privacy, safety, and health of the research participants are protected. IRB review of studies involving human participants is required by federal regulations of "all research involving human subjects conducted, supported, or otherwise subject to regulation by any Federal department or agency that takes appropriate administrative action to make the policy applicable to such research" (45 C.F.R. § 46.101). Federal regulation mandates that the IRB have at least five members with varying disciplinary backgrounds in order to ensure that its review of research protocols will encompass the institutional, legal, scientific, and social implications of the proposed research and will be complete and adequate (45 C.F.R. § 46.107).

Although in some cases monitoring by the principal investigator may be sufficient, a data safety monitoring board (DSMB) will be required. In many situations, such as a large multisite study, there is a need for an independent DSMB. As an example, the NIMH provides that all clinical trials funded through that Institute must, at a minimum, be monitored by both the principal investigator and an institutional review board. However, depending upon the size, complexity, and scope of the trial, an independent safety monitor or data safety monitoring board may be required as well [117]. NIMH guidance advises that multisite trials and most phase III clinical trials require monitoring by a DSMB.

An independent safety monitor (ISM) is an independent physician or other expert who is engaged to provide independent monitoring of a clinical trial [118]. This role is distinct from that of a medical monitor associated with the study. The ISM must not have any conflict of interest with either the study to be monitored or any member of the study team in order to ensure that he or she will maintain the objectivity necessary to ensure the safety of the trial participants and the integrity of the data. Although the ISM can be affiliated with the investigator's institution or the study site, he or she cannot be a collaborator, mentor, mentee, supervisor, supervisee, co-author, or a member of the investigator's department during the preceding 3 years.

A DSMB consists of individuals who are deemed to be expert in their respective fields and who are independent of the study to be monitored [118]. NIMH requires that a board have at least three members, who must include at least one content expert and one biostatistician. Additional members may include a bioethicist, pharmacologist, clinical trials expert, patient advocate, or community representative [114]. Members must be free of any professional or financial conflict of interests in order to assure objectivity. A member may be affiliated with the same institution as the investigator, but may not be a collaborator, co-author, supervisor, mentor, mentee, subordinate of the investigator, or a member of the investigator's institutional department during the previous 3 years [118]. The DSMB meets at predetermined intervals, such as semiannually or quarterly, but must in all cases meet at least once a year. They usually first meet in an open session that may include the investigators and the program officers associated with the funding source. Unlike the IRB, DSMB members may have access to the study data if required to evaluate safety concerns. Table 4.2 provides a comparison of IRB and DSMB functions.

Table 4.2 Comparison of IRB and DSMB functions

Function	IRB	DSMB
Review research protocol	√	√
Monitor rate of participant recruitment		√
Monitor performance of trial sites		√
Recommend study continuation or modification		√
Assess participant risk and benefit	√	√
Assess adequacy of participant protections	√	√
Recommend study termination due to unfavorable risk-benefit assessment or inability of study to answer study question		√
Recommend suspension or termination of one or more study arms based on concerns about participant safety or rate of enrollment		√
Recommend study termination based on efficacy findings		√
Review informed consent/assent process and associated forms	√	√
Monitor completeness of data		√
Evaluate safety of the participants as pre-specified in the DSMP		√
Evaluate efficacy of the treatments being tested as pre-specified in the interim monitoring plan of the protocol		√
Assess the presence of any early unanticipated therapeutic effects, side effects, or adverse consequences		√
Review final results	√	√

Sources: [114, 116]

Publication and Dissemination

Increasing efforts are being made to battle "helicopter research," whereby investigators from developed countries take samples and data from communities situated in less developed nations and return to their home institutions [120]. This practice contravenes the Declaration of Helsinki's admonition that "Researchers, authors, sponsors, editors and publishers all have ethical obligations with regard to the publication and dissemination of the results of research" [163]. Recently, the ethics working group of the Human Heredity and Health in Africa (H3Africa) Initiative issued guidelines for the ethical handling of samples for genomic studies to ameliorate the disempowerment of local researchers and communities that have collaborated in research. The suggestions include the imposition of an embargo period prohibiting scientists not involved in the conduct of the study from publishing from the data [120].

The Declaration of Helsinki notes the importance of such dissemination: "Researchers have a duty to make publicly available the results of their research on human subjects and are accountable for the completeness and accuracy of their reports" [163]. However, the frequent lack of feedback of research results to research participants and their community, apart from dissemination in scientific forums, is problematic [91]. Although feedback to participants may be challenging due to language differences, logistical issues, group dynamics, and the social and cultural constructions of knowledge, such feedback is critical to efforts to sustain trust in science and scientists.

Discussion of research findings with research participants even prior to their publication may serve a number of important purposes. First, the researchers can obtain approval for the use of specific quotes of case studies in situations in which anonymity cannot be guaranteed. Second, the participants may be able to provide insights to understanding the findings that the researchers may not have considered. Third, the researchers' framing of their findings may have serious implications for the participants and/or their larger community. As an example, findings related to a high prevalence of a mental illness or of substance use or dependence could exacerbate any stigmatization or marginalization that the community is already experiencing.

Concluding Thoughts

Clearly, there exists a critical need for mental health research in the global setting to enhance the suitability and availability of appropriate interventions and services and reduce the burden of suffering experienced by individuals, their family members, and their communities. Conduct of this research respectfully and ethically may be challenging due to differences in understandings and beliefs about what mental illness is and how it can be treated, less than optimal infrastructure for the conduct of research, translation difficulties, and varying levels of health literacy. In designing and conducting such research, researchers, their institutions, and the research sponsors must consider the level of risk, the nature and extent of the potential participants' vulnerability, and the extent to which individuals can ethically be asked to suffer for the potential benefit of others in the future. As findings in the extant literature demonstrate, what may appear to be informed consent does not ensure participant understanding and, by itself, is inadequate to protect the participants. Our excitement about the creation of new knowledge, our own hubris with respect to the impact of our discoveries, cannot blind us to the harms that we may cause or perpetuate, however unintentional they may be.

References

1. C.F.R. §§ 46.101, 46.107, 46.116 (2018).
2. Fed. Reg. 7149-7272 (January 19, 2017).
3. Fed. Reg. 28497-28520 (June 19, 2018).
4. Abdullahi v. Pfizer, Inc. ("Abdullahi IV"), 562 F.3d 1163 (2d Cir. 2009).
5. Adams, V., Miler, S., Craig, S., Samen, A., et al. (2005). The challenge of cross-cultural clinical trial research: Case report from the Tibetan Autonomous Region, People's Republic of China. *Medical Anthropology Quarterly, 19*(3), 267–289.
6. Addington, D. (1995). The use of placebos in clinical trials for acute schizophrenia. *Canadian Journal of Psychiatry, 40*, 171–175.
7. Adelekan, M. L., Makanjuola, A. B., & Ndom, R. J. (2001). Traditional mental health practitioners in Kwara State, Nigeria. *East African Medical Journal, 78*(4), 190–196.
8. Afolabi, M. O., Okebe, J. U., McGrath, N., Larson, H. J., Bojang, K., & Chandramohan, C. (2014). Informed consent comprehension in African settings. *Tropical Medicine & International Health, 19*(6), 625–642.
9. Agarwal, M. (2003). Voluntariness in clinical research at the end of life. *Journal of Pain and Symptom Management, 25*(4), 25–32.
10. Aghukwa, C. (2010). Medical students' beliefs and attitudes towards people with mental illness in southwestern Nigeria. *The Australian and New Zealand Journal of Psychiatry, 42*(5), 389–395.
11. Alenichev, A., & Nguyen, V.-K. (2019). Precarity, clinical labour and graduation from Ebola clinical research in West Africa. *Global Bioethics, 30*(1), 1–18.
12. Alexander, L. (2016). Deontological ethics. In: *Stanford encyclopedia of philosophy.* Available at https://plato.stanford.edu/entries/ethics-deontological/#DeoTheKan. Accessed 29 Feb 2020.
13. Allbutt, H., & Masters, H. (2010). Ethnography and the ethics of undertaking research on different mental health care settings. *Journal of Psychiatric and Mental Health Nursing, 17*, 210–215.
14. Alphs, L., Benedetti, F., Flieschhacker, W. W., & Kane, J. M. (2012). Placebo-related effects in clinical trials in schizophrenia: What is driving this phenomenon and what can be done to minimize it? *The International Journal of Neuropsychopharmacology, 15*, 1003–1014.
15. Annas, G. J., & Grodin, M. A. (Eds.). (1992). *The Nazi doctors and the Nuremberg Code: Human rights in experimentation.* London: Oxford University Press.
16. Anon. (2020). *Bucharest early intervention project.* Available at https://www.macbrain.org/beip.htm. Accessed 28 Feb 2020.
17. Anon. (n.d.). *Effects of early experience on brain-behavioral development.* Available at http://www.macbrain.org/effects2.htm. Accessed 26 Jan 2004.
18. Anon. (2008). The ethical neuroscientist. *Nature Neuroscience, 11*(3), 239. [editorial].
19. Appelbaum, P. S., Grisso, T., Frank, E., O'Donnell, S., & Kupfer, D. J. (1999). Competence of depressed patients for consent to research. *American Journal of Psychiatry, 156*(9), 1380–1384.

20. Appelbaum, P. S., Roth, L. H., & Lidz, C. (1982b). The therapeutic misconception: Informed consent in psychiatric research. *International Journal of Law and Psychiatry, 5*(3–4), 319–329.
21. Appelbaum, P. S., Roth, L. H., Lidz, C., Benson, P., & Winslade, W. (1982a). False hopes and best data: Consent to research and the therapeutic misconception. *The Hastings Center Report, 17*(2), 20–24.
22. Beecher, H. K. (1970). *Research and the individual: Human studies*. Boston: Little, Brown and Company.
23. Benson, P. R., Roth, L. H., Appelbaum, P. S., Lidz, C. W., & Winslade, W. J. (1988). Information disclosure, subject understanding and informed consent in psychiatric research. *Law and Human Behavior, 12*, 455–475.
24. Bentham, J. (1962). An introduction to the principles of moral and legislation. In *Utilitarianism and other writings*. New York: New American Library.
25. Berk, M. (2007). The place of placebo? The ethics of placebo-controlled trials in bipolar disorder. *Acta Neuropsychiatrica, 19*, 74–75.
26. Brandt, A. M. (1985). Racism and research: The case of the Tuskegee study. In J. W. Leavitt & R. L. Numbers (Eds.), *Sickness and health in America: Readings in the history of medicine and public health* (pp. 331–343). Madison: University of Wisconsin Press.
27. Brown, W. A. (1988). Predictors of placebo response in depression. *Pychopharmacology Bulletin, 24*, 14–17.
28. Burgess, L. J., Gerber, B., Coetzee, K., Terblanche, M., Agar, G., & Kotze, T. J. W. (2019). An evaluation of informed consent comprehension by adult trial participants in South Africa at the time of providing consent for clinical trial participation and a review of the literature. *Journal of Clinical Trials, 11*, 19–35.
29. Burke, N. J. (2014). Rethinking the therapeutic misconception: Social justice, patient advocacy, and cancer clinical trial recruitment in the US safety net. *BMC Medical Ethics, 15*, 68. https:www.biomedcentral.com/1472-6939/15/68.
30. Canadian Institutes of Health Research. (2014). *Ethical conduct for research involving humans (TCPS2)*. Available at http://www.pre-ethics.gc.ca/eng/policy-politique/initiatives/tcps2-eptc2/Default/. Accessed 2 Aug 2018.
31. Charney, D. S., Nemeroff, C. B., Lewis, L., Laden, S. K., Gorman, J. M., Laska, E. M., et al. (2002). National Depressive and Manic-Depressive Association consensus statement on the use of placebo in clinical trials of mood disorders. *Archives of General Psychiatry, 59*, 262–270.
32. Christakis, N. A., & Panner, M. J. (1991). Existing international guidelines for human subjects research: Some open questions. *Law, Medicine & Health Care, 19*, 214–221.
33. Christopher, P. P., Appelbaum, P. S., Truong, D., Albert, K., Maranda, L., & Lidz, C. (2017). Reducing therapeutic misconception: A randomized intervention trial in hypothetical clinical trials. *PLoS One, 12*(9), e0184224. https://doi.org/10.1371/journal.pone.0184224.
34. Council for International Organizations of Medical Sciences. (1993). *International ethical guidelines for biomedical research involving human subjects*. Geneva: Author.
35. Council for International Organizations of Medical Sciences. (2002). *International ethical guidelines for biomedical research involving human subjects*. Geneva: Author.
36. Council for International Organizations of Medical Sciences. (1991). *International guidelines for ethical review of epidemiological studies*. Geneva: Author.
37. Council for International Organizations of Medical Sciences. (2016). *International ethical guidelines for health-related research involving humans*. Geneva: Author.
38. Cox, A. C., Fallowfield, L. J., & Jenkins, V. A. (2006). Communication and informed consent in phase 1 trials: A review of the literature. *Support Care Cancer, 14*, 303–309.
39. Das, J., Do, Q. T., Friedman, J., McKenzie, D., & Scott, K. (2007). Mental health and poverty in developing countries: Revisiting the relationship. *Social Science & Medicine, 65*(3), 467–480.
40. DCCT Research Group. (1989). Implementation in a multicomponent process to obtain informed consent in the Diabetes Control and Complications trial. *Controlled Clinical Trials, 10*, 83–96.

41. Doak, L. G. A., & Doak, C. C. (1980). Patient comprehension profiles: Recent findings and strategies. *Patient Counselling and Health Education, 2*, 101–106.
42. Dunlop, B. W., & Banja, J. (2009). A renewed, ethical defense of placebo-controlled trials of new treatments for major depression and anxiety disorders. *Journal of Medical Ethics, 45*(6), 384–389.
43. Emanuel, E. J., & Miller, F. G. (2001). The ethics of placebo-controlled trials—a middle ground. *The New England Journal of Medicine, 345*(12), 915–919.
44. Emeka, O. C. N. (2015). Migration of international medical graduates: Implications for the brain-drain. *Open Medicine Journal, 2*, 17–24.
45. Emsley, R. (2017). On discontinuing treatment in schizophrenia: A clinical conundrum. *NPJ Schizophrenia, 3*, 4. https://doi.org/10.1038/s41537-016-0004-2.
46. Emsley, R., Chiliza, B., & Asmal, L. (2013b). The evidence for illness progression after relapse in schizophrenia. *Schizophrenia Research, 148*, 117–121.
47. Emsley, R., Chiliza, B., Asmal, L., & Harvey, B. H. (2013a). The nature of relapse in schizophrenia. *BMC Psychiatry, 13*, 50. http://www.biomedcentral.com/1471-244X/13/50.
48. Emsley, R., Fleischhacker, W. W., Galderisi, S., Halpern, L. J., McEvoy, J. P., & Schooler, N. R. (2016). Placebo control in clinical trials: Concerns about use in relapse prevention studies in schizophrenia. *British Medical Journal, 354*, i4728. https://doi.org/10.1136/bmj.i4728.
49. Etzioni, A. (1998). Introduction: A matter of balance, rights, and responsibilities. In A. Etzioni (Ed.), *The essential communitarian reader* (pp. ix–xxiv). Lanham: Rowman & Littlefield.
50. Fins, J. J. (2014). Orphans to history: A response to the Bucharest Early Intervention Project investigators. *Bioethics Forum.* Available at https://www.thehastingscenter.org/orphans-to-history-a-response-to-the-bucharest-early-intervention-project-investigators/. Accessed 29 Feb 2020.
51. Fins, J. J. (2013). Romanian orphans: A reconsideration of the ethics of the Bucharest Early Intervention Project. *Bioethics Forum.* Available at https://www.thehastingscenter.org/romanian-orphans-a-reconsideration-of-the-ethics-of-the-bucharest-early-intervention-project/. Accessed 29 Feb 2020.
52. Fitzgerald, D. W., Marotte, C., Verdier, R. I., Johnson, W. D., Jr., & Pape, J. W. (2002). Comprehension during informed consent in a less well-developed country. *Lancet, 360*, 1301–1302.
53. Freedman, B., Weijer, C., & Glass, J. K. C. (1996). Placebo orthodoxy in clinical research II: Ethical, legal, and regulatory myths. *The Journal of Law, Medicine & Ethics, 24*(3), 252–259.
54. Gilligan, C. (1982). *In a different voice: Psychological theory and women's development.* Cambridge, MA: Harvard University Press.
55. Goff, D. C., Falkai, P., Fleischhacker, W. W., Girgis, R. R., Kahn, R. M., Uchida, H., et al. (2019). The long-term effects of antipsychotic medication on clinical course in schizophrenia. *American Journal of Psychiatry, 174*(9), 840–849.
56. Grisso, T., Appelbaum, P. S., Mulvey, E., & Fletcher, K. (1995). Measures of abilities related to competence to consent to treatment. *Law and Human Behavior, 19*, 127–148.
57. Grisso, T., Appelbaum, P. S., & Hill-Fatouhi, C. (1997). The MacCAT-T: A clinical tool to assess patients' capacities to make treatment decisions. *Psychiatric Services, 48*, 1415–1419.
58. Henderson, G. E., Davis, A. M., King, N. M., Easter, M. M., Zimmer, C. R., Rothschild, B. B., et al. (2004). Uncertain benefit: Investigators' views and communications in early phase gene transfer trials. *Molecular Therapy, 10*, 225–231.
59. Hilts, P. J. (1994). Agency faults a U.C.L.A. study for suffering of mental patients. *New York Times.*
60. Hirschfeld, R. M. A. (1996). Placebo response in the treatment of panic disorder. *Bulletin of the Menninger Clinic, 60*(Suppl A), A76–A86.
61. Hornblum, A. M. (1998). *Acres of skin: Human experiments in Holmesburg Prison.* New York: Routledge.
62. Horng, S., & Grady, C. (2003). Misunderstanding in clinical research: Distinguishing therapeutic misconception, therapeutic misestimation, and therapeutic optimism. *IRB, 25*(5), 11–16.

4 Ethical Considerations in Global Mental Health Research

63. Horowitz, J. (1994). For the sake of science: When Tony Lamadrid, a schizophrenic patient and research subject at UCLA, committed suicide, it set off a national debate: What is acceptable in human experimentation and who decides? *New York Times.*
64. Hughes, V. (2013). *Detachment.* Available at https://aeon.co/essays/romanian-orphans-a-human-tragedy-a-scientific-opportunity. Accessed 29 Feb 2020.
65. Hyder, A. A., & Wali, S. A. (2006). Informed consent and collaborative research: Perspectives from the developing world. *Developing World Bioethics, 6*(1), 33–40.
66. International Conference on Harmonisation. (2001). Guidance E10: Choice of control group and related issues in clinical trials. Step 4 version. Author. Available at https://www.fda.gov/media/71349/download. Accessed 28 February 2020.
67. James B. (2002). U.S. study of Romanian children face European challenge. *New York Times.* Available at https://www.nytimes.com/2002/06/06/news/us-study-of-romanian-children-faces-european-challenge.html?auth=login-email&login=email. Accessed 29 Feb 2020.
68. Joffe, S., & Weeks, J. C. (2002). Views of American oncologists about the purposes of clinical trials. *Journal of the National Cancer Institute, 94*(24), 1847–1853.
69. Jonsen, A. R. (1995). Casuistry: An alternative or complement to principles? *Kennedy Institute of Ethics Journal, 5*, 237–251.
70. Kant, I. (1964 [1785]). *Groundwork of the metaphysic of morals. (Trans. H.J. Paton).* New York: Harper and Row.
71. Kass, N., & Hyder, A. (2001). Attitudes and experiences of U.S. and developing country investigators regarding U.S. human subjects regulations. In *Ethical and policy issues in international research: Clinical trials in developing countries* (Vol. II, p. B1–220). Bethesda: National Bioethics Advisory Commission.
72. Kass, N., Maman, S., & Atkinson, J. (2005). Motivations, understanding, and voluntariness in international randomized trials. *IRB, 27*(6), 1–8.
73. Keck, P. E., Jr., Welge, J. A., McElroy, S. L., Arnold, L. M., & Strakowski, S. M. (2000). Placebo effect in randomized, controlled studies of acute bipolar mania and depression. *Biological Psychiatry, 47*, 748–755.
74. Kessler, R. C., McGonagle, K. A., Zhao, S., Nelson, C. B., Hughes, M., Eshleman, S., et al. (1994). Lifetime and 12-month prevalence of DSM-III-R psychiatric disorders in the United States, Results from the National Comorbidity Survey. *Archives of General Psychiatry, 5*(1), 8–19.
75. Khan, A., Warner, H. A., & Brown, W. A. (2000). Symptom reduction and suicide risk in patients treated with placebo in antidepressant clinical trials: An analysis of the Food and Drug Administration database. *Archives of General Psychiatry, 57*, 311–317.
76. Kim, S. Y. H., Cox, C., & Caine, E. D. (2002). Impaired decision-making ability in subjects with Alzheimers disease & willingness to participate in research. *American Journal of Psychiatry, 159*(5), 797–802.
77. King, N. M., Henderson, G. E., Churchill, L. R., Davis, A. M., Hull, S. C., Nelson, D. K., et al. (2005). Consent forms and the therapeutic misconception: The example of gene transfer research. *IRB, 27*, 1–8.
78. Kipnis, K. (2003). Seven vulnerabilities in the pediatric research subject. *Theoretical Medicine, 24*, 107–120.
79. Krugman, S. (1996). The Willowbrook hepatitis studies revisited: Ethical aspects. *Reviews of Infectious Diseases, 8*, 157–162.
80. Levine, C., Faden, R., Grady, C., Hammerschhmidt, D., Eckenwiler, L., & Sugarman, J. (2004). The limitations of "vulnerability" as a protection for human research participants. *The American Journal of Bioethics, 4*(3), 44–49.
81. Levine, R. J. (1998). The 'best proven therapeutic method' standard in clinical trials in technologically developing countries. *IRB, 20*, 5–9.
82. Levine, R. J. (1985). The use of placebo in randomized controlled trials. *IRB, 7*(2), 1–4.
83. Lidz, C. W., Albert, K., Appelbaum, P., Dunn, L. B., Overton, E., & Pivovarova, E. (2015). Why is therapeutic misconception so prevalent? *Cambridge Quarterly of Healthcare Ethics, 24*(2), 231–241.

84. Loebel, A., Cucchairo, J., Siu, C., Daniel, D., & Kalali, A. (2010). *Signal detection in clinical trials: A post-study survey of schizophrenia trial sites.* Poster presentation, International Society for CNS Clinical Trials and Methodology 2010 Autumn Conference, October 13–14, Baltimore.

85. Loewy, E. H. (1996). *Textbook of health care ethics.* New York: Plenum Press.

86. Loue, S. (2004). Ethical issues in research: A Romanian case study. *Rev Română de Bioetică, 2*(1), 16–27.

87. Loue, S., & Loff, B. (2019). Teaching vulnerability in research: A study of approaches utilized by a sample of research ethics training programs. *Journal of Empirical Research on Human Research Ethics, 14*(4), 395–407.

88. Loue, S., Okello, D., & Kawuma, M. (1996). Research bioethics in the Ugandan context: A program summary. *The Journal of Law, Medicine & Ethics, 24,* 47–53.

89. LoVerde, M. E., Prochazka, A. V., & Byny, R. I. (1989). Research consent forms: Continued unreadability and increasing length. *Journal of General Internal Medicine, 4,* 410–412.

90. Luna, F. (2009). *Bioethics and vulnerability: A Latin American view.* Amsterdam and New York: Rodopi.

91. Macleod, C., Masilela, T. C., & Malomane, E. (1998). Feedback of research results: Reflections from a community-based health programme. *South Africa Journal of Psychology, 28*(4), 215–221.

92. Marshall, P. A. (2004). The individual and the community in international genetic research. *The Journal of Clinical Ethics, 15*(1), 76–86.

93. Marshall, P. A. (2006). Informed consent in international health research. *Journal of Empirical Research on Human Research Ethics, 1*(1), 25–42.

94. Marshall, P. A. (2001). The relevance of culture for informed consent in U.S.-funded international health research. In *Ethical and policy issues in international research: Clinical trials in developing countries* (Vol. II, pp. C1–C38). Bethesda: National Bioethics Advisory Commission.

95. Marshall, P., Thomasma, D. C., & Bergsma, J. (1994). Intercultural reasoning: The challenge for international bioethics. *Cambridge Quarterly of Healthcare Ethics, 3*(3), 321–328.

96. Mathews, D. J. H., Fins, J. J., & Racine, E. (2018). The therapeutic "mis"conception: An examination of its normative assumptions and a call for its revision. *Cambridge Quarterly of Healthcare Ethics, 27,* 154–162.

97. McKay, T., & Timmermans, S. (2009). The bioethical misconception: A response to Lidz. *Social Science & Medicine, 69,* 1793–1796.

98. McConville, P. (2017). Presuming patient autonomy in the face of therapeutic misconception. *Bioethics, 31,* 711–715.

99. McCormick, J. B. (2018). How should a research ethicist combat false beliefs and therapeutic misconception risk in biomedical research? *AMA Journal of Ethics, 20*(11), E1100–E1106.

100. McKay, T., & Timmermans, S. (2009a). The bioethical misconception: A response to Lidz. *Social Science & Medicine, 69,* 1793–1796.

101. McKay, T., & Timmermans, S. (2009b). Clinical trials as treatment option: Bioethics and health care disparities in substance dependency. *Social Science & Medicine, 69,* 1784–1790.

102. Michels, K. B., & Rothman, K. J. (2003). Update on unethical use of placebos in randomized trials. *Bioethics, 17*(2), 188–204.

103. Mill, J. S. (1998 [1863]). Utilitarianism. In J. P. Sterba (Ed.), *Ethics: The big questions* (pp. 119–132). Malden: Blackwell Publishers.

104. Miller, F. G. (2000). Placebo-controlled trials in psychiatric research: An ethical perspective. *Biological Psychiatry, 47,* 707–716.

105. Miller, F. G., & Brody, H. (2002). What makes placebo-controlled trials unethical? *The American Journal of Bioethics, 2*(2), 3–9.

106. Millum, J. (2013). Romanian orphans study: A bioethicist responds to ethical concerns. *Bioethics Forum.* https://www.thehastingscenter.org/romanian-orphans-study-a-bioethicist-responds-to-ethical-concerns/. Accessed 29 Feb 2020.

107. Millum, J., & Emanuel, E. J. (2007). The ethics of international research with abandoned children. *Science, 318*(5858), 1874–1875.
108. Molyneux, C. S., Peshu, N., & Marsh, K. (2004). Understanding of informed consent in a low-income setting: Three case studies from the Kenyan coast. *Social Science & Medicine, 59*(12), 2547–2559.
109. Moncrieff, J. (2006). Does antipsychotic withdrawal provoke psychosis? Review of the literature on rapid onset psychosis (supersensitivity psychosis) and withdrawal-related relapse. *Acta Psychiatrica Scandinavica, 2006*, 1–11. https://doi.org/10.1111/j.1600-0447.2006.00787.x.
110. Moser, D. J., Schulz, S. K., Arndt, S., Benjamin, M. L., Fleming, F. W., Berms, D. S., Appelbaum, P. S., & Andreason, N. C. (2002). Capacity to provide informed consent for participation in schizophrenia and HIV research. *American Journal of Psychiatry, 159*, 1201–1207.
111. Murali, V., & Oyebode, F. (2004). Poverty, social inequality and mental health. *Advances in Psychiatric Treatment, 10*, 216–224.
112. Mwangi, R., Ndebele, P., & Mongoven, A. (2017). Understanding therapeutic misconceptions and perceptions, and enrollment decision-making: A pediatric preventive malaria trial in rural Tanzania. *IRB, 39*(5), 8–18.
113. National Commission for the Protection of Human Subjects of Research. (1979). *The Belmont Report: Ethical principles and guidelines for the protection of human subjects of research.* Washington, D.C.: United States Department of Health, Education, and Welfare.
114. National Institute on Drug Abuse. (2018). *Guidelines for establishing and operating a data and safety monitoring board.* Available at https://www.drugabuse.gov/research/clinical-research/guidelines-establishing-data-safety-monitoring. Accessed 24 Feb 2020.
115. National Institutes of Health. (1979). Clinical trial activity. NIH guide for grants and contracts. 8(8):29. Available at https://grants.nih.gov/grants/guide/historical/1979_06_05_Vol_08_No_08.pdf. Accessed 29 Feb 2020.
116. National Institutes of Health. (1998). *NIH guide: NIH policy for data and safety monitoring.* Available at https://grants.nih.gov/grants/guide/notice-files/not98-084.html. Accessed 24 Feb 2020.
117. National Institute of Mental Health. (2015). *Data safety monitoring plan writing guidance: Guidance for developing a data and safety monitoring plan for clinical trials sponsored by NIMH.* Available at https://www.nimh.nih.gov/funding/clinical-research/data-and-safety-monitoring-plan-writing-guidance.shtml. Accessed 24 Feb 2020.
118. National Institute of Mental Health. (2015). *Policy governing independent safety monitors and independent data and safety monitoring boards.* Available at https://www.nimh.nih.gov/funding/clinical-research/policy-governing-independent-safety-monitors-and-independent-data-and-safety-monitoring-boards.shtml. Accessed 24 Feb 2020.
119. Ndebele, P., Mwaluko, G., Kruger, M., Oukem-Boyer, O. O. M., & Zimba, M. (2014). History of research ethics review in Africa. In M. Kruger, P. Ndebele, & L. Horn (Eds.), *Research ethics in Africa* (pp. 3–10). Stellenbosch: SUN Press.
120. Nordling, L. (2018). African scientists call for more control of their continent's genomic data. *Nature.* Available at https://www.nature.com/articles/d41586-018-04685-1. Accessed 29 Feb 2020.
121. Onyut, L. P., Neuner, F., Ertl, V., Schauer, E., Odenwald, M., & Elbert, T. (2009). Trauma, poverty, and mental health among Somali and Rwandese refugees living in an African refugee settlement—an epidemiological study. *Conflict and Health, 3*, 6. https://doi.org/10.1186/1752-1505-1183-1186.
122. Pailhez, G., Bulbena, A., López, C., & Balon, R. (2010). Views of psychiatry: A comparison between medical students from Barcelona and Medellín. *Academic Psychiatry, 34*, 61–66.
123. Perkins, D. O., Gu, H., Boteva, K., & Lieberman, J. A. (2005). Relationship between duration of untreated psychosis and outcome in first-episode schizophrenia: A critical review and meta-analysis. *American Journal of Psychiatry, 162*(10), 1785–1804.

124. Peterson, B. T., Clancy, S. J., Champion, K., & McLarty, J. W. (1992). Improving readability of informed consent forms: What the computers may not tell you. *IRB, 14*, 6–8.
125. Preziosi, M. P., Yam, A., Nidaye, M., Simaga, A., Simondon, F., & Wassilak, S. (1997). Practical experiences in obtaining informed consent for a vaccine trial in rural Africa. *The New England Journal of Medicine, 336*(5), 370–373.
126. Proctor, R. N. (1988). *Racial hygiene: Medicine under the Nazis*. Cambridge, MA: Harvard University Press.
127. Purdy, L. M. (1992). A call to heal. In H. B. Holmes & L. M. Purdy (Eds.), *Feminist perspectives in medical ethics* (pp. 9–13). Bloomington: Indiana University Press.
128. Reich, W. (2005). The power of a single idea. In M. Patrão Neves & M. Lima (Eds.), *Bioetica ou bioeticas na evolução das sociedades* (pp. 380–382). Coimbra: Grafica de Coimbra.
129. Resnik, D. B. (1998). The ethics of HIV research in developing nations. *Bioethics, 2*(4), 286–306.
130. Roberts, L. W., Laureillo, J., Geppert, C., & Keith, S. J. (2001). Placebos and paradoxes in psychiatric research: An ethics perspective. *Biological Psychiatry, 49*, 887–893.
131. Rothman, K. J., & Michels, K. B. (1994). The continued unethical use of placebo controls. *The New England Journal of Medicine, 331*, 394–398.
132. Saluja, S., Rudolfson, N., Massenburg, B. B., Meara, J. G., & Shrime, M. G. (2020). The impact of physician migration on mortality in low and middle-income countries: An economic modeling study. *BMJ Global Health, 5*, e001535.
133. Sherwin, S. (1992a). Feminist and medical ethics: Two different approaches to contextual ethics. In H. B. Holmes & L. M. Purdy (Eds.), *Feminist perspectives in medical ethics* (pp. 17–31). Bloomington: Indiana University Press.
134. Sherwin, S. (1992b). *No longer patient: Feminist ethics and health care*. Philadelphia: Temple University Press.
135. Siriwardhana, C., Adikari, A., Jayaweera, K., & Sumathipala, A. (2013). Ethical challenges in mental health research among internally displaced people: Ethical theory and research implementation. *BMC Medical Ethics, 14*, 13. http://www.biomedcentral.com/1472-6939/14/13.
136. Skiera, A.-S., & Michels, K. B. (2018). Ethical principles and placebo-controlled trials—interpretation and implementation of the Declaration of Helsinki's placebo paragraph in medical research. *BMC Medical Ethics, 19*(1), 24. https://doi.org/10.1186/s12910-018-0262-9.
137. Sorsdahl, K., Stein, D. J., Grimsrud, A., Seedat, S., Flisher, A. J., Williams, D. R., & Myer, L. (2009). Traditional healers in the treatment of common mental disorders in South Africa. *The Journal of Nervous and Mental Disease, 197*(6), 434–441.
138. Ssenbunnya, J., Kigozi, F., Lund, C., Kizza, D., & Okello, E. (2009). Stakeholder perceptions of mental health stigma and poverty in Uganda. *BMC International Health and Human Rights, 9*(1), 1. https://doi.org/10.1186/1472-698X-9-5.
139. Stewart, P. J., & Strathern, A. (2004). *Witchcraft, sorcery, rumors, and gossip*. Cambridge, MA: Cambridge University Press.
140. Sugarman, J., Popkin, B., Fortney, J., & Rivera, R. (2001). International perspectives on protecting human research subjects. In *Ethical and policy issues in international research: Clinical trials in developing countries* (Vol. II, pp. E1–E30). Bethesda: National Bioethics Advisory Commission.
141. Taub, H. A. (1986). Comprehension of informed consent for research: Issues and directions for future study. *IRB, 8*, 7–10.
142. Taylor, C. (1991). The harp that plays by itself. *Medical Anthropology, 13*, 99–129.
143. Taylor, K. M. (1992). Integrating conflicting professional roles: Physician participation in randomized clinical trials. *Social Science & Medicine, 35*(2), 217–224.
144. Taylor, K. M., Feldstein, M. L., Skeel, R. T., Pandya, K. J., Ng, P., & Carbone, P. P. (1994). Fundamental dilemmas of the randomized clinical trial process: Results of the 1,737 Eastern Cooperative Oncology Group investigators. *Journal of Clinical Oncology, 12*(9), 1796–1805.
145. Taylor, K. M., & Kelner, M. (1987). Interpreting physician participation in randomized clinical trials: The Physician Orientation Profile. *Journal of Health and Social Behavior, 28*(4), 389–400.

146. Tee, S. R., & Lathlean, J. A. (2004). The ethics of conducting a co-operative inquiry with vulnerable people. *Journal of Advanced Nursing, 47*(5), 536–543.
147. Temple, R., & Ellenberg, S. S. (2000). Placebo-controlled trials and active-control trials in the evaluation of new treatments part 1: Ethical and scientific issues. *Annals of Internal Medicine, 133*(6), 455–463.
148. ten Have, H. (2015). Respect for human vulnerability: The emergence of a new principle in bioethics. *Bioethical Inquiry, 12*, 395–408.
149. Thomas, S. B., & Quinn, S. C. (1991). The Tuskegee syphilis study, 1932 to 1972: Implications for HIV education and AIDS risk education programs in the black community. *American Journal of Public Health, 81*, 1498–1504.
150. Thong, I. S. K., Foo, M. Y., Sum, M. Y., Capps, B., Lee, T.-S., Ho, C., & Sim, K. (2016). Therapeutic misconception in psychiatry research: A systematic review. *Clinical Psychopharmacology Neuroscience, 14*(1), 17–25.
151. United Nations. *International covenant on civil and political rights. United Nations treaty collection.* Available at https://treaties.un.org/Pages/ViewDetails.aspx?src=TREATY&mtdsg_no=IV-4&chapter=4&clang=_en. Accessed 28 Feb 2020.
152. United States Department of Health and Human Services, Office for Human Research Protections. (2016). *Federal policy for the protection of human subjects ('Common Rule').* https://www.hhs.gov/ohrp/regulations-and-policy/regulations/common-rule/index.html. Accessed 17 Feb 2020.
153. United States Department of Health and Human Services, Office for Human Research Protections. (2017). *Revised common rule.* https://www.hhs.gov/ohrp/regulations-and-policy/regulations/finalized-revisions-common-rule/index.html. Accessed 22 Feb 2020.
154. Voinescu, B., Szentagotai, A., & Coogan, A. (2010). Attitudes towards psychiatry—a survey of Romanian medical residents. *Academic Psychiatry, 34*, 75–78.
155. Wang, H., Erickson, J. D., Li, Z., & Berry, R. J. (2004). Evaluation of the informed consent process in a randomized controlled trial in China: The Sino-US NTD Project. *The Journal of Clinical Ethics, 15*(1), 61.
156. Wassenaar, D. R. (2006). Commentary: Ethical considerations in international research collaboration: The Bucharest Early Intervention Project. *Infant Mental Health Journal, 27*(6), 577–580.
157. Weijer, C. (1999). Placebo-controlled trials in schizophrenia: Are they ethical? Are they necessary? *Schizophrenia Research, 35*, 211–218.
158. Welsome, E. (1999). *The plutonium files.* New York: Dial Press.
159. Wolinsky, H. (2006). The battle of Helsinki. *EMBO, 7*(7), 670–672.
160. World Health Organization. (2011). *Mental health atlas 2011.* Geneva: Author.
161. World Health Organization. (2005). *Mental health resources in the world.* Geneva: Author.
162. World Health Organization. (2007). *Ten statistical highlights in global public health, Part 1: World health statistics.* Geneva: Author.
163. World Medical Association. (2013). *WMA Declaration of Helsinki—Ethical principles for medical research involving human subjects.* https://www.wma.net/policies-post/wma-declaration-of-helsinki-ethical-principles-for-medical-research-involving-human-subjects/. Accessed 17 Feb 2020.
164. Young, D. R., Hooker, D. T., & Freeberg, F. E. (1990). Informed consent document: Increasing comprehension by reducing reading level. *IRB, 12*, 1–5.
165. MacQueen, K., Shapiro, K., Karim, Q., & Sugarman, J. (2004). Ethical challenges in international HIV prevention research. *Accountability in Research: Policies and Quality Assurance, 11*(1), 49–61.
166. Eckenwiler, L., Ellis, C., Feinholz, D., & Schonfeld, T. (2008). Hopes for Helsinki: Reconsidering "vulnerability." *Journal of Medical Ethics, 34*(10), 765–766.
167. Kahn, K., & Bryant, J.H. (1994). The vulnerable in developed and developing countries–A conceptual approach. In *Poverty, vulnerbility, the value of human life, and the emergence of bioethics* (pp. 57–63). Geneva: Council for International Organizations of Medical Sciences.

168. United Nations Development Program. (1999). *Human development report 1999*. New York: Oxford University Press.
169. Taylor, T. (1946). Opening statement of the prosecution, Dece,ber 9, 1946. In G.J. Annas, M.A. Gordon (Eds.). [1992]. *The Nazi doctors and the Nuremberg Code* (pp. 67–93). New York: Oxford University Press.
170. Vennell, V.A.M. (1995). Medical research and treatment: Ethical standards in the international context. *Medical Law International*, 2, 1–21.
171. Rosenthal, E. (1997). The International Covenant on Civil and Political Rights and the rights of research subjects. In A.E. Shamoo (Ed.). Ethics in neurobiological research with human subjects: *The Baltimore conference on bioethics* (pp. 265–272). Amsterdam: Overseas Publishers Association.
172. Stewart, D.P. (1993). United States ratification of the Covenant on Civil and Political Rights: The significance of the reservations, understandings, and declarations. *DePaul Law Review*, 42, 1183–1207.
173. Muss, H.B., White, D.R., Michielutte, R., Richards, F., Cooper, M..R., Williams, S., ...& Spurr, C.L. (1979). Written informed consent in patients with breast cancer. *Cancer*, 43, 1549–1556.
174. Lavelle-Jones, C., Byrne, D.J., Rice, P., & Cuschieri, A. (1993). Factors affecting quality of informed consent. *British Medical Journal*, 306(6882), 885–890.
175. Morrow, G., Gootnick, J., & Schmale, A. (1978). A simple technique for increasing cancer patients' knowledge of informed consent to treatment. Cancer, 42(2), 793–799.
176. de Melo-Martin, I., & Ho, A. (2008). Beyond informed consent: The therapeutic misconception and trust. *Journal of Medical Ethics*, 34(3), 202–205.
177. Taneja, V., Sriram, S., Beri, R.S., Sreenivas, V. Aggarwal, R., & Kaur, R. (2002). "Not by bread alone": The impact of a structured 90-minute play session on development of children in an orphanage. *Child Care, Health and Development*, 28(1), 95–100.
178. United Nations Children's Fund, Innocenti Research Centre. (2001). A decade of transition. Regional monitoring report no. 8. Florence, Italy: Author. https://www.unicef-irc.org/publicationspdf/monee8/eng5.pdf. Accessed 14 February 2021.
179. Groza, V., Ileana, D., & Irwin, I. (1999). *A peacock or a crow: Stories, interviews and commentaries on Romanian adoptions*. Lakeshore Communications.
180. Loue, S., Groza, V., & ARAS Working Group. (1998). HIV knowledge and attitudes in Iasi, Romania: A pilot study. *Journal of Health Management and Public Health*, 3(2).
181. Zeanah, C.H., Fox, N.A., & Nelson, C.A. (2012). Case study in ethics of research: The Bucharest early intervention project. *Journal of Nervous and Mental Disease*, 200(3), 243–247.

Part II

History, Culture, and Diagnosis

Ethics and Humanitarianism in Global Mental Health

Samuel O. Okpaku

Introduction and Background

Ethics in global health and global mental health have gained prominence in recent decades. There has been a general increased awareness for its consideration in the planning, execution, and outcomes of activities described as global mental health. This awareness has been justified by human rights issues, access to care, and the relationships between providers and users, donors and recipient entities, and a need for greater accountability.

Definitions

Ethics is defined by Merriam Webster as "rules of behavior based on ideas about what is morally good or bad", closely related to ethics is the term, humanitarianism [1]. Humanitarianism is defined by Merriam Webster dictionary "as the promotion of human welfare" [2] an accompanying graph depicts the volume of its usage over time [3]. It is suggested that its use has increased exponentially between 1900 and 1980, a period which encompasses World War I and World War II as well as major global civil unrests and catastrophes, e.g., Ethiopian famine and the Nigerian Biafran War. Global health and global mental health are movements whose roots are based on the process of globalization. There are multiple definitions of globalization, a process which was fueled by a confluence of factors including increased connectivity, easier communication, and a sense of recognition at one level that we are all together as for example in climate change. Most of the definitions have some common themes. These are facilitation of commerce

S. O. Okpaku (✉)
President, Center for Health, Culture, and Society, Nashville, TN, USA

Clinical Professor, George Washington University, Washington, DC, USA

© Springer Nature Switzerland AG 2021
A. R. Dyer et al. (eds.), *Global Mental Health Ethics*,
https://doi.org/10.1007/978-3-030-66296-7_5

and trade worldwide, access to a playing field, and humanitarianism [4]. In fact, international soccer has been seen as a model of globalization [5]. This was meant to highlight the breakdown of barriers in the recruitment of foreign players, the ease of labor migration, and the universal appreciation of soccer rules (In the use of this model, perhaps the unanticipated consequence was not foreseen. I am referring to the concentration of talented players in the major leagues and the corresponding dominance of these leagues in national and international soccer). This parallels some consequences of globalization which we will subsequently refer to. Amongst the definitions of globalization, the definition by Giddens is one of the most succinct and appealing to me. According to Giddens, globalization can be defined as "the intensification of worldwide-social relations which link distant localities in such a way that local happenings are shaped by events occurring many miles away and vice versa" [6]. Global health was defined by Koplan and colleagues as "an area of study, research and practice that places a priority on improving health and achieving equity in health for all people worldwide". Global health emphasizes transnational health issues, determinants, and solutions; involves many disciplines within and beyond the health sciences and promotes interdisciplinary collaboration; and is a synthesis of population-based prevention with individual-level clinical care [7].

Patel and Prince, borrowing from Koplan et al. and substituting "mental health" and "health" in Koplan's definition, arrive at their definition of global mental health [8].

I have since defined global mental health as a range of activities that meet some principle criteria. These are (1) universal and transnational criterion-the problem/issues should have a universal or transnational aspect. Examples will be the role of poverty in mental illness worldwide and stigma reduction worldwide. (2) Public health criterion-the problem should have a population basis, e.g., violence as a public issue. (3) Stakeholder's criterion-the composition of the stakeholders should have a population basis, e.g., violence as a public issue. (4) Problem ownership criterion-the problem should be owned by the recipient organization, institution, or country. (5) Team criterion-the teams engaged in the project should be multidisciplinary and multiparty.

Since global health and global mental health were driven by the globalization process, a discussion of the role of ethics in global mental health can benefit from a dimensional examination of globalization. These dimensions are:

Historical dimension–This dimension is very relevant in discussions about global health. Many countries in the developing world have until recently experienced a colonial past. The consequences of this for developing countries are increased suspicion and sensitivity towards actions of superpowers. "I fear donors when they bring gifts" (Trojan War). In fact, in some quarters, globalization has been described as "neo-colonization" [9]. In other words, globalization and its attendant processes can be seen as a back-door strategy to continue colonial domination.

Economic dimension–This dimension is a powerful one in a world system where there are now very few dominant financial markets. The powerful nations exercise great influence while the poorer ones are at risk of greater marginalization. Although the stated vision and goal of the International Monetary Fund and World Bank is the eradication of poverty worldwide and improved quality of life and well-being for all, there are examples of negative consequences of globalization in low- and middle-income countries (LMICs). There is an exacerbation of poverty in Africa where foreign direct investment (FDI) is falling [10].

Political dimension–This domain deals mostly with health, development, and security. In this domain are issues related to the prevention of pandemics and access to affordable pharmaceuticals (e.g., the availability of cheap antiviral medications) [11]. In this regard, Brazil declared the right to health as a human right. Also, poor health is linked to loss of economic and political viability [12].

Sociocultural dimension–The fourth theme in globalization is "a process of cultural mixing and hybridization across locations and identities" (Appadurai 1996) [13]. The internet, social media, and mass communications enable individuals to negotiate through different cultures and be subject to different sociocultural forces in real time.

Also an aspect of the definition of globalization is the confluence of several aspects of human endeavor and international relations. This is an ideal which was promoted by the Millennium Development Goals Achievement Fund (2005). In 2000, 80 heads of state signed the declaration and a commitment "to a collective responsibility to uphold the principles of human dignity, equality, and equity at the global level" [14]. Eight specific goals were to be achieved by year 2015. These goals were (1) End poverty and hunger, (2) Promote access to universal education, (3) Promote gender equality, (4) Improve child health, (5) Improve maternal health, (6) Combat HIV/AIDS, (7) Promote environmental sustainability, and (8) Promote global health.

The Millennium Development Goals were followed up by the UN Sustainable Development Goals [15]. There are 17 goals which include good health and well-being and no poverty. This has been buttressed by an emphasis on the social determinants of health. These are a set of economic and social factors which have an impact on individuals and or communities' health and well-being. The context in which global mental health is practiced is against a background of globalization and although the process remains a dominating contemporary force, the results so far have not been universally accepted. One of the concerns of globalization is highlighted by the frequent and regular protests of the International Monetary Fund meetings. Also consider the statement of the influential African group New Partnership for African Development (NEPAD). This is an African Union strategic framework for pan-African socioeconomic development. The group NEPAD stated,

> In the absence of fair and just global rules, globalisation has increased the ability of the strong to advance their interests to the detriment of the weak, especially in the areas of trade, finance, and technology. It has limited space for developing countries to control their own development, as the system makes no provision for compensating the weak. The conditions of those marginalized in this process have worsened in real terms. A fissure between inclusion and exclusion has emerged within and among nations [15]

Even an ex-president of the World Bank, James David Wolfensohn reflected as follows; "We cannot turn back globalisation. Our challenges to make globalisation an instrument of opportunity and inclusion—not of fear and insecurity. Globalisation must work for all" [16]. Meanwhile, some developed countries have taken into account health issues in terms of their foreign policy formulations. The Scandinavian countries have been very prominent in this regard. For example, in May 2003, the Swedish Parliament passed a bill—Shared Responsibility. The major theme of the bill was a policy for development that was multisectorial. It emphasized equity and sustainability for global development. It was driven from a human rights perspective and focused on poverty and poor countries [17]. Norway also passed a similar policy (Norwegian Ministry of Foreign Affairs 2012). The policy aimed to fight poverty, support and promote health services, reduce social inequalities worldwide, promote women's rights and gender equality, and help reduce disease burden [18].

For the US, the major policy objectives are (1) Health impact: improves the health and well-being of people around the world. (2) Health security: improves capabilities to prepare for and respond to infectious disease, other emerging health threats, and public health emergencies. (3) Health capacity: builds country public health capacity. (4) Organizational capacity: maximizes the potential of CDC's global programs to achieve impact.

The corresponding goals for the UK government were stated in a document Health is Global [19]. The policy objectives were better global health security, stronger, fairer, and safer systems to deliver health, more effective international health organizations, stronger, freer, and fairer trade for better health, strengthening the way we develop, and use evidence to improve policy and practice.

The Swiss government was a pioneer in interministerial agreements on health and her policies were directed at increasing stake holder's participation and the role of law and human rights [20]. The BRICS states which consist of Brazil, Russia, India, China, and South Africa have emphasized "health for all". These countries have expanding economies and may play a bigger role in health and foreign policy [21].

An underlying theme of these foreign policies includes equity, fairness, promotion of human rights, eradication of poverty, gender equality—all matters of ethics and equity in terms of policy orientations.

So, what are the ethical challenges to global mental health? We have suggested the five principal criteria required for an activity to be described as global mental health. Again, these are,

1. the universal and international criteria
2. the public health criteria
3. stakeholder's criteria
4. problem ownership criteria
5. the team criteria

The requirement of any one of these criteria taken against a background of the four dimensions of global mental health stated above point to a minefield of complex interactions in which ethical missteps may be made. Bearing in mind that the context in which the global mental health activity is being carried –be it a humanitarian crisis, a conflict situation, a research agenda, or a training and psycho-social intervention –the ethical priorities may vary. All of these are made more complex by the issues of local values, resources, and cultural criteria. The arrangement may be bilateral, multilateral, governmental, NGO's, or various permutations of these agencies. These issues are compounded by the salience of the context in which the intervention is to be carried out. In this regard, we must now pay close attention to the role of culture. One aspect of this is smart diplomacy –as opposed to muscle diplomacy –in negotiating foreign aid. Clarification of the above points is illustrated with the following examples:

1. Planning, Execution, and Monitoring of Foreign Aid

The planning and execution of foreign aid is a minefield of potential ethical violations. Foreign aid tends to be asymmetrical in terms of the power dynamics and benefits. Some aspects of this have been alluded to in my definition and criteria for global mental health in which I emphasized the need for problem ownership by the recipient country, organization, institution, or entity. In 2005, the Organization for Economic Co-operation and Development (OECD) developed a declaration aimed at the accountability of developed and developing countries for delivering, monitoring, and managing aid. This Paris Declaration (OECD 2005) had five principal objectives [22]. These were:

1. ownership—partner countries exercise effective leadership over their development policies and strategies, and coordinate development actions.
2. alignment—donors base their overall support on partner countries' national development strategies, institutions, and procedures.
3. harmonization—donor's actions are more harmonized, transparent, and collectively effective.
4. managing for results—managing resources and improving decision-making for results.
5. mutual accountability—donors and partners are accountable for development results.

In 2013 Sopko, a former US Special Inspector for Afghanistan Reconstruction suggested a template for making foreign aid in reconstruction more effective. His template has usefulness and relevance for other aid situations. His template of questions to be asked was as follows:

1. Does the project or program make a clear and identified contribution to national interests or strategic objectives of donor countries?
2. Does the recipient country want or need the project?
3. Has the project been coordinated with other donor implementing agencies, the recipient government and other international donors?

4. Are security conditions favorable to effective implementation oversight?
5. Are there adequate safeguards to detect, deter, and mitigate corruption?
6. Does the recipient nation have the financial resources, technical capacity, and political will to sustain the program?
7. Have the various stakeholders established meaningful and measurable metrics for determining success?

In addition, the World Health Organization has published a number of guidelines. The most important are (1) Ethics in epidemics, emergencies, and disasters. A training manual [23]. (2) Ethical standards and procedures for research. Again, here as a UN agency, the WHO cannot go beyond consultations and monitoring. The role of the above guidelines can be enhanced by state regulatory agencies as well as the ethical guidelines of professional organizations. And as suggested by Najan and Khan, we have to pay attention to the exclusion and inclusion of stakeholders, the growth of data collection, and information.

Lastly, we have to subscribe to the idea of a playing field that takes into account a fair playing ground and the asymmetrical nature of donor-recipient, patient and health giver, and developed country, and developing country arrangements.

2. Funding for Mental Health Services

Low income countries carry about 50% of the global burden of distress but according to WHO spend only 2% of global spending [21]. In many low resource countries, there may be less than ten psychiatrists for the total population and the mental health budget represents a small fraction of the total health budget. The UN target for international aid and spending is 0.7% of the country's GNP. In 2017, only five countries exceeded this target. They were Denmark (0.85%), the Netherlands (0.75%), Norway (1.05%), Luxenberg (0.95%), and Sweden (1.4%) [22]. It is an interesting commentary that although the US is the largest contributor percentage wise in total contribution, its GNP percentage is low. This aid is spread over nine categories that include health assistance. It is equally interesting that when the US population is surveyed as to how much the US government spends for foreign aid; the average response is 25%. In fact, it is less than 1% of the GNP [24].

3. Pharmaceutical Practices

An important area of ethical concerns in global mental health is that of pharmaceutical practices. Although 70% of the world's population lives in the developing world, it produces only 7% of pharmaceuticals that they use [25]. This disparity and other factors have resulted in a range of unethical issues ranging from dumping of expired medications, to overpricing, bribing of government officials, and the use of what will normally be used in the developed world. Also, when drugs are donated, it is not certain that they are delivered to targeted recipients. Another significant area of concern is in clinical trials. In 1996, there was a serious epidemic of cerebral meningitis in Kano State in Northern Nigeria. Legal action was taken by Kano State and the parents of some children who died during the Pfizer clinical trial. The allegations were that proper informed consent was not applied and that some children were given less than the recommended dose. Many of the children on the experimental antibiotic suffered brain damage, slurred speech, and paralysis. There were also allegations of inappropriate medical record keeping. Pfizer settled the case with monetary payments to the state and to the parents of some of the patients [26].

Another pharmaceutical ethical dilemma had to do with the ethical challenges observed in the HIV/AIDS epidemic, a condition affecting millions of Africans who died from lack of accessibility to care due to absence of effective drugs or stigma. An often cited ethical issue in the bioethical literature is the study of maternal and child transmission of HIV/AIDS. The drug AZT was already known to be effective in the treatment of HIV/AIDS. International studies were carried out with a placebo group and a short-term versus long-term protocol. There were two major criticisms to the studies. One was the unavailability of proven agent to sick pregnant women and the second criticism was that of a placebo group where there was already knowledge of an available effective agent (AZT) [27]. Another pertinent issue centers on the availability of psychotropics. Many jurisdictions in low and middle income countries have very little budgets for psychiatric medications even for old and tested medications such as these used in the treatment of psychosis and seizure disorders. Also, sometimes the continued supply of a donated medication or its supervision cannot be guaranteed. In my opinion, one of the worst imprisonments of the mind is a psychotic disorder or a very severe depression. A temporal relief is welcome and may lead to a better later functioning. In addition, nurses in developing countries pride themselves on their experience and competence and are able to supervise the administration of psychotropics in the absence of psychiatrists or family practitioners. Although adequate drug regulations and supervisory frameworks are necessary, sometimes in developing countries the administration of these functions may be too bureaucratic leading to diversion or deterioration of donated and nondonated medications in warehouses. Some of the above pharmaceutical practices especially relating to clinical trials in HIV/AIDS and the use of placebo controls have led to a significantly modified Declaration of Helsinki that was adopted in Edinburgh in 2000 and a modified version by the Council for International Organizations of Medical Sciences (CIOMS) [28].

4. Advocacy, Humanitarianism, and the Use of Photography

Advocacy and humanitarianism are important aspects of global mental health. It has been suggested that decreasing availability of funds, religious groups including conservative groups may play a more significant role in humanitarianism specifically in disasters and emergencies. In these circumstances, the quid pro quo arrangement for funding and proselytism is to be frowned upon. A major aspect of advocacy and humanitarianism is the promotion of awareness especially through the use of photographs and posters. Some individuals take exception to the use of images using a racial group such as Africans or Asians to represent the problem. Another aspect of this pernicious practice is the use of photography of patients in institutions. A few years ago, I encountered a young nurse who went to Africa and returned with pictures of individual patients in a mental hospital. This nurse, a US nurse, knows fully well that the practice will be unacceptable in the United States, but she had no hesitation to carry out this practice in a West African country. Her excuse was that the subject of the photos was asking her for an opportunity to move to the states. This practice is not new. In fact, Charcot [29] was criticized for manipulating his patients to take certain postures and attitudes to sustain his theory of hysteria. Photographing of mental patients is a strongly ethical issue. Individuals who support the practice frequently cite its usefulness in fundraising and raising awareness of the plight of mentally ill individuals. If photographs have to be taken for the sake of advocacy, there are indeed ways to ensure that the photographs do not give away the identity of the patients.

5. Research

Ethics like law has many gray areas especially as it relates to practice under different circumstances, e.g., routine intervention, emergency condition, and low resource conditions. The debate surrounding the clinical trials of AZT in the prevention of vertical transmission of HIV/AIDS is very illustrative of this. Other ethical issues in global mental health include the need for adequate informed consent in the appropriate local language, community and local leadership involvement, and sensitivity in data collection, and above all sharing of the research results. A frequent complaint from colleagues in developing countries is that they did not participate in the results of the research and may feel they have been unfairly exploited. The protocol to share the results with the community leaders should also be respected.

6. Brain Drain

The issues of Brain Drain, i.e., the migration of trained personnel from less developed countries to more advanced countries have been a perennial and vexing question. Because of the volume of this migration process, there has been considerable concern about the medical brain drain. It is estimated that between 27% and 30% of physicians in the major destination countries of Australia, the USA, the UK, and Canada are international medical graduates [30]. In addition, the phenomenon may be increasing despite attempts to curb it. On the surface there appears to be several factors for this phenomenon. These factors include easy migration of labor, population changes in high income countries, and some consequences of globalization. These are all ethical considerations. What appears to be forgotten at times is the impact of a colonial history in terms of training and certification. The lack of available post graduate training in some LMIC and the autonomous rights of individuals versus the community needs especially in situations of poor economic conditions, political upheavals, and lack of security for a satisfying professional life. Tankwench reported the following results from the American Medical Association 2011, (I) there were 17,376 physicians who were identified as having an African background, (II) about 2/3 were educated in medical schools in Nigeria and South Africa [31]. Also, Jenkins found that a large number of psychiatrists registered to practice in the destination countries were from LMIC [32]. Some of these may accept less desirable specialties and positions. It has also been reported that while in the UK, the ratio of psychiatrists to the population served rose from 5.9/100,000 in 2003 to 7.6/100,000 in 2013, the equivalent number in Africa was, i.e., 0.1/100,000 in 2014. Ndetei et al. have attempted to calculate the economic loss to a LMIC of training an individual who then migrates. It has been suggested that this investment should be compensated by the high income country [33]. Over many decades there have been a variety of attempts to deal with this ethical issue. For example, in the UK in the 70's, there was a plan for consultant physicians to encourage foreign medical graduates to return to their home lands upon completion of their courses. Some countries may delay the migration of newly trained doctors by insisting on a national service upon graduation. Other countries including the United States may approve restricted visas. South Africa now has a policy that bans the recruitment of doctors from other Sub-Saharan African countries. A more comprehensive strategy was developed by the World Health Organization. This is the WHO Global Code of Practice on the International Recruitment of Health Personnel [34]. The primary aim of the code is to encourage human capacity building buttressed in an enriched educational environment, strategic retention, and recruitment strategies.

7. Education and Training

In the last few decades, study abroad programs have expanded into the field of global health and mental health. In one survey, over 25% of the respondents reported having participated in global health experience [35]. Many residency programs in the US have partnership arrangements with African and South American mental health centers. Because of the nature of the field of mental health with confidentiality, low resources, and frequent relapses, there are many ethical issues surrounding training for global mental health. Many years ago at the annual global health meeting at Yale, I overheard a young medical student states that he carried out cardiac surgery. His boastful statements illustrate some of the critical ethical issues in global mental health training and education. Amongst these are matching clinical skills with participation in interventions, questions of care provided, the student expectation, and the expectation of the recipient centers, exploitation of limited human resources, and lack of professional standards. In planning these partnerships, it is imperative that the reciprocal expectations be clearly stated, what can the trainer, trainee, or the faculty member do and not do, and what are the bidirectional benefits? The experience may in some cases amount to a culture shock if it is the first time for the student or faculty from a high income country to be exposed to in some cases dire situations for which they had not been previously prepared. Adequate debriefing should be carried out at the end of such assignments. Partnership and training sites should develop a global mental health curriculum agenda and training with embedded issues of culture sensitivity. A middle aged African chief will consider it an insult to be instructed on family planning by a US health worker who is barely the age of his daughter. Familiarity with the professional codes of each discipline can also be helpful.

8. Ethical Implications for the Future of Global Mental Health

The future of global mental health is directly dependent on the status of globalization which in turn is dependent on relative peace and security as well as economic stability. The current global political situation is likely to make scholars somewhat nervous about the future of globalization. However, Hurst & Thompson suggested that native states will continue in terms of governance, to be the central loci in an increasingly complex globalized world [36]. Sponsored by international relief agencies, Khan and Najam explored the future of globalization by first identifying some drivers and applying those to some dominant areas [37]. The following drivers were selected (1) information and communications technology, (2) markets, (3) probability, and (4) policy orientation. The domains to which they applied the drivers to were (1) exclusion and inequality, (2) human insecurity, (3) health, (4) cultural & social environments, and (5) institutions and governance. Using a scenario analysis, a technique which the United Nations Environmental Program has suggested as the most suitable method for exploring complex and indeterminate systems such as social or planetary systems and which systems tend to have significant elements of "surprise, ignorance, and violation." Using this technique, Khan and Najan uncovered possible scenarios. These were "the Global Marketplace, the Managed Planet, and the Fortress World." Characteristics underlying in the Global Marketplace are the free market and political thinking. The corresponding characteristics for the Managed Planet are dominant policy issues and value systems. The Fortress World is characterized by a break from current policy institutions and value systems. Based on their model, the Fortress World will lead to increasing marginalization and poverty. Autocracies are predicted in this scenario. The researchers concluded that a combination of the Global Marketplace and the Managed Planet is the most desirable. In their recommendation to the international humanitarian group of agencies, they suggested a strategic approach in the selection of the key drivers that are relevant to their organization.

Khan and Najam recommended to the international relief agencies the need to,

1. participate in creating dominant belief systems
2. become policy actors and entrepreneurs
3. utilize information and communication technology (ICT)
4. Influence advances in ICT

In terms of the dominant areas they recommend a strong interest in the area of exclusion and inequality. The work of Khan and Najam points to a framework in an over globalized and complex world considering the issues related to poverty, climate change, migration, and the application of technological advances to global health and mental health. These issues become more relevant as we consider that religious groups are an important segment of the international relief groups and that their influences are likely to grow with shrinking funds from governmental agencies.

Discussion and Conclusion

The foregoing gives a background to important issues regarding ethical problems in global mental health. Country ownership of the problem, transparency, sustainability, research protocols, sharing of research data, and sustainability will remain as dominant themes. In terms of bribery and corruption, it is hoped that the various frameworks and guidelines stated above will be helpful. In this regard Bono, the entertainer and former US Congressman was optimistic about the use of informational technology to track funding and its use [38]. He was optimistic about the potential for the internet to enable tracking of corruption amongst politicians and civil servants. In addition, it is hoped that ongoing reforms at the UN and its agencies with respect to representations and diversity will respond to ethical situations. It will be ethical and useful for the policies of the World Bank and the International Monetary Fund to promote diversity of stakeholders and encourage an equal playing field.

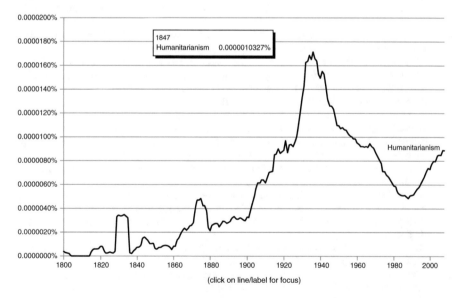

References

1. Merriam Webster: Definition of Ethics.
2. Humanitarianism Definition: Merriam Webster.

3. https://books.google.com/ngrams/graph?content=Humanitarianism+&year_start=1800&year_end=2010&corpus=0&smoothing=3&share=&direct_url=t1%3B%2CHumanitarianism%3B%2Cc0#t1%3B%2CHumanitarianism%3B%2Cc0
4. Okpaku, S. O. (2014). *History of global mental health in Essentials of Global Mental Health*. Cambridge: Cambridge University Press.
5. Milanovic, B. (2005). Globalization and goals: does soccer show the way? *Review of International Political Economy, 12*(5), 829–805.
6. Giddens, A. (1990). *The consequences of modernizing 1990*. Cambridge: Policy Press.
7. Koplan, J. R., Bond, T. C., Merson, M. H., et al. (2009). Toward a common definition of global health. *Lancet, 573*, 1993–1995.
8. Patel, V., & Prince, M. (2010). Global Mental Health, a new global health field comes of age. *JAMA, 303*, 1976–1977.
9. Akindele ST, Gidado TO, Olaopo OR (2002) Globalisation, its Implications and Consequences for Africa. http://globalization.icaap.org/content/v2.1/01_akindele_etal.html (accessed July 2013).
10. United Nations Conference on Trade and Development (UNCTAD) (2012) Global flows of foreign direct investment exceeding pre-crisis level in 2011, despite turmoil in the global economy. Global Investment Trends Monitor.
11. Safreed-Harmon K (2008) Human rights and HIV/AIDS in Brazil. GMHC Treatment Issues. http://www.gmhc.org/files/editor/file/ti_poz_0408.pdf (accessed July 2013).
12. United Nations General Assembly (2009) Global health and foreign policy: strategic opportunities and challenges. Note by the Secretary-General. (A/64/365). New York, NY: UN.
13. Appadurai A (1996) Modernity at Large: Cultural Dimensions of Globalization. Minneapolis, MN: University of Minnesota Press.
14. World Health Organization (2005) Health and the Millennium Development Goals. Geneva: WHO.
15. NEPAD. The New Partnership for Africa's Development (NEPAD) Abiya, Nigeria 2001. https://www.un.org/africa/osaa/reports/nepad.engeversion.pdf. Accessed July 2013.
16. Wolfensohn, J. D. The challenges of globalization: The role of the World Bank. Public Discussion Forum, Berlin, Germany, 2001. https://worldbank.org/wesite/external/topicsEX-TAID/OContentMDK:20025027-menuPK:336721–page: PK: 64020865–piPK; 149114–theSitelPK:336682,00 html. Accessed July 2013.
17. Swedish Ministry of Foreign Affairs, Federal Department of Home Affairs. (2006). *Swiss health foreign policy agreement on health policy objectives*. Berlin Swiss Government.
18. Norewegian Ministry Of Foreign Affairs. (2012). Global health on a foreign policy development. Meld. ST. 11 (2011--2012) Report in the Storting (white paper).
19. HM Government 2008: Health is Global a UK government strategy—2008—2013 London Department of Health.
20. Federal Department of Foreign Affairs, Federal Department of Home Affairs. (2006). *Swiss health foreign policy agreement on health policy objectives*. Berlin Swiss Government.
21. BRICS Health Ministry. (2011). *Beijing declaration*. BRICS Health Ministers Meeting Beijing, China.
22. OCED. The Paris Declaration on Aid Effectiveness: https://www.oecd.org/developmenteffec-tivenes/34428351.pdf. 2005. Accessed July 2013.
23. Sopko, J. U.S. reconstruction effort in Afghanistan Quad A segment presented at Simpson Center Washington, D.C. January 10, 2013, C-SPAN video library 2013 https://www.c-span-video.org/program/310312-1. Accessed July 2013..
24. UK among six countries to hit 0.7% UN one spending target https://www.theguardian.com<global development> January 4, 2019.
25. Medicinal Drugs in the Third World, *Cultural Survivor Quarterly Magazine* December 1987.
26. Wise, J. (2001). Pfizer accused of testing new drugs without ethical approval. bmj.com.
27. Luna, F. (2004). Bioethics Corruption and Research https://doi.org/10.1111/1467-8519.00155/.
28. International Ethical Guidelines for Health-Related Research cioms.ch; wp-content, 2017/01, WEB-CIOMS-Ethical G.

29. International Ethical Guidelines for Health-Related Research cioms.ch; wp-content, 2017/01, WEB-CIOMS-Ethical G.
30. Ioannidis JP. Global estimates of high-level brain drain and deficit. FASEB J. 2004;18(9):936–9. https://doi.org/10.1096/fj.03-13941fe. PMID: 15173104.
31. Tankwench, A.B.S.; Ozden, C.; & Vermund, S.H.: Physician emigration from sub-Shara Africa to the United States: analysis of the 2011 AMA physician masterfile PLoS Medicine 10, e1001513, CrossRef Google Scholar PubMed.
32. Jenkins, R., Kydd, R., Mullen, P., Thomason, K., Souley, J., Kuper, S., et al. (2010). International migration of doctors and its impact on availability of psychiatrists in low and middle income countries. *PLoS One, 5*(2), e9049. https://doi.org/10.1371/journal.pone.0009049.
33. Ndetei, D. M., Karim, S., & Mubhashar, M. (2004). Recruitment of consultant psychiatrists from low and middle income countries *International Psychiatry*, (6):15–18. Google search.
34. WHO Global Code of Ethics: www.globalcodeofethics.org
35. Global Health Career Interest among Medical and Nursing Students: Survey and Analysis.
36. Hurst, P., & Thompson, G. (1993). Globalization and the future of the nation state. *Economies et Societes, 24*, 408–442.
37. Khan, S., & Najan, A. The future of Globalization and its Humanitarian Impacts. Humanitarian Future Program 2009 https://www.humanitarianismfuture.org/wp.content/uploads/2013/06/ The Future of Globalization and its Humanitarianism—Impacts.pdf. Accessed 30 July 2015.
38. Bono. Webcast U2's Bono speaks at GU global social enterprise event Washington DC: Georgetown University; 2012, https://www.georgetown.enterprise.html. Accessed July 2013.

Counting What Counts: Epidemiologic Measurement and Generating Meaningful Findings

6

Bonnie N. Kaiser

Introduction

The collection of quantitative data is important for many aspects of global mental health research and practice. As mental health interventions become more widely available globally, quantitative data derived from screening tools inform who is in need of care – in other words, who should be referred to such interventions. Once individuals are connected to care, screening tools are often used to assess how well that care is working: are individuals' symptoms improving over time? In the case of controlled trials, we can also ask whether these improvements are greater than those seen in control or comparison groups. Additionally, epidemiologists, who study patterns of disease at the population level, use screening tools to identify risk and protective factors that are associated with mental health outcomes.

All of these aspects of global mental health research and practice rely on data, and the quality of our resulting inferences and decisions will only be as strong as the quality of our data. Additionally, if we do not measure any specific aspect – for example, a potential risk factor or outcome – we cannot make inferences about it or use it to guide our decision-making regarding research, programs, and resource allocation. This chapter focuses on potential problems or shortcomings with epidemiologic data, including the ethical challenges inherent in approaches to measurement. This focus on quantitative data is not to imply that it is the only type of data that matters. Qualitative data are likewise important for global mental health research and practice, and I describe ways that mixed-method approaches can strengthen our measurement and resulting decision-making. I approach the main ethical considerations as falling under (a) what we measure and (b) how we measure, with an exhortation to ensure that we remain focused on what matters most.

B. N. Kaiser (✉)
University of California San Diego, Department of Anthropology and Global Health Program,
La Jolla, CA, USA
e-mail: bnkaiser@ucsd.edu

© Springer Nature Switzerland AG 2021
A. R. Dyer et al. (eds.), *Global Mental Health Ethics*,
https://doi.org/10.1007/978-3-030-66296-7_6

What Matters to Measure?

When deciding what to measure, it can sometimes seem that the answers are obvious: for an intervention targeting a trauma-affected population, we'll measure post-traumatic stress disorder (PTSD); for a perinatal depression intervention, let's use a well-established screening tool such as the Edinburgh Postnatal Depression Scale. In reality, decisions regarding what to measure are often more complicated. As with all of the topics covered in this volume, there are usually myriad factors that go into decisions regarding what to measure, including addressing the needs of multiple stakeholders with potentially conflicting goals, and there are rarely straightforward answers. Here, I describe several conflicts or challenges that might arise in deciding what to measure in global mental health research and practice.

Whether intentional or not, global mental health researchers and practitioners are often most focused on measuring what matters to stakeholders in positions of power (e.g., research funding agencies or academic audiences), often to the neglect of populations who are most affected by a crisis or a new intervention. Being able to communicate to powerful stakeholders is often important: knowing what will convince funders to allocate additional resources to mental healthcare, building political will among global policy makers, and achieving buy-in from researchers or advocates in high-resource settings are all worthy goals. Outcomes that fit neatly into psychiatric diagnostic categories (e.g., depression, PTSD) are usually the most readily interpretable to such stakeholders [1]. However, as I describe below, psychiatric diagnostic categories are not the only possible outcomes of interest, and they are often not the best way to capture what matters most to those our interventions aim to serve.

Reflecting explicitly on how and why we make decisions about what to measure includes consideration of whose perspectives we are privileging and what alternatives might be considered. Social scientists have highlighted a number of problems to be aware of with our data collection systems. For example, Nigerian anthropologist and physician Adeola Oni-Orisan [2] studied maternal healthcare interventions in Nigeria and uncovered ways that decisions regarding what to measure are often politically driven. She found that program-design decisions were often motivated by the desire to most readily produce data that reflect well on the program. For example, facility-based maternal mortality programs were prioritized because they could easily produce data regarding improved outcomes, even though this choice conflicted with areas of greatest need, such as training traditional birth attendants (the preferred choice among women) in order to produce safer birth outcomes more broadly. Oni-Orisan also revealed how decisions regarding "what counts" – which data make it into reports and which do not – are also politically shaped, reflecting how our measures and resulting data are socially constructed in various ways. Similarly, anthropologist Ashley Hagaman's [3] ethnographic study of suicide reporting systems in Nepal demonstrated that community-based stigma, inaccessibility of reporting structures (e.g., police stations, death certificates), and misperceptions of suicide as illegal at both the institutional and community level combined to produce significant discrepancies between actual rates of suicide and what gets reported in national statistics. The result is massive underreporting of suicides and a missed opportunity to direct funds towards interventions and subpopulations that would have the highest impact.

By explicitly recognizing that we often solely measure what matters most to stakeholders like funders, politicians, and researchers, we can commit to also asking what matters most to the individuals and communities targeted by our interventions. Here, concepts from anthropology, cultural psychiatry, and cultural epidemiology can be useful. For example, we might focus on identifying relevant cultural concepts of distress, such as idioms of distress, which anthropologist Mark Nichter defines as "socially and culturally resonant means of experiencing and expressing distress in local worlds" (p. 405) [4]. Anthropologists and cultural psychiatrists have described a number of such idioms of distress, such as "thinking too much" or *nervios* [5, 6]. Significantly, cultural concepts of distress do not solely represent different local names for the same global experience – for example, although *nervios* shares common symptoms with anxiety, it is not merely a local equivalent of the psychiatric disorder. Instead, cultural concepts of distress often reflect constellations of symptoms that are related to culturally embedded ways of making sense of the person, the body, and expected social roles that do not translate at all across contexts [7].

Idioms of distress reference broader phenomena than solely psychopathology, so it is important not to equate the two [8]. However, where they do reference experiences locally recognized as requiring intervention, it is often precisely those experiences represented in idioms of distress that matter most for patients to see improvement. For example, I have spent my career as a medical anthropologist focusing on mental health in low-resource settings. Where I work in rural Haiti, psychologists are typically concerned with measuring change in depression symptoms over time, but they have been able to focus their clinical communication on relative improvement in "thinking too much" (Kreyòl: *reflechi twòp*), a key and meaningful outcome to many patients [21]. Focusing on idioms of distress can improve communication about interventions by reducing stigma, improving recruitment and participant buy-in, and improving adherence [5].

Additionally, mental health symptom burden does not necessarily translate into functional impairment for everyone. Focusing solely on mental health symptoms might not reflect what matters most to participants, such as assessing to what extent symptoms limit individuals' ability to fulfill important roles. Function impairment measures can gauge to what extent mental health symptom burden is associated with impaired ability to work, complete tasks, and fulfill socially expected roles. Paul Bolton and Alice Tang [9] designed a methodological approach to developing local function impairment measures that assess ability to care for oneself, one's family, and one's community, based on identifying locally meaningful tasks in each category. Including function impairment measures alongside symptom inventories can ensure that screening strategies identify those most in need of care.

What Matters About How We Measure?

After considering what to measure, a next critical consideration is how we ensure that we are measuring that construct in a valid way [11]. In other words, how do we ensure that we are measuring what we think we are measuring? There are many potential shortcomings and ethical trade-offs to be aware of, and a burgeoning literature deals with how to approach measurement development and validation cross-culturally. For example, many measurement tools used in epidemiologic or intervention research go through simple translation-back translation procedures starting from English tools. These translations are by definition completed by individuals fluent in English, and they often are professionals (e.g., doctors, NGO administrators) and may not best represent those groups our interventions intend to serve.

Without additional procedures to assess tools' functioning, we cannot know how (well) items are understood. There is the risk that participants' responses to assessment items in fact reflect a different question than we intended to ask. For example, in Nigeria, we found that an item intending to assess loneliness that was translated as "feeling there is only you in this life" was instead interpreted to mean that you are rich and can live alone in a gated complex with no one else [12]. In Nepal, anthropologist and psychiatrist Brandon Kohrt and colleagues found that the PTSD item "unable to have strong feelings" was interpreted as a desirable state; from a Buddhist perspective, no one should have strong feelings [13]. In my experience, respondents completing these tools will still respond to items, even when – as in these examples – they seem to be asking about a bizarre collection of experiences like being rich, having appropriate emotional detachment, and perhaps actually relevant items about mental distress. In situations like this, we are left with data that can be misleading or not useful [7].

A significant implication of measures with poor validity is that they are likely to lead us to mis-categorize individuals in terms of need for care, as well as result in inefficient use of already limited resources. For example, where a screening tool has poor specificity, it will result in a number of false positives, or individuals who are not in need of care but are categorized as needing care. Brandon Kohrt and colleagues [13] estimated that if an intervention costs $20 per individual to deliver, and a screening tool produces a high number of false positives (e.g., two false positives for every true positive), it could end up costing closer to $60 per individual in need of treatment. This is because for every individual actually in need of care who receives treatment, there are two individuals not in need of care who also receive treatment. Additionally, there is the obvious problem of failing to detect those individuals who are in need of care by mis-categorizing them as false negatives.

Fortunately, there are a number of procedures available for improving validity of screening tools. The use of rigorous cultural adaptation processes has been demonstrated to improve validity of measurement tools [14]. Cultural adaptation typically entails the use of qualitative or mixed methods that go beyond translation alone, to include focus group discussions and/or pilot testing with cognitive interviewing (i.e., asking participants how they understand questions or to "think aloud" as they decide how to respond). The focus of these methods is to assess and improve comprehensibility, acceptability, and relevance of items [15]. Beyond identifying problems with item meaning, there might be issues such as items being unacceptable to discuss (e.g., sexual interest on depression screeners, stigmatized behaviors on behavior disorder scales). Additionally, some items simply might not be relevant or experienced in a specific context, such as asking about having numerous speeding tickets (a potential indicator of antisocial behavior) in a population where no one drives cars [16]. It is important that cultural adaptation procedures also account for technical equivalence. For example, is delivering a screening tool verbally the same as having someone complete it individually in paper-and-pencil format? Are response options, such as those on a Likert scale from never to always, sufficiently well understood and equivalent cross-culturally? Insight regarding any of these potential problems can be gained through thorough discussion of tools so that they can be improved while striving to maintain equivalence to the original tool.

Cultural adaptation procedures can promote what some call ethnographic validity: they help to ensure that what we are measuring represents real, meaningful aspects of mental distress in a given context. Clinical or diagnostic validation techniques aim to ensure that our measures map onto psychiatric categories. These are both important goals and can help us to meet the needs of various stakeholders (see section "What Matters to Measure?"). The basic approach in diagnostic validity studies is to compare the results of our screening tools to a gold standard – typically a diagnostic interview conducted by a clinician. This allows us to identify the appropriate cutoff score above which individuals should be referred for care, and we can also assess the degree to which the screening tool matches findings of the gold standard.

There is a suite of challenges that comes with diagnostic validity studies. First, they require the availability of trained mental health specialists (e.g., psychiatrists, psychologists) who can complete diagnostic interviews. Because many global mental health settings have few if any specialists available, this can be a major limitation. Additionally, there is the ethical trade-off between devoting specialists' limited time fully to clinical care vs taking time to participate in validation studies, which ideally will improve accuracy of efforts to identify those in need of care and efficient use of resources. The shortage of specialist providers is also why interventions themselves often rely on screening tools rather than diagnosis for determining who is need of care [17]. Below, I describe alternatives for conducting validity studies where specialists are unavailable. A second limitation is that diagnostic validity procedures rely upon DSM- or ICD-based clinical assessments, which were themselves developed in a different cultural setting than where the validation study will occur. In general, such studies assume that employing local clinicians ensures ethnographic or on-the-ground validity, but using formal procedures to evaluate and culturally adapt diagnostic procedures is important.

Alternative approaches to validating assessment tools can account for both the limited availability of clinicians and the cultural bias of diagnostic tools. For example, Paul Bolton and colleagues [18] use an approach in which community leaders nominate individuals as distressed/needing care or not, and these categories are used for validation (in place of clinician diagnosis). Another approach, used by Leah Watson et al. [19] in Kenya, combines interviews conducted by lay individuals with ratings by clinicians. The ratings are based on interview transcripts and can therefore be conducted at a distance and more efficiently (in this case, by a team of Kenyan and US-based clinicians).

Another challenge that applies to both cultural adaptation and validation studies is that they are typically conducted in a single language. In multilingual and culturally diverse settings, this can create a challenge when screening tools are only available in one language: the result is that some people are screened in what is not their primary language or tools are translated on the fly, which raises questions regarding their validity. Alternatively, sometimes tools have been validated in multiple languages in the same setting, but the procedures were conducted independently, making them incomparable between languages (see section "Case Studies" for a suggested approach to resolve such problems).

A last (but certainly not least) concern regards what matters to have in place before we develop or use measures. Specifically, there is a need to establish some kind of referral system for those individuals that measures identify as in need of care. This is difficult to do when the development of assessment tools is linked – and occurring parallel – to efforts to design mental healthcare programs where they haven't previously existed. This parallel development often happens because measures are a fundamental part of such care delivery programs. At other times, measures are developed first in order to generate data regarding the burden of disease and areas of need in order to inform program development or support requests for program funding.

In such situations where measurement tools are used in the absence of local mental healthcare programs, there are several options for ensuring that some form of care is available for those indicating a high symptom burden, functional impairment, and/or suicidal ideation. In some cases, there are mental healthcare programs available in nearby regions, such that providing transportation is sufficient to connect individuals to care. In other cases, the only available care is through distant inpatient facilities that are not always appropriate depending on the condition. In such cases, drawing upon existing local resources is often the best way to ensure adequate support. For example, for individuals endorsing thoughts of suicide, safety plans can be developed in coordination with family members and neighbors [20]. These would typically include considerations of limiting access to lethal means, having someone accompany the individual at all times, and identifying ways to intervene with community supports to address the underlying causes. The case studies below both represent scenarios in which measurement tools were being developed prior to implementation of mental healthcare programming, which requires

Table 6.1 Questions to consider when making decisions regarding measurement tools

What to measure	How to measure
1. Whose perspectives and values are reflected in our selection of what to measure? Who is left out? 2. Have we considered what matters most to measure according to target communities? 3. Are there cultural concepts of distress that could be incorporated into our measures? 4. Do our measures include functional outcomes?	1. Does our team include anthropologists, care providers, and local community members? 2. What language/s should the measurement tools be in for the local context? 3. What cultural adaptation procedures are most appropriate and feasible for this context to ensure that items and response options are comprehensible, acceptable, relevant, and delivered in ways that are technically equivalent? 4. Are there specialists available to conduct diagnostic validation? Is it feasible and appropriate to have them devote time to a validation study (rather than patient care)? If not, are there alternate validation procedures that are feasible? 5. Are there sufficient referral procedures in place for participants expressing severe distress or suicidal ideation, drawing upon existing formal mental healthcare and/or community resources?

creative problem-solving to ensure that research participants are not placed at risk and that their needs can be addressed (Table 6.1).

Case Studies

Here I provide two case studies, from Nigeria and Haiti, that demonstrate several of the ethical challenges described above. I explain how we (teams of researchers, NGOs, and care providers) considered the various trade-offs and decided upon a course of action. These certainly do not represent the only way to resolve these ethical dilemmas; the aim is to provide concrete examples of the difficult decisions that have to be made in low-resource settings without existing formal mental healthcare.

Designing Screening Tools in Nigeria: Translating in Two Languages Simultaneously

The Gede Foundation is an NGO founded by Dr. Jennifer Douglas-Abubakar, a former first lady of Nigeria. Gede aims to promote research and service provision for stigmatized conditions like HIV and mental illness. One component of their work is providing care for orphans and vulnerable children (OVCs), as part of a program called Sustainable Mechanisms for Improving Livelihoods and Household Empowerment (SMILE). The SMILE consortium is a cooperative agreement between Catholic Relief Services and the US Agency for International Development, designed to scale up care and support services for OVCs in four Nigerian states plus the Federal Capital Territory. SMILE focused on providing a range of social services and more recently recognized the need to expand access to mental healthcare services, which are largely inaccessible in the rural areas outside the capital Abuja, where they work. Gede and SMILE identified as a promising avenue the training of community volunteers – who were already visiting OVCs to provide HIV support – to incorporate mental health into the services that they provide. There are challenges and ethical trade-offs inherent in such task-shifting approaches, particularly regarding increased availability of care balanced against concerns regarding quality of care, availability of supervision, and whether volunteers would be paid for what can become a significantly more time-consuming form of care. These issues are covered in other chapters (e.g., see Kohrt, Chap. 2). Here, I focus on the measurement challenges.

Gede Foundation saw that a fundamental aspect of developing a mental healthcare program was going to be developing screening tools to identify children in need of care. They gathered a team of US and Nigerian researchers, clinicians, and NGO collaborators to focus on measure development. There were several goals that were immediately apparent. Only screening tools – rather than full diagnostic assessments – could realistically be made available as part of the broader program being designed, due to a shortage of specialists. The tools would need to be short and easy to administer and interpret by community volunteers.

Other aspects were less immediately clear. For example, there are a number of mental, neurological, or substance use disorders that could have been selected, such as autism, developmental delays, epilepsy, or drug use. But some of these did not have an evidence base for community-based treatment in this context. Second, the only mental health screening tools that have been adapted for use in Nigeria are in English or Yoruba, which is spoken in the southwest part of Nigeria and would not be useful for the region around Abuja, where Gede works. However, there are not clear alternatives for this region, known as Federal Capital Territory. This area was intentionally developed in the 1980s at the meeting point of many ethnic and linguistic groups and is reflective of Nigeria's exceptional linguistic and ethnic diversity, with over 500 languages spoken (see Fig. 6.1 for a map of the most common languages). It would not be feasible to adapt screening tools for all languages for the region around Abuja, let alone the whole country. As always, there are a range of methodological and logistical decisions to make regarding adapting and validating assessment tools – including whether to validate at all, due to trade-offs in terms of time and resources that could instead be focused on care provision. Finally, knowing mental healthcare was not yet available in the communities where we focused our screening tool research, we needed to determine procedures for addressing needs of children identified as needing care.

Decision-Making [12]

In deciding how to manage the various ethical challenges faced in our work, we tried to balance existing evidence from global mental health as well as local and national needs. Somewhat unique to this research is that we were keenly aware of important mental health needs in other regions of the country. Specifically, the

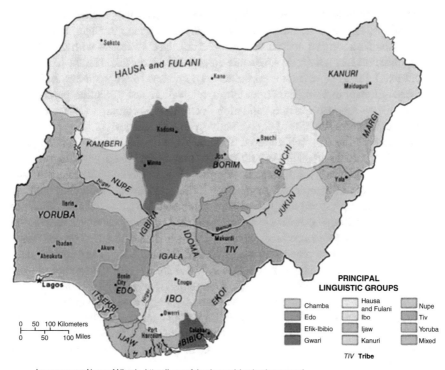

Image source: News of Nigeria, https://newsofnigeria.com/nigerian-languages/

Fig. 6.1 Primary linguistic groups in Nigeria. (Image source: News of Nigeria, https://newsofnigeria.com/nigerian-languages/)

ongoing Boko Haram insurgency in northeast Nigeria – although not affecting the immediate area of Gede's work – was a significant source of mental distress for a large number of Nigerians and was leading to internal displacement, including to Abuja.

To select disorders of focus, we drew upon research regarding burden of disease in other sub-Saharan African countries and conflict settings and local organizations' experiences, ultimately selecting depression, PTSD, and behavior disorders. We then identified commonly used and adapted screening tools for these disorders: Depression Self-Rating Scale (DSRS), Child PTSD Symptom Scale (CPSS), and Disruptive Behavior Disorders Rating Scale (DBDRS). As mentioned above, we intentionally did not select disorders such as autism or other developmental disorders, despite this being an important and underserved area in global mental health, because we knew this would not be feasible for our eventual program to address. Additionally, we selected PTSD rather than anxiety due to the anticipated high prevalence of trauma considering our target population of OVCs potentially affected by the Boko Haram insurgency.

Our selection of languages for the screening tools likewise aimed to achieve a balance of local and national needs. Pidgin is one of the most commonly spoken languages nationally, so we selected it in the hopes of having the widest applicability. Similarly, Hausa is the most commonly spoken language in Nigeria, including both in Abuja and in the northeast. We therefore selected Hausa with the goal of having the most reach for both Abuja and areas affected by Boko Haram. The selection of two languages raised novel challenges compared to other studies. Although we already aimed to complete both cultural adaptation and validation procedures, the use of two languages made validation even more important so that we could ensure that the tools functioned equivalently in both languages.

All stages of the research required close attention to equivalence between languages and efforts to reconcile any differences that might have arisen. Importantly, this required inclusion of trilingual (Pidgin, Hausa, English) members of the research team. For example, we began with initial translations, including both lay and professional perspectives. These were completed by trilingual individuals to encourage translations to be as similar as possible between Hausa and Pidgin. We next completed focus group discussions (FGDs), which each focused on one of the tools. Because FGDs were also gender and age (12–14, 15–17) segregated, doubling the number of languages meant doubling the number of FGDs required from 18 to 36. Although this was logistically demanding, it was important that we captured all relevant voices, particularly those that might not be heard in heterogeneous FGDs (e.g., girls, younger individuals). FGDs did not assume knowledge of English, so they were not focused on assessing translation of items. Instead, they assessed comprehensibility, acceptability, and relevance of items, as well as eliciting suggestions for better ways to ask questions.

After FGDs were completed, we made adjustments to items to account for problems identified, and we attended closely to any differences that arose between languages, attempting to use similar adaptations in both languages. However, maintaining equivalence was not always possible. For example, the PTSD item "unable to have strong feelings" was adapted in Hausa using the well-understood idiom of distress "having a dry heart" (*zuciyanka ya bushe*). We attempted to identify a similarly well-understood idiom of distress in Pidgin but could not. This item was ultimately more discriminant between cases and non-cases in Hausa than Pidgin. We then pilot tested the screening tools with 24 children, using cognitive interviewing to assess how children understood the items. This provides a different type of insight than FGDs, as children are not being asked to discuss the items hypothetically but to respond about themselves, which requires a different level of engagement. Piloting can therefore highlight different types of problems than FGDs.

Finally, we conducted a validation process with the three screening tools. This involved asking community organizations to recruit children who were either likely experiencing emotional or behavioral distress or were unlikely to be. The goal was to have a sample that includes people falling on both the higher and lower ends of the spectrum on the screening tools. However, we had difficulty recruiting enough children likely experiencing distress, which would have made it difficult to complete validation procedures. We hypothesized that, due to our affiliation with the SMILE program, community partners assumed that the children recruited had to be participants from the program – who were receiving support and likely had better functioning than others because they were attending school, as required by the program. We therefore emphasized to community partners who were coordinating recruitment that participants should not be limited to those already engaged in the SMILE program, which helped to address the problem.

Validation procedures consisted of having an enumerator work with children to complete the screening tools and then having a clinical psychologist complete a diagnostic interview guided by the Kiddie-Schedule for Affective Disorders and Schizophrenia (K-SADS). The clinicians categorized each child as a case or non-case for each condition (depression, PTSD, and behavior disorder – including oppositional defiant disorder and conduct disorder). Using these findings, we could identify which screening tool items discriminated by caseness (meaning scores were significantly different between cases and non-cases). By removing items that did not discriminate by caseness, we were able to produce shorter, easier-to-deliver screening tools that still had good psychometric properties. We identified the cutoff scores that produced the best accuracy in correctly categorizing cases and non-cases for each tool. Although this process was time-consuming, it provided the most confidence that our final screening tools would be well-understood and well-functioning and that they would validly reflect real experiences of distress as well as fit psychiatric diagnostic categories. A final concern regards referral of those identified as needing care, which is the focus of the next case study.

Addressing Mental Health Needs in Haiti: Research Prior to Development of Formal Mental Healthcare

In 2010, I began working in Haiti as part of a team of graduate researchers collaborating with a healthcare NGO (Fig. 6.2). Medical students who had completed short-term medical missions with the NGO were seeing patients with what they interpreted as mental illness that was not being addressed in any way in the clinical encounters. They suggested that there was a need for research exploring how

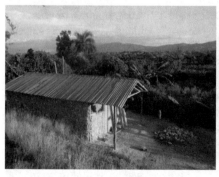 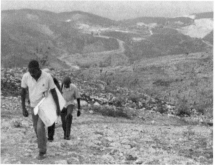

A home in rural Haiti   Data collection in rural Haiti

Fig. 6.2 (a) A home in rural Haiti. (b) Data collection in rural Haiti. (Photos by author)

mental illness is conceptualized, what care does exist, and how people seek care in relation to experiences of mental illness. Between 2010 and 2011, our team conducted broad, exploratory research examining these questions, which included identifying idioms of distress, assessing how they were interpreted by clinicians and lay individuals, examining care-seeking preferences and outcomes, culturally adapting and locally developing assessment tools, and applying those tools in community-based epidemiologic surveys [21–26]. An additional need that arose during the research was suicidal ideation, which was viewed by clinicians as indicating distress but not reflecting true intent to attempt suicide [27]. Community members, on the other hand, told numerous stories of neighbors and friends who had died by suicide.

Core to this research were efforts to identify individuals experiencing mental illness or suicidal ideation, whether through the assessment tools that we were developing and testing or through community members referring us to people experiencing mental illness for interviews. We knew that it would be unethical to purposely seek out individuals experiencing illness or disability in order to learn from them but then not provide some form of care to address their needs. At the same time, formal mental healthcare did not exist in the area where we worked. Typically, research like ours that takes place in higher-resource settings would establish referral systems with local mental health specialists. One of our goals was therefore to identify the best alternative referral systems and strategies, in the absence of local mental health specialists. Additionally, there are always concerns when asking about sensitive or potentially distressing topics, as is often the case in mental health assessment tools. Even for individuals not experiencing mental illness, discussing emotional or behavioral disorders can produce distress, and research and practice protocols should include appropriate approaches to respond.

Decision-Making

As described above, our study was situated in the ethically thorny context of needing to collect data to inform mental healthcare program development and therefore taking place prior to such care being available through the partner NGO. One of the complications was lack of clarity over time regarding the NGO's goal of using the screening information to seek funding, develop care delivery programs, or both. Our efforts to develop referral systems therefore centered on identifying various sources of informal mental healthcare, as well as more distant formal care options where needed. In terms of formal mental healthcare, the two options nationally available in the public sector were psychiatric hospitals, one of which had been severely damaged in the January 2010 earthquake and had not yet reopened. The other was known for overcrowding and human rights abuses, such that people knew of it but did not want to send family or friends there. Nevertheless, we debated whether this might represent a better option than nothing for severe cases.

Fortunately, at the same time that we were conducting our research, another NGO – Zanmi Lasante (ZL, Partners in Health) – was developing a mental healthcare program in the same region, about an hour from where we were working [28–31]. I call this fortunate, but the timing was not coincidental. Following the earthquake, there was a surge of humanitarian interest and intervention in Haiti, including a newfound focus on mental health needs. ZL (among others) secured funding to develop mental health services to address the stark lack of formal mental healthcare. They leveraged this funding into an approach focused on health systems strengthening, such that mental healthcare would be an integral part of all of their clinics and hospitals, even after the initial grant ran out. Due to our relative proximity to one of their clinical sites, we were able to coordinate a referral system such that people we identified as in acute need of care were connected to ZL's mental health team to schedule an appointment, and their transportation was subsidized. While this approach was moderately successful, we ran into the issue that individuals would connect to care providers and perhaps attend an initial appointment, but rarely did they attend follow-up visits. In this case, ZL used an innovative solution of a mental health mobile clinic [28], but in other settings, different solutions would likely be needed to keep people connected to care.

For people endorsing suicidal ideation, it was important to intervene in more immediate ways. We therefore developed a safety plan that drew together family and community resources to help prevent scenarios of self-harm or suicidal behavior. One of the key aspects of such safety plans is limiting access to means of attempting suicide. We learned through our research that local political leaders had previously taken such approaches, enacting community-wide interventions to reduce access to pesticides because it was a common means of suicide [27]. We first developed a series of follow-up questions for individuals who endorsed suicidal ideation on our survey. The questions assessed whether they had a plan and access to means, which indicate level of severity or risk for suicide. We then connected with the individual's closest family or community member and discussed strategies for ensuring that they were always accompanied, as well as ways to limit access to means. Individuals were also connected to ZL for care, as described above. Such approaches, which draw upon existing local resources, can be effective ways to provide some form of intervention for suffering individuals in the absence of formal mental healthcare [19].

Finally, in terms of addressing distress that could arise in the context of screening tool use, our focus was on ensuring that participants were in control. For researchers, it might feel that the best response to a distressed participant is ending the assessment (or interview), since that is what is causing the distress. However, this runs the risk of eliciting strong emotions and leaving them unprocessed, which might be worse for participants. Instead, it might be useful to provide a space for further discussion if desired or to provide a break for the participant before continuing. Of course, if they want to discontinue the assessment, that is what must happen. But it is important that researchers not allow their own discomfort (e.g., at having a participant become distressed) to solely determine what steps are taken but to ensure the participant remains in control.

Conclusion

This chapter has explored various ethical concerns that arise in the course of designing and utilizing measurement tools in global mental health research and practice. It is vital that such tools be routinely incorporated into global mental health programs in order to ensure that our work is effective, efficient, and ethical. Important recommendations arising out of the topics covered in this chapter include: (1) critically examine which stakeholders' goals are being met through selected measurement tools, and consider what might be of greatest value to other stakeholders, especially target communities; (2) form research teams for assessment tool development that include anthropologists, care providers, and representatives of the beneficiary community; (3) utilize rigorous cultural adaptation and validation techniques to ensure accuracy in identifying and referring individuals in need of care; (4) explore both diagnostic and ethnographic validity when designing validity studies, and consider using alternative validation approaches if needed where mental health specialists are not available; and (5) ensure that referral systems are in place for individuals identified as needing care, so that they are not used for knowledge production but left without support for identified needs. As with all global mental health research and practice, there are no easy answers when it comes to measurement. However, the above considerations can help us to ensure that what we measure and how we measure are optimally responsive and of greatest value to stakeholders who are most affected by our work.

References

1. Weaver, L. J., & Kaiser, B. (2014). Developing and testing locally-derived mental health scales: Examples from North India and Haiti. *Field Methods, 27*(2), 115–130.
2. Oni-Orisan, A. (2016). The obligation to count: The politics of monitoring maternal mortality in Nigeria. In V. Adams (Ed.), *Metrics: What counts in global health* (pp. 82–104). Durham: Duke University Press.
3. Hagaman, A. K., Maharjan, U., & Kohrt, B. A. (2016). Suicide surveillance and health systems in Nepal: A qualitative and social network analysis. *International Journal of Mental Health Systems, 10*(1), 46.
4. Nichter, M. (2010). Idioms of distress revisited. *Culture, Medicine and Psychiatry, 34,* 401–416.
5. Kaiser, B., Haroz, E., Kohrt, B., Bolton, P., Bass, J., & Hinton, D. (2015). Thinking too much: A systematic review of a common idiom of distress. *Social Science & Medicine, 147,* 170–183.
6. Guarnaccia, P., Lewis-Fernández, R., & Marano, M. R. (2003). Toward a Puerto Rican popular nosology: Nervios and ataque de nervios. *Culture, Medicine and Psychiatry, 27,* 339–366.
7. Kohrt, B., & Hruschka, D. J. (2010). Nepali concepts of psychological trauma: The role of idioms of distress, ethnopsychology and ethnophysiology in alleviating suffering and preventing stigma. *Culture, Medicine and Psychiatry, 34*(2), 322–352.
8. Kaiser, B. N., & Jo Weaver, L. (2019). *Culture-bound syndromes, idioms of distress, and cultural concepts of distress: New directions for an old concept in psychological anthropology.* London: SAGE Publications Sage UK.
9. Bolton, P., & Tang, A. M. (2002). An alternative approach to cross-cultural function assessment. *Social Psychiatry and Psychiatric Epidemiology, 37*(11), 537–543.

10. van Ommeren, M. (2003). Validity issues in transcultural epidemiology. *The British Journal of Psychiatry, 182*, 376–378.
11. Kaiser, B. N., Ticao, C., Anoje, C., Minto, J., Boglosa, J., & Kohrt, B. A. (2019). Adapting culturally appropriate mental health screening tools for use among conflict-affected and other vulnerable adolescents in Nigeria. *Global Mental Health, 6*, e10.
12. Kohrt, B., Jordans, M. J. D., Tol, W. A., Luitel, N. P., Maharjan, S. M., & Upadhaya, N. (2011). Validation of cross-cultural child mental health and psychosocial research instruments: Adapting the Depression Self-Rating Scale and Child PTSD Symptom Scale in Nepal. *BMC Psychiatry, 11*(1), 127.
13. Ali, G.-C., Ryan, G., & De Silva, M. J. (2016). Validated screening tools for common mental disorders in low and middle income countries: A systematic review. *PLoS One, 11*(6), e0156939.
14. van Ommeren, M., Sharma, B., Thapa, S., Makaju, R., Prasain, D., Bhattarai, R., et al. (1999). Preparing instruments for transcultural research: Use of the translation monitoring form with Nepali-speaking Bhutanese refugees. *Transcultural Psychiatry, 36*(3), 285–301.
15. Flaherty, J. A., Gaviria, F. M., Pathak, D., Mitchell, T., Wintrob, R., Richman, J. A., et al. (1988). Developing instruments for cross-cultural psychiatric research. *The Journal of Nervous and Mental Disease, 176*(5), 257–263.
16. Reynolds, C. F., 3rd, & Patel, V. (2017). Screening for depression: The global mental health context. *World Psychiatry, 16*(3), 316.
17. Bolton, P. (2001). Cross-cultural validity and reliability testing of a standard psychiatric assessment instrument without a gold standard. *The Journal of Nervous and Mental Disease, 189*, 238–242.
18. Watson, L. K., Kaiser, B. N., Giusto, A. M., Ayuku, D., & Puffer, E. S. (2019). Validating mental health assessment in Kenya using an innovative gold standard. *International Journal of Psychology, 55*(3), 425–434.
19. Murray, L. K., Skavenski, S., Bass, J., Wilcox, H., Bolton, P., Imasiku, M., et al. (2014). Implementing evidence-based mental health care in low-resource settings: A focus on safety planning procedures. *Journal of Cognitive Psychotherapy, 28*(3), 168–185.
20. Kaiser, B., Kohrt, B., Keys, H., Khoury, N., & Brewster, A.-R. (2013). Strategies for assessing mental health in Haiti: Local instrument development and transcultural translation. *Transcultural Psychiatry, 15*(4), 532–558.
21. Kaiser, B. N., McLean, K. E., Kohrt, B. A., Hagaman, A. K., Wagenaar, B. H., Khoury, N. M., et al. (2014). Reflechi twop-thinking too much: Description of a cultural syndrome in Haiti's Central Plateau. *Culture, Medicine and Psychiatry, 38*(3), 448–472.
22. Keys, H., Kaiser, B., Kohrt, B., Khoury, N., & Brewster, A.-R. (2012). Idioms of distress, ethnopsychology, and the clinical encounter in Haiti's Central Plateau. *Social Science & Medicine, 75*(3), 555–564.
23. Khoury, N., Kaiser, B., Brewster, A.-R., Keys, H., & Kohrt, B. (2012). Explanatory models and mental health treatment: Is Vodou an obstacle to psychiatric treatment in rural Haiti? *Culture, Medicine and Psychiatry, 36*(3), 514–534.
24. McLean, K., Kaiser, B., Hagaman, A., Wagenaar, B., Therosme, T., & Kohrt, B. (2015). Task sharing in rural Haiti: Qualitative assessment of a brief, structured training with and without apprenticeship supervision for community health workers. *Intervention, 13*(2), 135–155.
25. Wagenaar, B., Hagaman, A., Kaiser, B., McLean, K., & Kohrt, B. (2012). Depression, suicidal ideation, and associated factors in rural Haiti. *BMC Psychiatry, 12*, 149.
26. Wagenaar, B., Kohrt, B., Hagaman, A., McLean, K., & Kaiser, B. (2013). Determinants of care seeking for mental health problems in rural Haiti: Culture, cost, or competency? *Psychiatric Services, 64*, 366–372.
27. Hagaman, A., Wagenaar, B., McLean, K., Kaiser, B., Winskell, K., & Kohrt, B. (2013). Suicide in rural Haiti: Differences in clinical and lay community perceptions of prevalence, etiology, and religious implications. *Social Science & Medicine, 83*, 61–69.
28. Fils-Aime, J. R., Grelotti, D. J., Therosme, T., Kaiser, B. N., Raviola, G., Alcindor, Y., et al. (2018). A mobile clinic approach to the delivery of community-based mental health services in rural Haiti. *PLoS One, 13*(6), e0199313.

29. Legha, R., Eustache, E., Therosme, T., Boyd, K., Reginald, F.-A., Hilaire, G., et al. (2015). Taskshifting: Translating theory into practice to build a community based mental health care system in rural Haiti. *Intervention, 13*(3), 248–267.
30. Raviola, G., Eustache, E., Oswald, C., & Belkin, G. S. (2012). Mental health response in Haiti in the aftermath of the 2010 earthquake: A case study for building long-term solutions. *Harvard Review of Psychiatry, 20*(1), 68–77.
31. Raviola, G., Severe, J., Therosme, T., Oswald, C., Belkin, G., & Eustache, E. (2013). The 2010 Haiti earthquake response. *Psychiatric Clinics of North America, 36*, 431–450.

Where Ethics and Culture Collide: Ethical Dilemmas in Grief Work Following the Easter Sunday Attacks in Sri Lanka

7

Nilanga Abeysinghe and Evangeline S. Ekanayake

Counselling in Sri Lanka: Development Through the Decades

Although there has been a state acceptance of the need for counselling services since the 1950s in Sri Lanka, services have not been regulated over the years. As a result, an array of different set of quality standards in service delivery and counsellor training have been proposed and been in operation among several counselling associations that have been formed over the last couple of decades.

The development of the mental health sector in a country takes place in response to the socio-economic and political milieu and needs of a nation [16]. This was evident in the development of the sector in Britain and also in the USA following the Second World War and the Vietnam War. Considering the situation in Sri Lanka, along with the socio-political and economic changes in a post war reality after, a three-decade-long civil war, two youth insurgencies, 2004 Asian Tsunami have contributed heavily to the development of mental health services and its later evolution to its current shape.

The concept of mental illness prevailed for over 2000 years in Sri Lanka as part of the Ayurvedic (traditional) medicine (Neki, 1973, cited in [7]). However, contemporary mental health care emerged during the British colonial era as a speciality in Sri Lanka and continues as a speciality in allopathic medicine [7]. A landmark of this development was the establishment of the first "lunatic asylum" as it was called then, in 1846 (Wambeek, 1866 cited in [7]). Ever since, Sri Lanka has had mental health services as part of the state medical services.

The mental health sector in Sri Lanka has expanded beyond medication-based care and evolved to incorporate counselling support along with psychiatric care for little over two decades. This is partly evident when we consider the increase in the number of counselling positions in the state service since 2005 [14, 15]. Despite the sweeping developments in mental health services, it is noteworthy that the country

N. Abeysinghe (✉) · E. S. Ekanayake
Faculty of Graduate Studies, University of Colombo, Colombo, Sri Lanka

© Springer Nature Switzerland AG 2021
A. R. Dyer et al. (eds.), *Global Mental Health Ethics*,
https://doi.org/10.1007/978-3-030-66296-7_7

has one of the highest rates of suicide attempts and deliberate self-harm rates in the world [9]. As such, though the country claims a steep development in the mental health sector, it is still shackled by a serious lack of staff to deal with the demand for services [6]. Despite the three-decade-long war and other adverse events that warranted the development and services of the psychosocial sector, we are yet to actively explore how best society and individuals need to be helped out of their collective and individual trauma. Hence, as mentioned above, the ethical challenges we face need to be addressed in service delivery and training of professional counsellors and psychosocial workers using counselling skills. Based on our experience over the years, we see the need for training in ethics to be continuously modified with reflective practice in relation to the standards identified in the global mental health sector.

Below we provide a detailed account of one of the more recent national level disasters which seriously impinged upon the wellbeing of the nation and its mental health services. This was the 2019 Easter Bombings in Sri Lanka that claimed over 250 lives, leaving us wiht rich learning on how the counselling community was engaged and the dilemmas therein. We attempt by this to highlight some of the challenges of a professionalized national counselling system.

The Easter Bombing in Sri Lanka

The 21st of April, Easter Sunday of 2019, has left a grim scar in the minds of Sri Lankans, especially the Catholic and Christian communities as several churches and hotels became the deadly targets of suicide bombers who claimed to be associates of the Islamic State of Iraq and Syria (ISIS). The 9 suicide bombers killed over 250 lives and threw in to chaos the day-to-day life of the Sri Lankans who were just rebuilding after the three-decade civil war (1983–2009) between the Liberation Tigers of the Tamil Eelam (LTTE) and the Sri Lankan government. Over the months following the Easter Bombings, many attempts were taken to reinstate normalcy, to strengthen security and to support the direct victims and the many indirect victims of the unfortunate incident.

This example is based on the personal experiences of the authors in relief and support work done in the aftermath of the Easter suicide bombings in Sri Lanka. It sets the cultural, political and religious context of the relief and support work and provides a profile of key actors in the scene in order that the nature of the ethical dilemmas that followed may be better understood. This is a personal reflection of events that took place on that morning and the months that followed.

Easter morning of 2019, I was getting ready for this special day of resurrection. It was 9.05 am when I received my first call after which I would forever remember this day as one of death and destruction. A close friend called me from a hotel in the city to ask if I knew what was happening, as the hotel they were in was suddenly placed under security lockdown with little explanation. She said they had felt tremors of a blast minutes before and there were speculations that the surrounding hotels were under attack. I quickly switched on all media and was instantly flooded by the horrors of the suicide bombs that had just ripped through three churches packed with Easter worshippers and three hotels all surrounding the one my friend was calling from. As I offered to pick my friend up as she was too shaken to drive, news kept flooding in, and gruesome first-hand clips from the scenes of the massacre in the churches were already clogging WhatsApp.

As I drove downtown towards the hotels, the streets were eerily empty with a few nervous drivers (like myself) speeding on their missions, police cars on alert and screeching ambulances flying past. News poured in. Seven suicide bombers claiming to be ISIS associates had targeted three churches holding Easter mass and three hotels which were hosting Easter Brunch. This was a first. We had survived 27 years of armed conflict and many suicide bombs by the LTTE fighting the Sri Lankan army for a separate state. After a bloody end to those battles, we had known a silencing of guns for 10 years.

I was stopped at a barricade close to the hotel. The armed forces were out again. If I had nearly forgotten what it was like to be searched and questioned by tense armed guards at checkpoints, I was quickly reminded. Easter Sunday of 2019 took Sri Lanka by complete surprise, shook her to her core again and left her reeling.

Ethno-religious Tensions

During the last decade, since the end of the civil war, unfortunately, we could not build the necessary strong bridges between ethnic and religious groups in Sri Lanka. As a result, there was always some tension between the different religious groups that were fuelled by hate speech and lack of active peacebuilding among dividing factions. It is in this milieu that the Easter Sunday attacks took place, and it did not take much time for the suspicions against the "other" to rise up and flood through social media. Tension between the Muslim community and the non-Muslims heightened suspicion, and fear towards each other continued to this day. Thus, psychosocial work including counselling support to victims had to be carried out in this fragile atmosphere of racial and religious tension.

An Invitation to Support Grieving Families

The weeks after the attack, we saw three different entities converge upon the carnage to offer emergency assistance and psychosocial support to the hundreds of injured and bereaved: Civil society activists including the mental health and psychosocial community, the government health and mental health apparatus and the Catholic churches' relief and rehabilitation mechanism. The ensuing coordination and collaboration challenges have their own story to tell and lessons to teach. However, the Catholic Church emerged as the overarching shepherd of the wounded and bereaved taking the lead in coordinating all initiatives from burying the dead, supporting the bereaved, to organizing teams to visit every home in the affected villages and meet with every family, conduct psychosocial needs assessments and do referrals to the government services. The churches coordinating apparatus called on professionals initially from the church and then from a wider professional community to help them organize psychosocial interventions. Interventions were offered to children, young people, parents who had lost children and even those in religious orders who had been directly affected. Many hundreds of bystanders in the different locations who helped to clear debris, identify and carry bodies, who by virtue of living among the families that were bereaved were also subjected to vicarious trauma and were also offered support.

Fast forward a month. Emergency interventions change gear. The wounded return home from hospitals. Extended family members who rallied around returned to their own lives. The hard cold realities of empty spaces and silenced voices begin to hit. The bitterness of grief sets into the village.

Among the many, we describe below the work done with one of the girls' schools just outside the village hardest hit by the bombings. It has a vibrant school community led by a selflessly dedicated and dynamic principal, a nun herself. It was the school that lost the highest number of girls in the attack, and the principal moved the school to throw a net of support and comfort around the grieving families belonging to her school community. With a background in counselling herself, the Principal Rev. Sister realised that the parents who lost their children in her school needed additional support and made a request to my colleagues and I to offer grief support. Seven families had lost their girls between ages 7 and 15. Twenty-seven members of these seven families signed up for the grief support groups.

The Work of Grief Accompaniment: The Stage is Set

I, together with two of my colleagues, offered a series of four to six sessions of group support. A session consisted of a half-day combination of small group sharing together with other interactive activities and individual short sessions as well. Our sessions would start at 9.00 and end at 1.00 with a fellowship lunch. After which, we offered individual sessions, designed to assist in our threefold theme "Recognising Grief", "Respecting Grief" and "Releasing Grief".

The Rev. Sister Principal had secured a venue belonging to a Catholic seminary because the parents were as yet unable to come to the school premises due to the recency and rawness of their loss. The rector of the seminary provided a room free of charge and all conveniences including a beautifully laid-out garden for our use. Other activities too were taking place in the premises of the seminary. One such activity was that of a team of musicians including a Buddhist monk who wanted to make a song on reconciliation as their response to the heightened race-related tensions in the country and had come to seek the support of the rector. But we had to push on to our own programme. The first in the series was itself a reverting exercise in grief work. We were to meet for the second session in 2 weeks. And that's where the rest of our story unfolds.

An Interruption: "A Play Within a Play"

It was the second day of the series. Everyone arrived on time (this is not usual for a Sri Lankan audience). There was a palpable increase in the tempo and energy levels as compared to the first meeting – almost an anticipation!

This was the space in which parents could simply not be "parents" and be themselves. People could leave their roles and responsibilities at the door if they wished and enter as their bare self. They did not have to act, pretend or hold back. There were no doorbells to answer, no incessant media prying for their scoops, no neighbors with an excess of sympathy gushing, no distraught kids clinging…this room, this day, this group was where they could sulk to the depths or cry to high heaven or shake with fury, and it was all ok.

The session started as usual. We, the three facilitators greeted every participant as he or she walked in and spent a moment individually touching base with each one before everyone was seated. Instrumental music was played in the background as everyone greeted each other, found their seats and got comfortable. The highlights of the last session were presented. A simple question starts the first round of group sharing.

"What was last week like? What has changed? What are you doing differently?" And then "how has your grief journey taken you this week?"

Each familiar voice shares… some bolder than before, some as shaky and weak soft and faltering as before and some with the slightest, faintest but definite hint of a new resolve in their voice. "K" is one of the most articulate. Her pain surfaces in searing words, "God has snatched and uprooted the entire tree of my life …" she says, bitter anger pouring down her face. "He has left nothing for me!" No one speaks; no one is surprised. In one clean swipe, that day K lost all she had: her husband, her son and her daughter. One remains silent. She hasn't cried and speaks little. She is here too.

Having ended the first session, there was a sense of relief mixed with a new closeness for having reached such depths of shared pain in such an encounter. A guided relaxation session in the green grass and shady trees helped everyone gear up for the next session which was an exercise in mapping one's grief and following how and where it impacted on the different areas of one's life. Sheets of demy paper were distributed, and coloured pens, cards and stationery were being passed around. The group was getting ready to make their individual maps of grief when suddenly a group of people immerged at the glass door of the class. It was the group of musicians and the monk we had noticed before. They are accompanied by the rector of the seminary. They appeared as they wanted to come in.

While my colleagues continue with the activity, I slip out together with the Rev. Sister Principal of the hosting school to engage the group at the door. The rector of the seminary speaks first.

"This group is here to make a song about reconciliation". He smiles looking at us for approval. I remember to look appreciative and smile back as he introduces the monk mentioning his name.

"This is Rev... Thero (*an honorific term addressing the monk*), a famous musician himself..." – by now I am nodding in acknowledgement, but I must have betrayed my query, why are you here? But, as I keep thinking, someone from the musicians group speaks up.

"We heard that you were doing some work with grieving parents, we came to see them and greet them". A long awkward pause follows. My mind is racing. It's in turmoil. A million arguments crisscross my brain and those agonizing seconds as I debate within myself.

"What? Stop the group now at this stage? An interruption will destroy our momentum".

"This is a monk you are talking to, it is not politically expedient to refuse him entrance". My mind rages on "They are here on a mission of reconciliation. How can you not support them? How can you deny them a moment?"

"But the group is in a very vulnerable and raw stage. Unexpected unauthorized entrances will surely not be proper at this stage?"

"But what about do-no-harm? And cultural sensitivity? This group says they merely want to greet the group and go on their way…"

I look desperately to the Rev. Sister and the rector (this was the moment I was to regret later, when I needed to have stood firm and not looked around for acquiescence). But I did look. And I found that acquiescence, and I went along with an uneasy decision to open the doors and let an outside team enter the sacred space of our grief support group.

In a few painful minutes, we nearly lost what we had struggled so much to build: the trust of a wounded group of people, the sense of safety and security we had created among us, a level of comfort and a rhythm and a momentum.

The musicians and the saffron-robed monk enter followed by the Rev. Sr. Principal and the Rev. Fr. Rector. It's a high-powered gathering. All put down their demy papers, coloured cards and half-constructed sentences and stand up. The monk sits down. He isn't about to confine himself to a greeting. He is getting into a full-blown sermon. "K" in her passion and pain engages with her words and begins to weep bitterly again. From the corner of my eye, I see a cameraman getting in position to shoot, and I instinctively move sharply and ask him to lay his camera aside. He obliges. We got that one right. But the drama continues, the monk preaches, "K" weeps, and the others stand in a confused silence. Until "A", another group member of all people who never cried all this while, starts to cry. My colleague takes her out. It is only then that I find my voice. I know now if I hadn't known it before that this group is disintegrating and we have to move fast to reverse what's happening. A few quick moves and words and it's all over. The intruding team is gently whisked off. A short chocolate break, a word of apology, and we are on the roads again. We nearly lost it, but only nearly.

The Dilemma Discussed: "Whose Fault Was It?"

It's an hour's drive back into the capital; we, the facilitators of the grief-group, let our hair down and release the stress of the day as we travel.

"I just don't believe this happened! How dare they just walk in on us like that? Didn't they know what this group was about?"

"Well, how would they (the Buddhist monk and the musicians) know I suppose if the Catholic priest (the rector) didn't tell them? He should have known better".

"Maybe the Catholic priest (rector) was just offering us the premises and didn't really know too much about what we were actually doing with this group, other than that we are trying to help".

"Well then the Rev. Sister who invited us should have been firm and told them no... She knew what we were about? Or, was that our assumption that she had a clear idea about how a grief counselling group is conducted? Or, is it something we never gave thought about?"

"Oh dear, I suppose they did not want to offend the Buddhist priest and perhaps he too didn't really see the issues. I was at the door. I suppose I should have just told them it was not possible to barge in mid-way. I'm just starting to kick myself for letting this happen".

"But you are a visitor too using the premises, they should not have put you and all of us in that situation of having to stop a Buddhist monk, and a group of song-writers just saunter into an on-going grief group".

"To be honest, I was taken totally by surprise, and though I knew this was not admissible, I guess especially being a Christian, I didn't want to be the one to stop a Buddhist monk from coming in, as he said to share condolences".

"Well, he didn't just share condolences did he? That would have been ok, for them to say a brief word if they thought they had to and move on, but they seated themselves and started delivering speeches!". My mind tries to free myself from the responsibility as a facilitator for letting this happen. But it keeps coming back to me.

There was also what they said about making a song about reconciliation and it all sounded so justifiable that I didn't want to stand in their way and thereby create more conflict in an already tensed situation. Anyway, we just didn't have the presence of mind or the courage of our convictions to avert what happened. Looking back, what I really found amazing is that it was actually our participant "A" who found a way to break into the unfolding chaos and stop it. Initially, when I saw her cry, I didn't realise why. I thought she was finally moved to weep for her loss...But I was so wrong.

Yes, we took her outside to give her some space, and then she was bursting with articulate anger! She was angry with everyone! And she did so with her tears. That was amazing! She never cried with her grief all this time, but when someone threatened the group process, she cried... And those were not tears of sadness/those were tears of protest! Yes, that's what made it so amazing.

Mental health practitioners engaging in counselling services in low- and middle-income countries (LMICs) such as Sri Lanka continue to struggle with ethical dilemmas as they try to deal with the cultural values of the people and the ethical standards introduced to them in their formal education and training, while we lack a formal code of ethics to guide us or a statutory body to monitor and guide the professional practice. The above was a classic example of how and when this could hit us hard while we become helpless, potentially harming our clients - the very group we try to help, and the profession itself. The above example reflects the nature of collision between culture and ethical standards in counselling we face as practitioners and trainers in Sri Lanka. In this chapter, we try to focus on our struggles and highlight transferable learning from our context.

Need for Standardized Training and Supervision

As mentioned previously, the mental health sector in Sri Lanka experienced an expansion as the number of counsellors in the country, especially in the state sector, rapidly increased over a period of less than two decades. Despite this improvement, the counsellors in Sri Lanka, even in the state sector, are not regulated by a statutory body. Several groups of counsellors have formed associations with the aim of self-governing. However, it is not mandatory for a practitioner to seek membership in any association as these memberships do not seem to have any weight in the job market. Hence, at this point in time the counsellors are not legally bound or controlled by any authority, or they are not bound by the ethical guidelines of a counsellor association in which they hold membership.

In addition, there is also a dearth in qualified clinical supervisors in the country to meet the needs of the increased number of practicing counsellors. Thus, although counsellors have learnt about the importance of supervision during their initial or ongoing training as they study the codes of ethics for counsellors (e.g. American Psychological Association, 2017 [2]; Australian Counselling Association, 2019 [3]) and other ethical guidelines for practitioners providing counselling services, most counsellors reported that it is very difficult to find a suitable supervisor [14, 15]. This is probably a situation that is common in other LMICs and even in the rural areas of high-income countries (HICs) that must be addressed with efficient and creative ways. Referring back to the personal experience in our example, if we had the opportunity to discuss similar dilemmas that arose in other instances during supervision, we may have had the opportunity to use that knowledge to deal better in such vulnerable and challenging moments. If we have supervision at this moment of time, some of us may have the opportunity to discuss it with our supervisees and colleagues so that they would handle such situations differently, ensuring better services for their clients.

Peer Supervision as a Way Forward

With the intention of supporting the counselling community, a "peer supervision model" was introduced for state sector counsellors in 2016, as an alternative measure to address the shortage of expert supervisors. We initiated this following two detailed studies [14, 15] and a needs assessment prior to introducing Continuing Professional Development (CPD) training programmes for a group of state sector counsellors in 2015. The group identified the lack of clinical supervision as an ongoing issue faced by the counsellors working in different areas in the country. Although this was introduced to the state sector counsellors, the situation remains to be equally bad or worse among private sector counsellors working on their own. However, due to the shortage of formal data and the absence of a formal mechanism to address any deficit in mental health care, attempts to address this issue were limited to the state sector counsellors. Upon exploring alternatives to deal with the ground realities, peer supervision was introduced as a feasible alternative.

This was taken as an ongoing project after an initial 3-day residential workshop. Counselling officers throughout the country were supported with training and continued monitoring on carrying out peer supervision at district level. Although this was successful to some extent, as a whole the counselling officers did not use the peer supervision model as expected. Thus, it is evident that most counsellors in Sri Lanka practice without clinical supervision. Discussions with counsellors on the topic did not indicate a lack of knowledge or awareness about the value of clinical supervision. Yet, lack of resources was always mentioned as a reason for not being able to receive supervision, and most of them perceived the peer supervision as an inadequate alternative since they did not feel they received any useful results from these sessions. This could also be due to the absence of a structure to guide the peer supervision and feedback process [1].

In addition, counsellors also felt threatened or ashamed to share their perceived weaknesses with peers during supervision. This situation has been observed in other contexts too [4, 12]. As discussed by Pugh [12], the dual relationship experienced in peer supervision settings, where one is expected to be the supervisor and the supervisee in the same relationship, probably led to its unsuccessfulness as they struggled in giving and receiving objective feedback. Hence, to address this, it will be important to go beyond introducing a model of accessible supervision and enable the participants with acceptable and user-friendly tools and structures of receiving and providing feedback objectively. This probably is the situation in other LMICs too. Thus, the shortage of practitioners with sufficient training and tools/structures to provide objective supervision to peers significantly contributes to the issue as much as the shortage of expert supervisors.

Cultural Beliefs: "You Can Deal with Any Problem Because You Are a Counsellor"

In Sri Lanka, culturally personnel in helping professions are put on a pedestal. As a result, mental health workers are considered expected to be unrealistically psychologically balanced individuals at all times. They are perceived as capable of withstanding any tragic experience as they are "mental health workers", and in some instances, "mental health experts". This false belief seems to linger in the minds of the laymen as well as the counselling practitioners themselves. As a result, comments such as the following are made by the laymen: "Can't you handle it even though you are a counsellor yourself!" Most counsellors we interviewed discussed the difficulties of getting professional help when we asked to whom they could turn when they are faced with situations similar to what their clients turn to them. Most of them simply mentioned that it is not easy to even turn to their own family and friends as possible sources of support, let alone professional help. Thus, we feel the need to acknowledge this ethical and cultural dilemma related to counselling practitioners' help-seeking behaviours in personal or professional dilemmas.

What we found in Sri Lanka indicated that they not only find it challenging to access supervision that is necessary for continued professional development and self-improvement, but also seem even to lack access to professional mental health support when needed. Could this be addressed through overall education and by exploring feasible mechanisms for supervision that is provided by experienced counsellors who are not peers that could eventually end up struggling with dual relationships? Evidence from HIC may suggest so. But how feasible would it be in LMICs? Some practitioners in the urban settings are overcoming this issue through online/tele supervision from overseas supervisors. This might not be feasible for all counsellors due to lack of necessary contacts or lack of other resources. However, online/tele supervision might be an option to be explored within the country/region for practitioners in LMICs as telecommunication becomes more accessible. This is something we would suggest for Sri Lankan counsellors in rural areas as well as in countries with limited access to clinical supervision. This has been explored in areas where there is a shortage of supervisors either due to geographical characteristic such as travel distance in places like India or Australia or when working in specialty areas such as in art therapy [5, 11, 13, 17]. In addition, we emphasize that it might contribute to the success of the supervision process if it is facilitated with tools that could assist the objective evaluation and feedback process [8]. This might include counsellor assessment tools such as the Enhancing Assessment of Common Therapeutic Factors (ENACT) or ENACT-SL in the Sri Lankan context [1, 10] or any other tool that allows the supervisor and the supervisee to have a better understanding of the aspects that contribute to therapy outcomes.

Counsellor Training

As discussed before, mental health awareness is considerably increasing in Sri Lanka as it is the case worldwide. The number of people seeking mental health support has continued to increase over the past few dacades, which could be partially attributed to this increasing awareness. Hence, the trainers are faced with challenges to ensure that students are able to handle contemporary issues presented by their clients and use of modern technology in the process [8, 17]. In addition to this sophistication in approaches to counselling, the example shared at the beginning of this chapter emphasizes the need to be conscious and vigilant in diverse circumstances to ensure ethical practice while being considerate of the ground realities such as culture, security concerns, social hierarchies, and even technology, such as video cameras and other recording devices. Thus, in counsellor training it is important to address how ethical concepts in mental health care collide with cultural norms, developing social phenomena and the needs in relation to other aspects of the society such as racial and religious tensions and conflict. This sort of active, collaborative and critical assessment training will be essential for current and future practitioners to fulfil their duties ensuring the well-being of clients in terms of basics such as confidentiality, use of technology or other aspects of an evolving society.

Lessons Learned

Finally, at the end of the day, to reflect on what we learnt from our experience with the grief-therapy group, we discussed it over some coffee and cookies in a favorite spot of our team. The long but refreshing and reassuring discussion led us to the following points to ponder upon.

- Working with vulnerable individuals or groups in a volatile environment warrants a thoughtful selection of a location. Even when free accommodation or venues are given, the free offer must not carry with it a sense of obligation to step beyond the boundaries of good practice.
- People who are well-meaning may not always do what is in the best interest of those who are injured and may need to be made aware or given boundaries.
- It is not only important to have principles of confidentiality, but they need to be communicated to those whom we work alongside, especially when they are from different perspectives and backgrounds.
- When one is caught between respect for religious/cultural dignitaries and respect for the vulnerability of the wounded and one needs to choose between hurting the already injured and offending the powerful, as people helpers we must perhaps err on the side of the vulnerable for that is our mandate.
- However urgent the need and however much in haste we are, let's take the time to communicate our parameters and principles and maintain a sound understanding of the ethical guidelines that are for the safety of the clients.

References

1. Abeysinghe, N., Kohrt, B. A., & Galappatti, A. (2020). *Common factors in counselling in Sri Lanka – what works and what helps? Perceptions of counsellors and clients.* Unpublished manuscript.
2. American Psychological Association. (2017). Ethical principles of psychologists and code of conduct (2002, amended effective June 1, 2010, and January 1, 2017). https://www.apa.org/ethics/code/?_ga=2.265330886.876423061.1594952363-1266296820.1594952360
3. Australian Counselling Association. (2019). Code of Ethics and Practice of the Association for Counsellors in Australia. ACA.
4. Bailey, R., Bell, K., Kalle, W., & Pawar, M. (2014). Restoring meaning to supervision through a peer consultation group in rural Australia. *Journal of Social Work Practice, 28*(4), 473–495.
5. Deane, F. P., Gonsalvez, C., Blackman, R., Saffioti, D., & Andresen, R. (2015). Issues in the development of e-supervision in professional psychology: A review. *Australian Psychologist, 50*(3), 241–247. https://doi.org/10.1111/ap.12107.
6. Ekanayake, E. S., & Abeysinghe, N. (2019). Drawing in or ruling out "Family?" The evolution of the family systems approach in Sri Lanka. In L. L. Charles & G. Samarasinghe (Eds.), *Family systems and global humanitarian mental health approaches in the field.* Cham: Springer.
7. Gambheera, H. (2013). The evolution of psychiatric services in Sri Lanka. *South Asian Journal of Psychiatry, 2*(1), 25–27.

8. Goss, S., & Anthony, K. (2003). *Technology in counselling and psychotherapy: A practitioner's guide*. Basingstoke: Palgrave Macmillan.

9. Kinpe, D. W., Metcalfe, C., & Gunnell, D. (2015). WHO suicide statistics – a cautionary tale. *The Ceylon Medical Journal, 60*(1), 35.

10. Kohrt, B. A., Jordans, M. J. D., Rai, S., Shrestha, P., Luitel, N. P., Ramaiya, M. K., et al. (2015). Therapist competence in global mental health: Development of the ENhancing Assessment of Common Therapeutic factors (ENACT) rating scale. *Behaviour Research and Therapy, 69*, 11–21. https://doi.org/10.1016/j.brat.2015.03.009.

11. Orr, P. P. (2010). Distance supervision: Research, findings, and considerations for art therapy. *The Arts in Psychotherapy, 37*(2), 106–111. https://doi.org/10.1016/j.aip.2010.02.002.

12. Pugh, R. (2007). Dual relationships: Personal and professional boundaries in rural social work. *British Journal of Social Work, 37*(8), 1405–1423.

13. Singla, D. R., Ratjen, C., Krishna, R. N., Fuhr, D. C., & Patel, V. (2019). Peer supervision for assuring the quality of non-specialist provider delivered psychological intervention: Lessons from a trial for perinatal depression in Goa, India. *Behaviour Research and Therapy*. https://doi.org/10.1016/j.brat.2019.103533.

14. The Asia Foundation. (2015). *Mapping study of the work and capacity of counselling assistants of the Ministry of Child Development and Women's Affairs*. Colombo: TAF.

15. The Asia Foundation. (2015). *Mapping study of the work and capacity of the counselling assistants of the Ministry of Social Services and counselling officers of the Ministry of Child Development and Women's Affairs*. Colombo: TAF.

16. Woolfe, R. (2012). Risorgimento: A history of counselling psychology in Britain. *Counselling Psychology Review, 27*(4), 72–78.

17. Wright, J., & Griffiths, F. (2010). Reflective practice at a distance: Using technology in counselling supervision. *Reflective Practice, 11*(5), 693–703. https://doi.org/10.1080/1462394 3.2010.516986.

Public Mental Health in Low-Resourced Systems in Uganda: Lay Community Health Workers, Context and Culture

Byamah B. Mutamba

Introduction

This chapter is informed by the experience of implementing a non-randomized, community health worker (CHW)-led intervention within the government health system, to address mental health issues associated with nodding syndrome (NS), a mysterious neuropsychiatric illness affecting children in northern Uganda. Using health systems, clinical psychiatry, social science, and public health perspectives, I argue for not only "why" but also "how" we should involve government CHWs in task sharing of public mental health care in low-resourced publicly funded health systems. Lessons learned from this and other studies are highlighted to suggest an agenda for integration of mental health interventions into LMIC government health systems, specifically the roles and utilization of lay community health workers (LCHWs) within health systems in low- and middle-income countries. Outcomes from research studies that employed varied methods including a systematic literature review and qualitative and quantitative methods, including key intervention outcomes relating to the contextualization and effectiveness of group interpersonal therapy (IPT-G) intervention for caregivers and their children affected by nodding syndrome, are discussed [1–3]. In addition, I emphasize the "dual mental health" benefits (for both caregivers and their children affected by neuropsychiatric conditions) of a psychological treatment contextualized for delivery within routine health care, as important consideration for intervention research in child and adolescent mental health [4].

Utilization of an implementation framework to contextualize evidence-based PT (IPT-G) within a low-resourced government health system provides new insights/perspectives for the "translation of research to practice" field [5]. It builds on the increasing evidence in global mental health about task-sharing delivery of PTs with

B. B. Mutamba (✉)
Community Mental Health, YouBelong Uganda, Kampala, Uganda

Butabika Hospital, Kampala, Uganda

© Springer Nature Switzerland AG 2021
A. R. Dyer et al. (eds.), *Global Mental Health Ethics*,
https://doi.org/10.1007/978-3-030-66296-7_8

LCHWs [6] and the need to work within a health system platform to sustainably address the mental health gap in LMICs [4].

To draft the agenda, I re-envision the four phases of the Replicating Effective Programs (REP) implementation science framework [7] that I used to implement IPT-G delivered by LCHWs [4]: (i) pre-conditions, (ii) pre-implementation, (iii), implementation, and (iv) maintenance and evolution as a guide to integration of mental health research and practice into routine health services.

Pre-conditions: Culture, Context, and Syndemics

As government health systems in LMICs work to respond to a large and growing burden of disease attributable to mental, neurological, and substance use (MNS) disorders, there are major issues to address to ensure that interventions are effective and sustainable for diverse cultural groups within the context of their local social, economic, political, and health systems context. Despite attention to cultural adaptation of interventions, contextual adaptation has received limited attention and is rarely discussed outside of some arenas of implementation science. In this section, I suggest that pre-conditions necessary for implementation of an effective public mental health intervention require a syndemic model which is an important heuristic to address these limitations.

In Mendenhall and colleagues' [8] work on the concept of syndemics, they harken back to the anthropological tent that design and implementation of mental health (and other) interventions for vulnerable populations is influenced by how one perceives what causes disease/illness. Therefore a reframing is required to move from viewing diseases in isolation to a syndemic model that considers the clustering of two or more diseases and the complex interplay between the biological, social, and psychological aspects of those diseases within an environment that precipitates and maintains the disease clustering in the first place [8]. A syndemic approach is informed by the need to institute accessible, affordable, and available health systems and policies that address these mutually exacerbating conditions. Social, cultural, and economic factors are central to understanding health and the nature of the health system is seen as shaping the health profile of a population. Syndemic thinking, which originated in medical anthropology, follows the tenet that no biological process occurs in isolation of social, experiential process—a central tenet of medical anthropology. Moreover, the pathophysiology of a condition is always in transaction with other health conditions, disorders, diet, environmental exposures, and other biological determinants [9–11].

Therefore, formative research to determine the pre-conditions for a mental health intervention must take into account all these elements ranging from cultural explanatory models to human resources in health systems to socio-biological-psychological illness interactions and other contextual factors. My work on nodding syndrome reflects some of these elements in a syndemic approach. The individual, family, and community experience of nodding syndrome in northern Uganda exemplifies the disease burden and gap in health care associated with mental, neurological, and

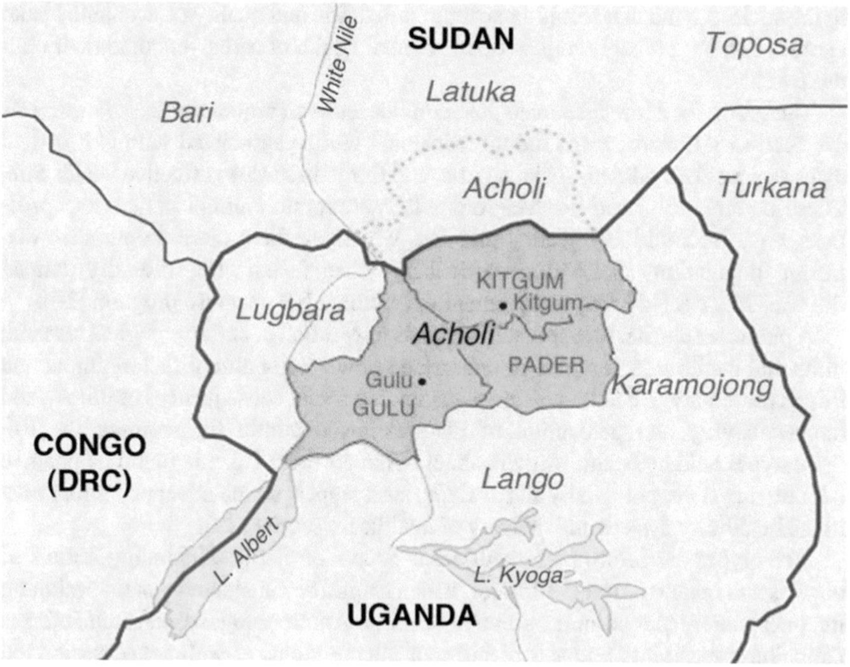

Fig. 8.1 Nodding syndrome-affected areas in northern Uganda (Downloaded from Wikipedia) (https://link.springer.com/article/10.1007/s00401-018-1909-9)

substance use (MNS) disorders in LMICs [1, 2, 12–14]. A heavy burden of care, high levels of stigmatization and social exclusion, extreme psychological distress, physical exhaustion, and economic hardships, characterize the objective and subjective burdens experienced by caregivers of children with nodding syndrome living in resource-poor, post-war northern Uganda [1] (Fig. 8.1). In a setting with limited access to primary healthcare services, the "strange presentation," perceived causes/illness explanatory model, and caregiver burden associated with NS inform and guide health-seeking behavior in the affected community. A combination of biomedical/western medicines and traditional remedies (traditional rituals, traditional medicines, and spiritual healing) is routinely sought by caregivers [12, 14].

The health-seeking experiences and trajectories also reveal several barriers to accessible and affordable primary health care for NS in a low-resourced setting: (1) health system-related factors which included inadequate skills of healthcare providers, coupled with negative attitudes, the need for repeated visits to health facilities which required travelling long distances, a limited access to safe modes of transport, shortage of medicines, congestion, and long waiting times at health facilities, and (2) other contextual factors including poverty and illness fatigue [12]. Some caregivers were reported to sometimes neglect the health needs, feeding, and personal hygiene of their children, a reflection of the caregiver burden [1, 12, 14]. Negative stereotypes/attitudes toward NS held by primary health workers not only contribute to the social stigma that forms a barrier to utilization and quality of available health care [2, 12], but probably impact on the mental health of caregivers (and their children) [1].

Therefore, for a low-resourced post-conflict setting, community-based initiatives are necessary to address the multidimensional burden associated with NS: patient distress, caregiver burden, social stigma, and limited access to effective health care. These community-based interventions will incorporate cultural beliefs and practices, e.g., the traditional healing practices which are the preferred option for distressed populations in LMICs, particularly when faced with culturally defined illnesses like NS [15], and complement the national NS response program [16].

A public mental health approach demands integration of anthropological research in mental health interventions to understand how socio-cultural factors impact on illness presentation, health-seeking behavior, the social consequences of illness, and the availability and perception of the treatments within the community [10]. Stereotypes held by health workers about NS in northern Uganda found no positive but only negative, potentially stigmatizing stereotypes, which adversely affect trust in the healthcare system and delivery of healthcare services [2].

Stereotypes are informed by cultural concepts of distress, including idioms of distress and other cultural syndromes, which should be considered when developing treatment interventions in a particular locality. Anthropological research informs the cultural feasibility and acceptability of interventions, as well as measuring the impact of health services from the perspective of providers and beneficiaries [10]. Implementing psychosocial interventions, e.g., coping strategies, should be adapted to local needs and concerns and the local culture [17]. Idioms of distress are grounded in a community's culture and form a medium of communicating culturally defined distress. The formative phase of the IPT-G for NS study therefore necessitated investigation of cultural aspects (explanations, practices) of NS and their incorporation into the training of health workers and CHWs to deliver IPT-G for NS [5].

Whereas alternative and local healers understand and utilize this cultural explanatory medium to provide psychological care, this cultural responsiveness is lacking in conventional mental health service delivery [18]. One view holds that improving access to culturally responsive care in LMICs may require mutual training and supervision programs so that alternative healers become part of the public mental health system [15, 18]. However, unifying the two schools of practice to deliver mental health care seems to be an undertaking that is not likely to bear fruit soon. A more feasible alternative is to use lay community health workers.

Community health workers represent the perspectives of both alternative and conventional practitioners and could provide a useful alternative vehicle to design and scale up culturally feasible and acceptable public mental health services [10]. Because of their connections within communities, premised on elements such as trust and reciprocity, the use of community actors that are part of a national health system is gaining ground [19]. Reviews of the extant literature indicate effectiveness of non-specialist health worker-led community-based mental health interventions [3, 20] and specifically the role of CHWs in the delivery of psychological and psychosocial interventions [3]. The evidence for CHW-led psychological interventions in LMICs was however lacking with respect to contextual factors and delivery of care processes. This would limit translation and/or scaling up of similar initiatives into routine health services to provide useful process and implementation data for LCHW-led interventions in LMIC settings [3]. The lack of accessible and contextually evidence-based mental health services for the caregivers and their children affected by NS was an evident gap in the NS national response strategy in northern Uganda [5, 16].

Toward building on existing resources and strengthening of health systems in LMICs that are feasible and cost-effective, a syndemic model, if comprehensively implemented, can provide integrated health care that will enable CHWs to identify a more complex array of social, psychological, and physical symptoms. This approach will not only enhance their capabilities but will also prevent overburdening community health workers with extra tasks by reducing the geographical area of operation [9].

The neuropsychiatric symptoms, probable infectious cause, and social and cultural attributions of NS make one ask the question: is NS a syndemic? Is it a combination of illnesses, a form of co-morbidity, or a syndemic interaction between psychiatric, neurological, and infectious disease processes maintained by an enabling environment? "A syndemic interaction is the co-occurrence of social and health conditions, including social–psychological, social–biological, and psychological–biological interactions, which worsen the condition of the person or population afflicted" [11]. NS has been described as a progressive epileptic encephalopathy with varied mental, neurologic, and physical signs [21]. It affects previously normal developing brains characterized by bouts of repetitive head nodding and is sometimes associated with epileptic seizures. It is complicated by multiple physical and functional disabilities (cognitive decline, delayed sexual and physical growth, wasting or stunting) and psychiatric manifestations [21, 22]. Its manifestation as a syndrome in a post-conflict environment suggests that a syndemic approach, typically taking into account the social context as enabling the adverse disease interactions leading to an exacerbated burden of disease, could help explain its development and presentation. The emergence of NS occurred within a context of multiple biological-psychological and social/environmental risk factors including changing political and economic conditions, shifting ecological and environmental conditions and breakdown of public health protective measures [21, 22]. These conditions are similar to those evidenced to enable other syndemic interactions [11]. War and conflict, as was the situation preceding NS, are traumatic biosocial events that compromise existing conditions and healthcare access, thereby increasing the likelihood of disease clustering and syndemic interaction [9, 11, 23]. One could argue that the prolonged Lord's Resistance Army-led insurgency disrupted social and health systems resulting in minimal preventative interventions for the population, e.g., mass distribution of ivermectin reduced hence communal recognition and treatment of *Onchocerca volvulus*-infected individuals decreased (Figs. 8.2 and 8.3). This facilitated multiplication of the intracellular *Wolbachia* microbe which in turn might have resulted in the neuro-inflammatory reaction postulated to cause NS. A

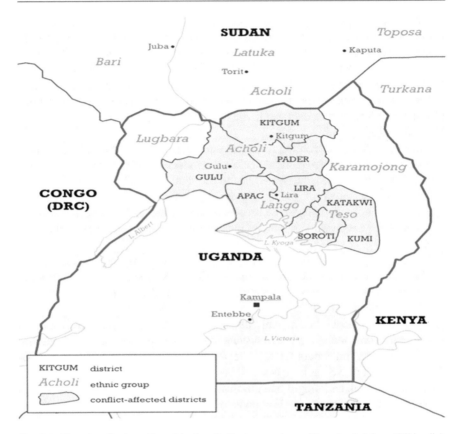

Fig. 8.2 Ugandan districts affected by Lord's Resistance Army (Downloaded from Wikipedia). https://commons.wikimedia.org/wiki/File:Ugandan_districts_affected_by_Lords_Resistance_Army.png

syndemic approach explores the health effects of identifiable disease interactions and the social, environmental, or economic factors that promote such interaction and worsen the complex outcomes of those diseases in populations [11, 24]. Such interactions are amplified in populations that face extreme structural, political, and social vulnerabilities, such as refugees or displaced persons [8]. As was the case for war affected, onchocerciasis infected populations with limited health services in northern Uganda.

NS could therefore fulfill the criteria for a syndemic: a synergistic relationship between health problems exacerbating the burden of disease within the context of persistent social and economic inequalities that affect the health of a population [9]. Recognition of NS as a syndemic has important policy implications for the design and implementation of interventions that target both disease-disease interactions and disease context interactions. A syndemic/integrative care approach may be best suited to task sharing, the requirement of holistic health or trans-diagnostic models notwithstanding [9].

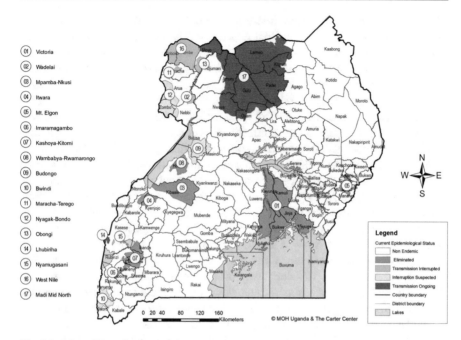

Fig. 8.3 Map of Uganda showing the status of onchocerciasis in 2017

A syndemic care model enhances capabilities of community health workers through task-sharing initiatives. This will necessitate integrated health care and the strengthening of health systems that will translate into provision of simplified care by CHWs using integrated treatment protocols rather than separate algorithms for different diseases [9, 15]. Lay community health workers therefore provide an important resource for mental health service delivery within a task shifting model [6, 25, 26], but this may best be utilized within an integrated care system that recognizes the complex coexistence of social and medical conditions [9, 27]. A public health system provides a platform for increased access, scale-up, and sustainability of CHW-led syndemic interventions in LMICs [4, 25].

Pre-implementation: Moving Away from "Efficacy-Thinking" in Global Health

Given my argument for a syndemic approach in the prior section, it is not surprising that I question the utility of "efficacy-thinking" in intervention research. In traditional research paradigms, efficacy of interventions is tested under controlled conditions to establish whether an intervention works before moving it to real-world conditions. Following this, one is expected to evaluate if a known efficacious intervention can demonstrate comparable effectiveness in a particular setting [28]. However, from an anthropological perspective, one can challenge presumptions that efficacy trials are separable from real-world conditions. Whether or not an intervention is successful in an efficacy trial depends on the real-world conditions under which it is tested, which include cultural assumptions of practitioners and patients; the health system in which it is evaluated; the social, economic, and political conditions surrounding the trial; and myriad other factors. Therefore, I propose that efforts into efficacy trials are misplaced from the perspective of often ignoring the contextual factors of the trial that influence the outcomes. Rather, all mental health trials should be framed in terms of effectiveness considering that they ought to take into account implementation science, social and anthropological considerations of factors such as context, culture, and syndemic interactions. A syndemic approach recognizes all treatments and their outcomes as inseparable from the context in which they exist, i.e., biology does not exist outside of social context. Therefore, one cannot expect treatments such as medications to work universally across context, and definitely not psychotherapies. If the "myth" of efficacy trials in global health were challenged, we—as a field—could move toward approaches in which interventions are evaluated directly in the context under which we ultimately plan for them to be delivered. This does away with an unnecessary "efficacy to effectiveness" step and misuse of resources that slows the progress toward tackling global public health challenges. The case of IPT-G in Uganda further illustrates this point; the evidence generated by Bolton and others in 2003 [29] is, 17 years since completion, yet to be integrated into mainstream health services because of a lack of contextualization [5]. I postulate that had the IPT-G trial been conducted within the government health system, it would have reduced the time to scale up.

The significant and rising proportion of children in the world's population, together with the increasing public health burden of child and adolescent mental health problems, particularly in LMICs, warrants specific public mental health attention to expansion of effectiveness trials for low-resourced settings [30, 31]. The comparative lack of child and adolescent prevention and treatment services will require not only an increase in targeted services but innovative approaches to address the diverse challenges experienced by this vulnerable group [32]. Moreover, child mental health is especially sensitive to the familial, educational, community, and broader social context as illustrated in ecological-transactional theories [23, 33, 34].

To address this gap in mental health services, we aimed to contextualize an evidence-based PT within the Uganda health system. Having reviewed the evidence base on PTs previously trialled in Uganda, IPT-G was selected [5]. The aim was to inform routine mental health care in line with implementation science principles [35, 36] and inform scale-up. Appropriate dissemination and implementation (DI) research is critical to translating global mental health research knowledge into effective and sustainable scale-up of psychological treatments in LMICs [6, 37]. Contextualization of IPT-G would identify barriers and facilitators to effective delivery of the treatment within routine care. In addition, this process allows for potential modifications to the clinical intervention to facilitate integration within mainstream health service delivery [38]. Pursuant to our suggestion of doing away with efficacy trials and the recognition of an already existing bank of evidence-based PTs, hybrid designs have been suggested as a way to quickly move from establishing intervention effectiveness to achieving public health impact. Hybrid designs have a dual focus in assessing both clinical effectiveness and implementation outcomes [39]. Contextualization is integral to hybrid interventions "which focus on process evaluations during a clinical effectiveness trial to inform subsequent 'real-world' implementation of the intervention" [39]. Though large RCTs provide further evidence of effectiveness and scale-up of PTs delivered by LCHWs within health systems in LMICs [3, 4], it may be pragmatic to generate evidence for effectiveness and implementation using well-designed non-randomized studies in the initial stages of interventions [3] especially in situations where randomization is not practical as was the case for IPT-G for NS [4].

Because we aimed to recommend an implementation strategy for delivery of PTs in the health system, the REP framework, a prescriptive implementation strategy, was our choice [5, 7, 40]. During pre-implementation, we engaged with various community and government stakeholders including administrators, health officials, and affected populations to contextualize IPT-G. This involved a number of activities including selection of study sites in consideration of on-going NS programming within the study district, revision of IPT-G structure, delivery agents and content (focused on NS-specific needs), and training and supervision of VHTs and facility-based health workers to provide IPT-G in line with government policies, NS treatment guidelines, human resources availability, and caregiver mental health needs [5].

Involvement of stakeholders and decision-makers is key to scale-up and sustainability of EBTs, ensuring that they are locally relevant and address aspects of existing systems [41]. Relationship with formal health services is known to be a key determinant of the effectiveness and sustainability of a community health worker program [42].This is in addition to other contributory factors to effectiveness of LCHW-led interventions: health system factors such as supervision of LCHWs; national political and socioeconomic factors; and community factors related to leadership, infrastructure, and community empowerment [42]. How best to train, utilize, supervise, and integrate LCHW-led PT delivery within health systems requires additional implementation research [43]. Although results from IPT-G for NS informed the WHO Mental Health Gap Action Programme (mhGAP) pilot in Uganda, a larger randomized study using a hybrid 3 design which aims at "testing of an implementation strategy while observing and gathering information on the clinical intervention's impact on relevant outcomes" [39] is a necessary next step in generating further evidence of effectiveness, utility for uptake, and scale-up of PTs within the public health system.

Use of an implementation framework requires modification to suit the particular setting(s) as we found during implementation of IPT-G for NS. To enable contextualization of IPT-G within the public health system, we modified the REP framework, e.g., setting up a stakeholder guidance group in the pre-implementation as opposed to a community working group (CWG) because of logistic and health system factors [5].Therefore, implementation frameworks should be guiding templates/ guidelines, but not a hard and fast rule of how to implement, given the varying health system contexts in LMICs. "The selection of implementation framework(s) should not be based solely on the healthcare innovation to be implemented, but include other aspects of the framework's orientation, e.g., the context and end-user, as well as the degree of inclusion and depth of analysis of the implementation concepts. The resulting generic structure provides researchers, policy-makers, health administrators, and practitioners a base that can be used as guidance for their implementation efforts" [40].

Implementation: Pluripotent Interventions

Another issue that requires rethinking in global mental health is how we frame outcomes based on clinical trials rationales. The clinical trial approach emphasizes the need for a single primary outcome, and demonstration of evidence is considered if there is a change in that single outcome. However, if one is considering a syndemic approach, then it would be important to consider a host of potential interrelated changes in multiple areas of health as well as socioeconomic conditions and the functioning of the health system. The potential to address multiple outcomes as well as increase access to health care makes group interpersonal therapy, delivered by CHWs within health systems in LMICs, a useful social intervention [19].

We designed and implemented IPT-G for NS with the hypothesis that a community-based PT would have dual mental health benefits for caregivers and children affected by NS. Our findings support the increasing evidence that community-based interventions can be delivered to family members, particularly caregivers, not only to improve their mental health but also of the (child) patient [4, 30]. Compared with children of caregivers who received treatment as usual, children whose caregivers received IPT-G had significant reduction in depression symptoms at both study time points [4].

Implementation of a controlled trial of IPT-G for NS resulted in positive effects for both beneficiaries and the providers and presented a model for how PTs can be adapted for government health systems in low-resourced settings. This study added to the evidence base of LCHW-led psychotherapeutic interventions that can be delivered effectively and with fidelity in routine health systems and whose effects [on the primary depression outcome] are sustained after the intervention [44]. Integration within government health system structures may provide the right platform for sustainable service provision within a public mental health framework.

A key finding of IPT-G for NS was the "dual" health benefits of this intervention demonstrated by significant reduction in the number of caregivers and children with depression [4]. This lends emphasis to the two-generation (mother and child) intervention model that incorporates caregiver mental health strategies into child and adolescent mental health interventions [45]. The mental health of caregivers plays an important role in mediating child mental health and behavioral outcomes [46–48]. Caregivers' mental health problems determine the family environment by influencing factors such as connectedness, parenting practices, access to services, and availability of social support [49].

A focus on strengthening the capabilities of their caregivers significantly impacts the healthy development and life prospects of vulnerable young children more than interventions that focus on the child's health alone [45]. The relationship between child and adult mental health is well described in post-conflict settings [47] particularly the role of caregiver mental health [50]. The effects of war on families include displacement, separation, and emotional distress leading to various psychological sequelae. These impact on interpersonal relationships such that adults in a post-conflict setting are unable to carry out their caring and nurturance roles for young children [51]. Morris and others found that depressed mothers in northern Uganda showed impaired monitoring and nurturance of young children [52]. Similarly, we found that the psychological, social, physical, and economic distress experienced by caregivers of children with NS affected the care provided to their sick children [1]. Targeting the relationship between caregiver and child mental health should form the basis for child and adolescent mental health interventions in LMICs, key among these being caregiver treatments [50, 51, 53].

There is evidence to show that parent-mediated interventions improve the mental health of the ill child [54–56]. This growing body of evidence serves to highlight the need for two-generation psychosocial interventions, which extend beyond the individual child, to account for the dynamic between caregiver and child mental health [45, 50, 51]. Addressing caregiver and child mental health dynamics will require interventions that are culturally meaningful and contextually relevant [50].

Although not an a priori hypothesis, we found that the group approach resulted in benefits for both providers and intended beneficiaries. This was evidenced by improved hygiene and humane methods of care for the children, a sense of group cohesion among caregivers who continued to meet after completion of the intervention for peer support and financial gain (*Bol Cup*), and reduced incidences of domestic violence reported among attendee caregivers. In addition, improved personal relationships and self grooming and reduced alcohol use among the village health team members (VHTs) demonstrate the potential for IPT-G to positively impact on social, health, and potentially economic outcomes [4, 5].With the added evidence of cost-effectiveness, IPT-G is a potentially worthwhile investment for the Uganda health system [57].

Employing the REP framework helped to identify key intervention components and processes relevant to key stakeholders and to contextualize IPT-G within routine care settings, a key step in translating an evidence-based treatment from search to practice [35]. The impact of IPT-G for NS on a range of outcomes suggests that trials be designed to investigate multiple interrelated outcomes rather than a single [primary] outcome. Using a syndemic approach, future PT trials should develop more holistic approaches to determine effectiveness on health, social, and economic outcomes at individual and system levels, as well as the relationship between multiple outcomes. This will require inclusion of specific research questions on how an intervention impacts the providers and the health system when delivered within a health system, in addition to evaluation of impact on the primary [intended] beneficiaries. For example, do the IPT-G providers incorporate these skills into other routine health activities? Does the system itself change over time as CHWs take on more roles of delivering psychological treatments, what is the impact on the CHWs' lives, and what are the socioeconomic benefits at beneficiary, family, and community level? These are areas that will require further exploration over time.

Maintenance and Evolution Phase: Key Considerations for Public Mental Health in LMICs

Our implementation of IPT-G for NS demonstrates how a PT initially delivered through a highly structured, supervised, and well-funded NGO can also be effective when adapted for use in the real-world conditions of low-resourced government health systems. We began initial activities for the maintenance and evolution phase in collaboration with the MOH during their efforts to integrate IPT-G into WHO mhGAP nationwide scale-up [5].

There remains little evidence to inform transportation of EBTs to service provision settings with maintenance of fidelity in dissemination and implementation programs [58]. Initiatives to scale up PTs [6] would benefit from systematic reporting on treatment elements and implementation processes [39]. My take is that successful integration of evidence-based PTs into routine health systems will require systematic contextualization of EBTs that takes into account the various contextual factors [5, 59]. Development of a standardized contextualization tool for the country's health system, and the use of hybrid interventions to determine both effectiveness [and cost-effectiveness] and implementation outcomes, could inform the scale-up of PTs within health systems in LMICs [39]. IPT-G for NS brings to the fore key considerations when using lay health workers in the contextualization of evidence-based PTs in LMICs [5] that are consistent with the literature: "recruitment from the local community; participatory training, modification of the PT to address their skill set, contextual issues and barriers; supervision provided by persons with more expertise in mental health using structured protocols for supervision and integrating the intervention with routine health care or existing community delivery systems"; [60] and sustaining NSP-delivered treatments by motivating NSPs and developing compensation mechanisms [6].

Systematic contextualization can be complemented by a "learning health systems" approach that is premised on bidirectional learning from research and practice-based evidence to improve health care [61]. For instance, there continue to be concerns in the field about how nonprofessional providers with limited education learn and use the multiple elements for a range of client problems. This will require more evaluation of non-specialist provider competencies in clinical decision-making, supervision mechanisms, amount of resources, and delivery platforms, e.g., groups or individuals necessary for psychological treatments to work in LMICs [30, 62, 63], more and different training for holistic health models as opposed to singular diseases [9, 27], and more evidence for the effectiveness of integrative task-sharing models to detect syndemic problems and deliver syndemic care [9].

Using evidence from research and practice, mechanisms can be put in place to address training and supervision requirements to assure competency and quality of non-specialists delivering psychological interventions. LCHWs and their immediate supervisors will require more support, supervision, and monitoring to prevent work-force distress and address challenges associated with delivery of interventions [30, 64], which could be improved through a learning health systems approach. Specialist supervisors of CHWs including psychiatric nurses, psychiatric clinical officers, psy-chiatrists, psychologists, and psychiatric social workers do not routinely provide PTs at primary or community health care levels. They will therefore require training in the delivery of culturally adapted and contextualized PTs within a task shifting framework in Uganda and LMICs.

In low-resourced settings, task shifting to LCHWs needs to occur within a stepped care approach supported by adequate infrastructure and a specialist referral and supervisory structure, consistent with applied public health principles. Stepped care has been shown to be cost-effective in the short and long term for mental health programming [65]. Learning health systems can better uncover which patients require more intensive care and when to refer them. Training of the village health teams (VHTs) in Uganda was thought to have improved identification and referral of people with mental disorders who otherwise would not have gained access to the healthcare system [25]. Our findings suggest that CHWs, supervised by primary health workers and specialists, can not only increase access to but deliver evidence-based mental health care within low-resourced health systems [5].

The increasing public health burden of MNS disorders necessitates an integrated public health response especially in under-resourced LMICs [30, 66]. A public mental health approach gives attention not only to the individual but also to larger systems that affect an individual and helps in strengthening available psychological resources. It is also in keeping with individual and community values that "place others' needs above one's own" [67]. Developing public mental health services (prevention, detection, and treatment of mental health problems) in low-resourced settings requires assessment of available local social supports [67] and an under-standing of the vicious cycle of social determinants and MNS disorders [30, 67]. Addressing most of the social determinants of health will require interventions out-side the health system, such as the social and economic sectors. However, health interventions that facilitate community member's participation like IPT-G not only improve access to and quality of health services but also address social determinants of health [63]. Improved social support and decreased stigma were significant out-comes of the IPT-G for NS study, and these facilitated continued engagement between caregivers that resulted in shared economic activities [5].

The continued engagement between caregivers was also facilitated by the VHTs who volunteered to keep carrying out their group facilitation roles as "concerned" members of the community. LCHWs are usually ordinary people who are part of the local community and possess local knowledge about healing and healing systems. Involving them in mental health programs makes them agents of change because the impact on their lives outlasts the program life, with effects at individual and com-munity levels [10]. LCHWs reported that the experience of delivering IPT-G to caregivers of children with NS had also impacted their health and social life [5]. Public mental health initiatives in LMICs that engage LCHWs through task sharing will require collaborative stepped care within a health systems platform [30, 68]. This would also require customization, refining the skills and delivery packages for different members of the health workforce within a task shifting model and standardizing and coordinating roles and tasks [9, 59, 68] to support delivery of syndemic care for mental health problems in these settings.

Policy Implications for LCHW-Led Public Mental Health in LMICs

Findings from the group interpersonal therapy intervention for caregivers and their children affected by NS and the individual, family, and community experience of nodding syndrome in northern Uganda highlight a number of considerations in the design and implementation of public mental health interventions in LMICs:

1. The need to include emic and etic perspectives of illness or disease [10, 14]. They provide insight into the ways larger social and cultural factors impact on those who are ill, the social consequences of their illness, what treatments are available to the community, and their perception of the treatments [10]. IPT-G may potentially be an effective intervention for PTSD, anxiety disorders, and other common mental disorders for both caregivers and their children, but this will require evaluations involving not only larger population samples but the development and validation of local, culturally sensitive measures/tools. Communication and stigma reduction activities related to culturally defined illnesses like NS should be incorporated into public mental health interventions to enhance understanding and promote treatment-seeking [69]. Future research should explore both clinical and non-clinical forms of treatment, including traditional healing and social interventions [10, 18, 69], and how the two approaches can inform treatment interventions delivered by LCHWs.
2. LCHWS remain a valuable resource for increasing access to evidence-based PTs to vulnerable populations in LMICs. They are able to carry on a variety of roles, deliver effective mental health interventions within low-resourced settings [3], represent western and non-western healing practices, and act as agents of change. Because of these attributes, community health workers improve a range of health and social outcomes and are an important link between communities and government services [63]. Not only can they provide formal care, but they may help to incorporate traditional/cultural idioms of distress into PT delivery. Health systems vary across LMICs, and the performance of LCHW-led interventions is greatly influenced by contextual factors, making contextualization a prerequisite step for uptake of interventions within health systems [5, 63]. Because they (LCHW) too are beneficiaries of the PT provided, they are potential agents of social inclusion and economic activity. Task sharing of PT delivery necessitates substantial training across the range of practitioners including mental health professionals. Specialists will require not only skills in planning, training, supervision, and advocacy [41] but also technical skills in PT delivery within primary or community settings, so as to develop a training and supervision workforce in the public health system of LMICs. Incorporating LCHWs into public mental health initiatives, specifically PT delivery, will require extending their capabilities as

frontline health workers to include a minimum skill package on the basis of local resources and their abilities [60, 62, 70]. It has been suggested that the common elements approach, using an internal stepped care model delivery system, would enable LCHWs to provide a range of PTs based on severity and type of problems of the client [62]. Although this approach reduces the need for different groups of LCHWs to provide multiple PTs and loss of clients to referrals, it necessitates the LCHWs to have a minimum set of capabilities, adequate training and supervision, and which health systems in LMICs may not be capable of. Consistent supervision and skill-based training of LCHWs adapted to local needs is important for skill retention and program success [70] as illustrated by IPT-G for NS [4, 5]. And with these additional roles for LCHWs, should come adequate certification, remuneration, and formal recognition within the health system [5, 63].

3. Public mental health interventions led by LCHWs in low-resourced government systems could use a syndemic approach that bridges social policies and clinical care to address the confluence of mutually exacerbating conditions and instituting strong health systems that are accessible, affordable, and available for vulnerable populations [9]. A syndemic approach requires that relevant policies and systems to enable provision of "holistic" care at the point of access are instituted; this demands further research on how syndemic treatments can be delivered within low-resourced health systems.

4. The unavailability and lack of access to child and adolescent services for MNS disorders in Uganda remains an enduring challenge, particularly for psychological treatments, family therapy, and specialized first-line treatments [32]. As noted by Okello et al. (2014), these challenges are more pronounced for children in post-conflict settings necessitating the use of public health approaches to deliver culturally adapted and contextualized psychosocial interventions [71]. Employing the dual or two-generation approach interventions that target the mental health and capabilities of caregivers as well as the children could, to a large extent, address this gap in routine mental health services for children and adolescents in low-resourced settings [4]. This remains a complex challenge [45] that demands further implementation research involving larger populations of children and their caregivers in low-resourced health systems to inform effectiveness, scalability, and sustainability of these approaches. A syndemic approach using hybrid 3 design methods [39] will be an important next step in informing scale-up of IPT-G for NS in the Uganda public health system.

References

1. Nakigudde, J., Mutamba, B. B., Bazeyo, W., Musisi, S., & James, O. (2016). An exploration of caregiver burden for children with nodding syndrome (lucluc) in Northern Uganda. *BMC Psychiatry, 16*(1), 255.
2. Mutamba, B., Abbo, C., Muron, J., Idro, R., & Mwaka, A. (2013). Stereotypes on Nodding syndrome: Responses of health workers in the affected region of northern Uganda. *African Health Sciences, 13*(4), 986–991.
3. Mutamba, B. B., van Ginneken, N., Paintain, L. S., Wandiembe, S., & Schellenberg, D. (2013). Roles and effectiveness of lay community health workers in the prevention of mental, neuro-

logical and substance use disorders in low and middle income countries: A systematic review. *BMC Health Services Research, 13*(1), 412.

4. Mutamba, B. B., Kane, J. C., de Jong, J. T., Okello, J., Musisi, S., & Kohrt, B. A. (2018). Psychological treatments delivered by community health workers in low-resource government health systems: Effectiveness of group interpersonal psychotherapy for caregivers of children affected by nodding syndrome in Uganda. *Psychological Medicine, 48*, 2573–2583.

5. Mutamba, B. B., Kohrt, B. A., Okello, J., Nakigudde, J., Opar, B., Musisi, S., et al. (2018). Contextualization of psychological treatments for government health systems in low resource settings: Group interpersonal psychotherapy for caregivers of children with nodding syndrome in Uganda. *Implementation Science, 13*(1), 90.

6. Singla, D. R., Kohrt, B. A., Murray, L. K., Anand, A., Chorpita, B. F., & Patel, V. (2017). Psychological treatments for the world: Lessons from low-and middle-income countries. *Annual Review of Clinical Psychology, 13*, 149–181.

7. Kilbourne, A. M., Neumann, M. S., Pincus, H. A., Bauer, M. S., & Stall, R. (2007). Implementing evidence-based interventions in health care: Application of the replicating effective programs framework. *Implementation Science, 2*(1), 42.

8. Mendenhall, E. (2017). Syndemics: A new path for global health research. *Lancet, 389*(10072), 889–891.

9. Mendenhall, E., Kohrt, B. A., Norris, S. A., Ndetei, D., & Prabhakaran, D. (2017). Non-communicable disease syndemics: Poverty, depression, and diabetes among low-income populations. *Lancet, 389*(10072), 951–963.

10. Kohrt, B. A., & Mendenhall, E. (2016). *Global mental health: Anthropological perspectives*. Routledge New York, NY, USA.

11. Singer, M., Bulled, N., Ostrach, B., & Mendenhall, E. (2017). Syndemics and the biosocial conception of health. *Lancet, 389*(10072), 941–950.

12. Mwaka, A. D., Okello, E. S., Abbo, C., Odwong, F. O., Olango, W., Etolu, J. W., et al. (2015). Is the glass half full or half empty? A qualitative exploration on treatment practices and perceived barriers to biomedical care for patients with nodding syndrome in post-conflict northern Uganda. *BMC Research Notes, 8*(1), 386.

13. Gumisiriza, N. K. (2015). *The prevalence of the different subtypes of Nodding syndrome and their associated features as seen in northern Uganda*. Kampala: Makerere University.

14. Van Bemmel, K., Derluyn, I., & Stroeken, K. (2014). Nodding syndrome or disease? On the conceptualization of an illness-in-the-making. *Ethnicity & Health, 19*(1), 100–118.

15. Wagenaar, B. H., Kohrt, B. A., Hagaman, A. K., McLean, K. E., & Kaiser, B. N. (2013). Determinants of care seeking for mental health problems in rural Haiti: Culture, cost, or competency. *Psychiatric Services, 64*(4), 366–372.

16. Idro, R., Musubire, K. A., Byamah, M. B., Namusoke, H., Muron, J., Abbo, C., et al. (2013). Proposed guidelines for the management of nodding syndrome. *African Health Sciences, 13*(2), 219–225.

17. de Jong, J., & Reis, R. (2013). Collective trauma processing: Dissociation as a way of processing postwar traumatic stress in Guinea Bissau. *Transcultural Psychiatry, 50*(5), 644–661.

18. de Jong, J. T. (2014). Challenges of creating synergy between global mental health and cultural psychiatry. *Transcultural Psychiatry, 51*(6), 806–828.

19. Amurwon, J., Hajdu, F., Yiga, D. B., & Seeley, J. (2017). "Helping my neighbour is like giving a loan…"–the role of social relations in chronic illness in rural Uganda. *BMC Health Services Research, 17*(1), 705.

20. Van Ginneken, N., Tharyan, P., Lewin, S., Rao, G. N., Meera, S., Pian, J., et al. (2013). Non-specialist health worker interventions for the care of mental, neurological and substance-abuse disorders in low-and middle-income countries. *Cochrane Database of Systematic Reviews, 11*, CD009149.

21. World Health Organization, editor. (2012). *International scientific meeting on nodding syndrome*. Meeting Report UKaid, CDC, The Republic of Uganda, Kampala: WHO.

22. Idro, R., Opar, B., Wamala, J., Abbo, C., Onzivua, S., Mwaka, D. A., et al. (2016). Is nodding syndrome an Onchocerca volvulus-induced neuroinflammatory disorder? Uganda's story

of research in understanding the disease. *International Journal of Infectious Diseases, 45,* 112–117.
23. de Jong, J. T., Berckmoes, L. H., Kohrt, B. A., Song, S. J., Tol, W. A., & Reis, R. (2015). A public health approach to address the mental health burden of youth in situations of political violence and humanitarian emergencies. *Current Psychiatry Reports, 17*(7), 60.
24. Hart, L., & Horton, R. (2017). Syndemics: Committing to a healthier future. *Lancet, 389*(10072), 888–889.
25. Petersen, I., Ssebunnya, J., Bhana, A., & Baillie, K. (2011). Lessons from case studies of integrating mental health into primary health care in South Africa and Uganda. *International Journal of Mental Health Systems, 5*(1), 8.
26. Murray, L. K., Dorsey, S., Haroz, E., Lee, C., Alsiary, M. M., Haydary, A., et al. (2014). A common elements treatment approach for adult mental health problems in low-and middle-income countries. *Cognitive and Behavioral Practice, 21*(2), 111–123.
27. Tsai, A. C., Mendenhall, E., Trostle, J. A., & Kawachi, I. (2017). Co-occurring epidemics, syndemics, and population health. *Lancet, 389*(10072), 978–982.
28. Patel, V., & Prince, M. (2010). Global mental health: A new global health field comes of age. *JAMA, 303*(19), 1976–1977.
29. Bolton, P., Bass, J., Neugebauer, R., Verdeli, H., Clougherty, K. F., Wickramaratne, P., et al. (2003). Group interpersonal psychotherapy for depression in rural Uganda: A randomized controlled trial. *JAMA, 289*(23), 3117–3124.
30. Patel, V., Chisholm, D., Parikh, R., Charlson, F. J., Degenhardt, L., Dua, T., et al. (2016). Addressing the burden of mental, neurological, and substance use disorders: Key messages from disease control priorities. *Lancet, 387*(10028), 1672–1685.
31. Patel, V., Flisher, A. J., Hetrick, S., & McGorry, P. (2007). Mental health of young people: A global public-health challenge. *Lancet, 369*(9569), 1302–1313.
32. Uganda MoH. (2017). Child and adolescent mental health policy guideline. In USE MHAS (Ed.), (p. 11–2). Uganda.
33. Tol, W. A., Jordans, M. J., Kohrt, B. A., Betancourt, T. S., & Komproe, I. H. (2013). Promoting mental health and psychosocial well-being in children affected by political violence: Part I– Current evidence for an ecological resilience approach. In *Handbook of resilience in children of war* (pp. 11–27). Springer, New York. 2013.
34. Tol, W. A., Jordans, M. D., Reis, R., & de Jong, J. (2008). Ecological resilience. In *Treating traumatized children: Risk, resilience and recovery* (p. 164). Springer, New York.
35. Proctor, E. K., Landsverk, J., Aarons, G., Chambers, D., Glisson, C., & Mittman, B. (2009). Implementation research in mental health services: An emerging science with conceptual, methodological, and training challenges. *Administration and Policy in Mental Health and Mental Health Services Research, 36*(1), 24–34.
36. Proctor, E., Silmere, H., Raghavan, R., Hovmand, P., Aarons, G., Bunger, A., et al. (2011). Outcomes for implementation research: Conceptual distinctions, measurement challenges, and research agenda. *Administration and Policy in Mental Health and Mental Health Services Research, 38*(2), 65–76.
37. Murray, L. K., Tol, W., Jordans, M., Sabir, G., Amin, A. M., Bolton, P., et al. (2014). Dissemination and implementation of evidence based, mental health interventions in post conflict, low resource settings. *Intervention, 12*, 94–112.
38. World Health Organization, UNICEF. (2014). *Implementation research toolkit.* World Health Organization.
39. Curran, G. M., Bauer, M., Mittman, B., Pyne, J. M., & Stetler, C. (2012). Effectiveness-implementation hybrid designs: Combining elements of clinical effectiveness and implementation research to enhance public health impact. *Medical Care, 50*(3), 217.
40. Moullin, J. C., Sabater-Hernández, D., Fernandez-Llimos, F., & Benrimoj, S. I. (2015). A systematic review of implementation frameworks of innovations in healthcare and resulting generic implementation framework. *Health Research and Policy and Systems, 13*(1), 16.
41. Eaton, J., McCay, L., Semrau, M., Chatterjee, S., Baingana, F., Araya, R., et al. (2011). Scale up of services for mental health in low-income and middle-income countries. *Lancet, 378*(9802), 1592–1603.

42. Haines, A., Sanders, D., Lehmann, U., Rowe, A. K., Lawn, J. E., Jan, S., et al. (2007). Achieving child survival goals: Potential contribution of community health workers. *Lancet, 369*(9579), 2121–2131.
43. Wainberg, M. L., Scorza, P., Shultz, J. M., Helpman, L., Mootz, J. J., Johnson, K. A., et al. (2017). Challenges and opportunities in global mental health: A research-to-practice perspective. *Current Psychiatry Reports, 19*(5), 28.
44. Petersen, I., Hancock, J. H., Bhana, A., & Govender, K. (2014). A group-based counselling intervention for depression comorbid with HIV/AIDS using a task shifting approach in South Africa: A randomized controlled pilot study. *Journal of Affective Disorders, 158*, 78–84.
45. Shonkoff, J. P., & Fisher, P. A. (2013). Rethinking evidence-based practice and two-generation programs to create the future of early childhood policy. *Development and Psychopathology, 25*(4pt2), 1635–1653.
46. Beardselee, W. R., Versage, E. M., & Gladstone, T. (1998). Children of affectively ill parents: A review of the past 10 years. *Journal of the American Academy of Child and Adolescent Psychiatry, 37*(11), 1134–1141.
47. Betancourt, T. S. (2011). Attending to the mental health of war-affected children: The need for longitudinal and developmental research perspectives. *Journal of the American Academy of Child and Adolescent Psychiatry, 50*(4), 323–325.
48. Betancourt, T. S., Yudron, M., Wheaton, W., & Smith-Fawzi, M. C. (2012). Caregiver and adolescent mental health in Ethiopian Kunama refugees participating in an emergency education program. *The Journal of Adolescent Health, 51*(4), 357–365.
49. Elbedour, S., Ten Bensel, R., & Bastien, D. T. (1993). Ecological integrated model of children of war: Individual and social psychology. *Child Abuse & Neglect, 17*(6), 805–819.
50. Panter-Brick, C., Grimon, M. P., & Eggerman, M. (2014). Caregiver—child mental health: A prospective study in conflict and refugee settings. *Journal of Child Psychology and Psychiatry, 55*(4), 313–327.
51. Betancourt, T. S., McBain, R. K., Newnham, E. A., & Brennan, R. T. (2015). The intergenerational impact of war: Longitudinal relationships between caregiver and child mental health in postconflict Sierra Leone. *Journal of Child Psychology and Psychiatry, 56*(10), 1101–1107.
52. Morris, J., Jones, L., Berrino, A., Jordans, M. J., Okema, L., & Crow, C. (2012). Does combining infant stimulation with emergency feeding improve psychosocial outcomes for displaced mothers and babies? A controlled evaluation from northern Uganda. *The American Journal of Orthopsychiatry, 82*(3), 349–357.
53. Morris, J., Belfer, M., Daniels, A., Flisher, A., Villé, L., Lora, A., et al. (2011). Treated prevalence of and mental health services received by children and adolescents in 42 low-and-middle-income countries. *Journal of Child Psychology and Psychiatry, 52*(12), 1239–1246.
54. Rahman, A., Divan, G., Hamdani, S. U., Vajaratkar, V., Taylor, C., Leadbitter, K., et al. (2016). Effectiveness of the parent-mediated intervention for children with autism spectrum disorder in South Asia in India and Pakistan (PASS): A randomised controlled trial. *Lancet Psychiatry, 3*(2), 128–136.
55. Stadnick, N. A., Stahmer, A., & Brookman-Frazee, L. (2015). Preliminary effectiveness of project ImPACT: A parent-mediated intervention for children with autism spectrum disorder delivered in a community program. *Journal of Autism and Developmental Disorders, 45*(7), 2092–2104.
56. Shaw, D. S., Connell, A., Dishion, T. J., Wilson, M. N., & Gardner, F. (2009). Improvements in maternal depression as a mediator of intervention effects on early childhood problem behavior. *Development and Psychopathology, 21*(02), 417–439.
57. Siskind, D., Baingana, F., & Kim, J. (2008). Cost-effectiveness of group psychotherapy for depression in Uganda. *The Journal of Mental Health Policy and Economics, 11*(3), 127–133.
58. McHugh, R. K., Murray, H. W., & Barlow, D. H. (2009). Balancing fidelity and adaptation in the dissemination of empirically-supported treatments: The promise of transdiagnostic interventions. *Behaviour Research and Therapy, 47*(11), 946–953.

59. Atun, R., de Jongh, T., Secci, F., Ohiri, K., & Adeyi, O. (2009). Integration of targeted health interventions into health systems: A conceptual framework for analysis. *Health Policy and Planning, 25*(2), 104–111.
60. Patel, V., Chowdhary, N., Rahman, A., & Verdeli, H. (2011). Improving access to psychological treatments: Lessons from developing countries. *Behaviour Research and Therapy, 49*(9), 523–528.
61. Greene, S. M., Reid, R. J., & Larson, E. B. (2012). Implementing the learning health system: From concept to action. *Annals of Internal Medicine, 157*(3), 207–210.
62. Murray, L., & Jordans, M. (2016). Rethinking the service delivery system of psychological interventions in low and middle income countries. *BMC Psychiatry, 16*(1), 234.
63. Agyepong, I. A., Sewankambo, N., Binagwaho, A., Coll-Seck, A. M., Corrah, T., Ezeh, A., et al. (2017). The path to longer and healthier lives for all Africans by 2030: The Lancet Commission on the future of health in sub-Saharan Africa. *Lancet, 390*(10114), 2803–2859.
64. Padmanathan, P., & De Silva, M. J. (2013). The acceptability and feasibility of task-sharing for mental healthcare in low and middle income countries: A systematic review. *Social Science & Medicine, 97*, 82–86.
65. Thornicroft, G., & Patel, V. (2014). *Global mental health trials*. Oxford, UK.
66. De Jong, J. 2011. (Disaster) ublic mental health. *Post-traumatic Stress Disorder*. 217–262.
67. Song SJ. Globalization and mental health: The impact of war and armed conflict on families. 2015.
68. Patel, V., Belkin, G. S., Chockalingam, A., Cooper, J., Saxena, S., & Unützer, J. (2013). Grand challenges: Integrating mental health services into priority health care platforms. *PLoS Medicine, 10*(5), e1001448.
69. Kaiser, B. N., Haroz, E. E., Kohrt, B. A., Bolton, P. A., Bass, J. K., & Hinton, D. E. (2015). "Thinking too much": A systematic review of a common idiom of distress. *Social Science & Medicine, 147*, 170–183.
70. Belkin, G. S., Unützer, J., Kessler, R. C., Verdeli, H., Raviola, G. J., Sachs, K., et al. (2011). Scaling up for the "bottom billion": "5 x 5" implementation of community mental health care in low-income regions. Psychiatric Services, 62, 1494–1502.
71. Okello, J. (2014). *War, trauma, attachment and risky behaviour in adolescents in Northern Uganda*. Ghent University, Ghent, Belgium.

Suicide Outside the Frame of Mental Illness: Exploring Suicidal Behaviors in Global and Cultural Contexts

Rida Malick and James L. Griffith

Introduction

In his 1942 philosophical essay *Le Myth De Sisyphe*, Albert Camus, Algerian-French philosopher, starts his piece with the following:

> "There is but one truly serious philosophical problem, and that is suicide. Judging whether life is or is not worth living amounts to answering the fundamental question of philosophy. All the rest–whether the world has three dimensions, whether the mind has nine or twelve categories–comes afterwards. These are games; one must first answer" – [7]

In the first section of this essay, titled 'An Absurd Reasoning,' Camus is arguing that the question on whether to live or die is the most critical and all other questions can be addressed once that is answered. Suicide and self-harming behaviors have long been a perplexing concept, given that it contradicts the fundamental biological drive that all living creatures are motivated by self-preservation and gene transmission via reproduction [23]. While human beings, like all living creatures, are inherently driven to survive, they are also a solution oriented and a problem solving species [32].

Close to one million people worldwide die by suicide each year which accounts for more than all armed-conflict, war, and other forms of interpersonal violence combined [23, 41]. This means that one is more likely to die by their own hand than someone else's [23]. Death by suicide occurs once every 40 seconds and for every adult who dies by suicide, there are more than 20 others attempting the act [41]. About 85% of these global suicides occur in lower and middle income countries due to inadequate resources and poor infrastructure to implement sufficient preventative measures [38].

R. Malick (✉) · J. L. Griffith
Department of Psychiatry and Behavioral Sciences, The George Washington University, Washington, DC, USA
e-mail: malickr@email.gwu.edu; jgriffith@mfa.gwu.edu

© Springer Nature Switzerland AG 2021
A. R. Dyer et al. (eds.), *Global Mental Health Ethics*,
https://doi.org/10.1007/978-3-030-66296-7_9

When discussing suicidal behaviors, we are referring to a range of behaviors that can exist on a spectrum. The spectrum of suicidal behaviors includes fatal or completed suicides, highly lethal but failed attempts, self-injurious behaviors, self-mutilating acts, impulsive acts, and in its most simple form, suicidal ideation. These behaviors can be further classified by method, lethality, cognitive impairment, and other descriptive features [5]. In psychiatric training within the United States, suicide is often taught as and learned as a symptom of mental illness, most commonly depression but also others such as bipolar disorder and schizophrenia. In fact, 90–95% of those who die by suicide have a diagnosable mental illness [24]. However, in other parts of the world, these rates drop significantly. In India and China for example, only 35–40% of those who die by suicide have a diagnosable mental illness [39]. While suicidal behaviors are typically thought of as a combination of a mental illness plus a stressful life event, not all mental disorders present with suicidal ideation and not all stressful life events lead to suicidal thoughts. While a diagnosable psychiatric illness is arguably the strongest risk factor for suicidal behaviors, it is a risk factor only and not a requirement. Other significant risk factors include anhedonia, hopelessness, poor emotional regulation, alcohol or substance abuse, poor impulse control, psychosis, and personality disorder. Therefore, suicide is a behavior that can exist outside the frame of mental illness and can exist against the background of various cross-cultural settings.

This chapter will explore the various human motivations towards suicidal behaviors that do not necessarily fit into the frame of mental illness in global society both historically and currently and the ethical implications. There are numerous motivations for suicidal behaviors across cultures including but not limited to honor, shame, humiliation, preservation of dignity, political motivations, protest, and more. As stated earlier, humans are solution-oriented beings, and while we are not required to agree with the solution, suicide for many contemplating it can be seen as a solution to a deeply painful problem [32]. Genuine curiosity and nonjudgmental inquiry about the dilemma suicide would be solving for a suffering individual can serve as a gateway to understanding their anguish and producing alternative "solutions."

Genetics and Neurobiology of Suicide: A Brief Overview

In addition to psychological stressors, genetic and biological factors are critical to understanding suicidal behaviors. The stress-diathesis model of suicidal behaviors demonstrates its importance. Diathesis refers to the components of the body itself that makes it react in specific ways to external stimuli [20]. External stimuli or life stressors then interact with predisposing biological factors to produce disease in already susceptible individuals. Family, twin, and adoption studies show that both suicide attempts and completed suicides are genetic in nature [30]. Heritability of suicide is about 21–50%, whereas the heritability of suicidal ideation and behavior is about 30–55% [17]. This was commonly attributed to the heritability of mental illness; however, there are studies that show the heritability for suicidal behavior remains even after controlling for mood and psychotic disorders [23]. Genetic transmission of suicide attempts is distinct from genetic transmission of psychiatric disorder [6]. Suicidal behaviors therefore have a distinct genetic background that does not depend on the presence of concomitant psychopathology [17].

There are three major systems that play a crucial role in suicidal behaviors, the hypothalamic pituitary axis or the HPA axis, the noradrenergic system, and the serotonergic system. The system most consistently linked with suicidal behaviors is the serotonergic system. Suicidal behaviors are linked to alterations in serotonergic function that are independent of the serotonergic dysfunction associated with major depressive disorder [21]. In both suicide and more lethal but nonfatal suicides, lower levels of the serotonin metabolite 5-hydroxyacetic acid (5-HIAA) are seen in the cerebrospinal fluid (CSF). Meta-analysis showed below median levels of 5-HIAA in CSF in major depressive disorder has a 4.5 times higher odds ratio for suicide compared to those with major depressive disorder with above median levels of the metabolite [22]. Additionally, lower 5-HIAA in CSF is seen in those who attempt suicide with depression, schizophrenia, and personality disorder compared to those with the same exact disorder without attempts [20]. Anatomical studies show a reduction in serotonin transporter binding in the ventromedial prefrontal cortex and anterior cingulate. These regions are associated with decision making, willed-action, and mood and impairment can lead to impulsivity and disinhibited behaviors. Findings of serotonergic impairment are independent of psychiatric illness and appear to share a common feature of being related to complete and nonfatal suicide attempts [20].

The HPA axis has a bidirectional relationship with both the serotonergic and norepinephrine system [22]. The HPA axis is responsible for stress regulation with the help of corticotropin-releasing hormone (CRH) neurons. These neurons extend to the raphe nucleus, which controls serotonin transmission to various parts of the brain containing CRH. Stress additionally activates the locus coeruleus which is the major source of norepinephrine to the brain. It is thought that hyperactivity of both the HPA and norepinephrine system seen in suicidal patients may be related to severe anxiety secondary to a heightened stress response. Stress can lead to abnormalities in the HPA and norepinephrine system which can then have downstream effects on the serotonergic system [22]. Alterations in the serotonergic system can lead to impulsivity, aggression, and disinhibited behaviors while alteration in the norepinephrine system can also lead to aggression and may be related to helplessness, hopelessness, and pessimism over time [8].

Suicidal Behaviors and Motivations: Cross-Cultural Analysis

Suicidal behaviors are not always a sequelae of mental illness and thus it is imperative to understand motivations that go beyond treatment of mental illness. This section of the chapter will further explore some of the motivations for suicidal behaviors across cultures including but not limited to honor, shame, humiliation, preservation of dignity, political motivations, and protest. Although distinct, many of these motivations are woven throughout the fabric of the same narrative and bleed together.

Roles and Groups

While society has many distinct roles and groups, this section will focus on the roles of gender with a specific focus on the role of women. Gender gaps are evident in suicide data worldwide and the gender disparity is typically dictated by cultural context [35]. In 2015, suicide surpassed maternal mortality as the leading cause of death among girls age 15–19 globally [26]. It is thought that strict gender roles may account for higher suicide rates among this demographic. Gender refers to a social construct and culturally defined behaviors and expectations assigned to each biological sex [35]. Socialization and conformation to culturally prescribed gender roles have been implicated in states of well-being for both men and women [35, 40]. By following their gender roles, women (and men) are able to protect their personal and family reputations. The expectation for a woman is typically that of a "good" and "virtuous" woman which generally equates to sexual chastity and loyalty [25].

The historical practice of *Sati* is a grim demonstration of this strict adherence to one's prescribed role within society. Sati refers to the expectation that a widow would walk into the funeral pyre of her husband and die alongside her husband [2]. Once a woman's husband died, she became vulnerable to accusations that her devotion was inadequate. The practice of Sati was a way to prove her devotion. The act has been described in the Hindu epic Mahabharata which is one of the key religious scriptures in Hinduism. The practice originates from a religious anecdote in which the Hindu Goddess Parvati self-immolates when her father insults her husband. This practice of suicide was viewed through the lens of Dharma which refers to one's sense of duty and law and was believed to lead to good karma and more favorable reincarnation. In addition to benefits for the self, Sati was believed to have benefits those close to the widow as well. People highly valued the blessings from a widow on her way to becoming Sati. The act was seen as a way of exalting the status of the family including both the widow's family and her in-laws which served as reason to encourage a woman to carry the act through. Therefore, it can be seen as a complex amalgamation of personal devotion and coercion [2].

Sati was abolished by the British while India was under colonial rule in the early 1800s; however, the practice resurfaced back to the spotlight more recently when 18 year old RoopKanwar performed Sati in 1987 in a small village in Rajasthan, India. While police were informed, they did not intervene to prevent or stop the act [2]. The incident created immense public outrage, and splits public opinion most notably across urban and rural lines, gender lines, and traditional and modern lines. There was controversy on whether she chose to do it herself or was drugged and forced to go into the funeral pyre. Regardless of the ultimate truth, the outrage surrounding these events led to the Rajasthan Prevention of Sati Act in 1987 which forbids the act of sati and encouragement or glorification of sati, punishable by death, life imprisonment or a fine [28]. Interestingly, the law specified that it did not matter whether a woman was choosing to become sati of her own volition.

The impact RoopKanwar left on her small village almost 30 years later gives us a glimpse into why a woman may choose this route not only for herself but also for those she leaves behind. Those in the village believe she did it of her own choosing.

The story goes that after she saw her husband's dead body, she cried and then began dressing up like a new bride [37]. When her family asked her what she was doing she disclosed her choice to commit Sati and was unable to be persuaded otherwise. A shrine for RoopKanwar exists and many consider her to be an omnipresent spirit in the village. The youth grow up hearing the story of her act. One young boy who grew up hearing the tale states "Sometimes, I also go in the evening to light an incense stick there [Kanwar's cremation site/shrine]. It is just a matter of faith." One relative of the family, Mangu Singh, said "She was my nephew's wife, but now she is like my mother. It was a choice which she made and we have immense respect for her" [37].

Another suicidal behavior seen in the context of social roles and gender roles is honor suicides. There is a Pakistani folk saying that roughly translates to "When wealth is lost nothing is lost; when health is lost something is lost, when honor is lost everything is lost" [16]. Honor suicides occur today mostly in the Middle East in countries such as Turkey, Jordan, and Pakistan. Women who have been perceived to dishonor their families commit suicide to alleviate the shame it brought to their families, which is not entirely voluntary [25]. Interestingly, the practice of honor suicides has grown as legislation against honor killings grows harsher. Traditionally, a male in the family would be expected to kill the woman who had dishonored the family. The result is two-fold –the male upholds his own masculinity and restores family honor. Ironically, there is a strong disdain for death in the society which earns the male perpetrator greater respect –having to endure killing someone is worse than death itself [16]. Now that penalties against honor violence are increasing, families encourage the girl to kill herself so they do not lose a second male child to the justice system [3].

Derya, a 17 year old girl in Eastern Turkey, received a text message from her uncle reading *"You have blackened our name. Kill yourself and clean our shame or we will kill you first"* [3]. Derya had fallen in love with a boy and news of her love affair was spreading throughout the community. Derya soon began to receive similar text messages from multiple male family members, sometimes up to 15 times a day and it felt like a death sentence. She said *"My family attacked my personality, and I felt I had committed the biggest sin in the world. I felt I had no right to dishonor my family, that I have no right to be alive. So I decided to respect my family's desire and to die."* Derya had three failed suicide attempts before she was able to escape. While laws have changed, culture is slower to follow.

It is important to have insight into the desperation associated with these acts both for someone like Derya and her family. In cases of besmirched honor, if the act is not completed that dishonor can extend beyond the immediate family to the entire lineage, or community [16]. In Eastern Turkey, in situations in which families did not want their loved one to die, some said incessant gossip and immense social pressure drove them to it [3]. For Derya, who has now escaped, had counseling and is hopeful for her future, she said regarding her story "You can either escape by leaving your family and moving to a town, or you can kill yourself." This gives us a glimpse into the anguish and torment she experienced when she felt this was truly the only path to solving her affliction.

While honor killings and sati are certainly distinct, they both show the significance of roles, groups, and social organizations within a community. The social role dominates over the person as an individual. Molding into one's role is considered more important than the desires, hopes, and dreams of the individual. If one does not fit into the role as prescribed, as seen in Derya's case, consequences of ostracization follow. In RoopKanwar's case, she did follow the rules of her social role and even in her death she continues to be revered and part of her group. It is likely that living as a widow in the case of sati or with a broken reputation in the case of honor suicides, may be so horrendous for not just you but your family, and those close to you, that glorification and restoration of reputation after death may be preferable and an unfortunate option on the table.

Honor and Shame

As stated earlier, many of these motivations bleed together and will present within the same narrative. The themes of honor and shame are present in many suicide narratives. Cultures of honor place a strong emphasis on upholding and defending honor and reputation not just of oneself but also of the entire family [25]. Cultures that place a high priority on honor tend to have strict values and expectations for societal roles such as gender roles and tend to be hypersensitive to threats to reputation. When failure occurs or reputation is significantly threatened, death is a considerable option.

This is exemplified in the ritualistic suicide practice developed in the twelfth century for the Japanese elite samurai warrior class known as *seppuku* ("cutting the stomach") or *harakiri* ("belly cut"). Typically performed in the battlefield, the purpose was to achieve an honorable death by avoiding the dishonor of surrendering to the enemy [27]. Embracing death signified a devotion to the principles of loyalty, duty, honor, and self-sacrifice. While *seppuku* was primarily performed in wars to avoid enemy capture and surrender, it was considered a way to protest or express grief over the death of a leader [1]. It eventually became a form of capital punishment for samurai warriors. The act was usually preceded by a large ceremony where the samurai would read a short "death poem." While the practice of *seppuku* fell out of favor and was outlawed in the 1870s, a similar emphasis on honor was observed with kamikaze pilot tactics in World War II [25, 27]. Japanese pilots chose death in the service of their country over surrender by using their own planes as missiles demonstrating the strong emphasis on honor and sacrifice in Japanese culture.

While many of these practices may seem foreign or "exotic", the concepts underlying them are prevalent in the United States as well. This is an important point to emphasize because while global mental health may seem far away at times, it is also occurring within our own backyard in our day to day clinical experiences. These motivations for suicidal behaviors exist across cultures and are not confined to any one culture – what differs may just be the frequency in which you see it. Honor cultures are known to have elevated levels of interpersonal violence or violence against others [25]. In these cultures, one is expected to be able to perceive threats and respond to them in an "honorable" manner. Osterman and Brown did a study in the United States to see whether this meant that these cultures also have high levels of *intra*personal violence of violence against the self. In this study, Western and Southern states were classified as high honor culture states with the exception of Hawaii and Alaska. States with high honor culture have significantly higher male and female suicide rates than nonhonor states most significantly observed in nonmetropolitan areas among whites. Another interesting finding was that individual endorsement of honor ideology was positively associated with depression. In the United States, the gender disparity in suicides is higher among men. For men in honor culture, failure to prove masculinity, either as a provider or defender, can affect both private sense of self worth and public reputation [25]. These cultures are associated with higher levels of interpersonal violence against others, especially for the purposes of restoration of honor and thus, honor cultures might thus regard violence against self or suicide as a logical response to damaged honor as well.

Preservation of Dignity

Suicide in order to preserve dignity serves as the basis for a relatively well-accepted yet controversial form of suicide–physician's assisted suicide (PAS). PAS or "medical aid in dying" refers to when a physician provides a mean for end of life such as by writing a prescription whereas euthanasia or "mercy killing" refers to when a physician intentionally and directly takes a patient's life in order to alleviate suffering [29]. Psychological anguish and suffering associated with end of life and terminal illness includes loss of health, mobility, ability to care for self, including ability to feed self, incontinence, loss of role within family [32]. While it remains a controversial topic, for those in favor, it is considered a legitimate and rational time to consider ending life, and putting an end to extended psychological torment while preserving self-dignity. The "right to die" or "death with dignity" movements aim to uphold patient autonomy and self-determination and put an end to unbearable suffering [27]. Interestingly, a recent retrospective analysis of suicides in the geriatric population showed that older adults who die by suicide do not have a known mental health condition [33]. Understanding alternative ways to identify risk outside the frame of mental illness are crucial in many of these cases.

Political Protest

In some cases, suicide is used as a communicative act or protest. When people have power or status in society, they may be able to make choices or express their views in socially acceptable ways [19]. However for those without power or resources or for those who feel voiceless, suicide may present as their last option to garner attention with the purposes of getting a message across.

In October 1963, a Buddhist monk named Thich Quang Duc, lit himself on fire in the middle of a busy Saigon intersection in South Vietnam [31]. Arguably one of the most famous instances of self-immolation in history, this was done in order to protest Ngo Dinh Diem's rule of South Vietnam in which he was supportive of the Catholic minority and discriminating against the Buddhist monks. Photographer Malcolm Browne's photo of the Buddhist monk lighting himself on fire was seen around the world and brought widespread attention to the policies of the government. Journalist David Halberstam who witnessed and reported on the story later recalled in one of his books "Flames were coming from a human being; his body was slowly withering and shriveling up, his head blackening and charring. In the air was the smell of burning flesh... Behind me I could hear the sobbing of the Vietnamese who were now gathering. I was too shocked to cry, too confused to take notes or ask questions, too bewildered to even think" [31]. John F. Kennedy commented "no news picture in history has generated so much emotion around the world as that one" [36]. The photo was seen around the world and brought attention to the policies of the government and the Buddhist monk's sacrifice played a pivotal role in public opinion against the South Vietnamese regime.

Self-immolation as a catalyst for large political movements is present in our more recent history as well as demonstrated by the initiation of the Arab Spring. On December 17, 2010, a young 26-year old man named Mohamed Bouazizi who pushed a fruit and vegetable cart for a living ignited a movement he likely did not forsee. Bouazizi's father died when he was 3-years old. He was the oldest of his family of eight and they depended on him financially. He had been working since he was a 10-year old boy. The evening before he lit himself on fire, he looked at his mother and said "With this fruit I can buy some gifts for you. Tomorrow will be a good day" [15].

Bouazizi's job did not make him much money. He would often get harassed by officials, such as police officers, market inspectors, sometimes demanding bribes to leave him alone, stealing his fruit, or treating him with indignity [15]. On this particular day, he was being harassed by police officers. One particular policewoman, FeydaHamdi, attempted to take multiple crates of apples from his cart. He attempted to stand up for himself by blocking her but was pushed to the ground by two other officers who then took his scale. The policewoman Hamdi then slapped Bouazizi across the face among a crowd of witnesses. He was humiliated, crying out of frustration and shame. "Why are you doing this to me? I'm a simple person, I just want to work." This sense of humiliation is important to note because it distinguishes his emotions on this particular work day. Bouazizi was angry and attempted to file a complaint at the governor's office. However he was denied and unable to do so. Later in the day, he set himself on fire outside the governor's office. Bouazizi did not die immediately–he was initially hospitalized–however, the impact of his act was certainly immediate.

This incident led to widespread anger and public outcry throughout the country about various issues including economic and financial hardship and regime and systematic corruption. On December 28th, President Ben Ali visited Bouazizi in the hospital with a camera crew in order to quell public sentiment; however, this was not effective. On January 4th Bouazizi passed away and by January 14th the protest movement had grown tremendously, leading to Ben Ali's forced resignation as president. Bouazizi became the face of the prodemocracy movement. Many demonstrators carried signs and banners with his image. His act is credited as being the catalyst for the Arab Spring which eventually found its way to other countries such as Bahrain, Egypt, and Syria and spread fear across regimes and monarchies throughout the Middle East. Right after, there were similar cases of self-immolation throughout the Arab world during the Arab spring. In Tunisia alone, self-immolation events tripled in the 5 years after the revolution started [4]. In 2017, with a population of 11 million people, public protest was the second most common form of suicide in Tunisia.

Immolation which means sacrifice and has come to mean self burning is certainly self-destructive which is how we typically see suicidal behaviors. However, it is also seen as sacrificial [11]. It is an individual gesture that speaks for collective distress and is thus viewed as an act of martyrdom or altruistic suicide. Altruistic suicide refers to Emile Durkheim's theory of suicide that it is determined by ones relationship to culture and society [13]. Altruistic suicide is often seen in societies that place less value on the individual and are completed with the intention of a greater good for the group or a higher purpose [27, 34]. Fire symbolizes purification and self-immolation may represent a collective desire for rebirth, resurrection, and change [11].

Conclusion

Suicide is a behavior that can exist outside the frame of mental illness. There are numerous reasons that could motivate a person to contemplate suicide including fitting into a role, group or social organization, honor, shame, humiliation, preservation of dignity, and political acts. While these motivations may or may not occur within the setting of psychopathology, they share the common theme of feeling as if death is the best solution to the dilemma at hand.

Suicide outside the frame of mental illness brings up several ethical challenges. Suicide is an act of self harm meant to inflict injury or death while we as physicians are tasked with promoting and protecting life [12]. While suicidal behaviors certainly can occur in the setting of psychiatric illness, one would say it may be rational under specific circumstances. Within the Western biomedical model, the "death with dignity" and "right to die" movements argue that requesting death is logical given unbearable suffering and this would be means of respecting patient autonomy. However this question becomes convoluted when explored further. While medical comorbidity is certainly a risk factor, the proportion of suicide victims suffering from terminal illness is approximately two to four percent [27]. Additionally, a majority of those with terminal illness independent of depression do not wish to die. Legislation on PAS and euthanasia varies internationally. Some countries allow only PAS whereas others also allow euthanasia. In Switzerland, both physicians and nonphysicians are able to perform passive voluntary euthanasia which makes it a popular destination for "suicide tourism" for those wishing to die from neighboring countries [27]. How would finances and profits from potential industry and tourism affect the way we handle or assess death? In the Netherlands, those with mental disorders are able to request PAS and in Belgium, it extends to those who are mentally incompetent which brings up the ethical dilemma of voluntariness and consent. The other main ethical challenge is that while acceptance of death with dignity appears to be a mainstream in the West, this then begs the question of who decides when is it rational or logical to want death? Are we then infringing upon autonomy if we also impede death in "rational" cases of suicide aside from PAS?

Culture is not a single variable but rather multiple dynamic variables that affect all aspects of a person's experience. These experiences incorporate economic, political, religious, psychological, and biological events and can differ within the same ethnic or social group based on differences in age, gender, political association, and more [18]. "Unbearable suffering" is a subjective process and is not defined by any one person or culture. While different cultures construe personhood differently, "unbearable suffering," across cultures, often describes the experience of one's intactness as a person under threat of destruction, whether that threat is physical pain, political injustice, exclusion from one's family or community, God's judgment, or some other threat [9, 10]. From this perspective, suicide can be regarded as a re-assertion of oneself as a person, a refusal to submit to circumstances, a violent turn towards assertive coping. Through suicide, a person can choose to die as one would have chosen to live, but cannot, due to life's circumstances.

Justification for PAS depends on the presence of a terminal illness; however, death is technically an endpoint for all human beings and it is not always clear how terminal an illness is going to be [27]. Perhaps a young girl who felt she has dishonored her family faces a similar prolonged psychological anguish and torment, shame, feelings that death will not only be a better option for herself but for her family and she will relieve them of the burden of her dishonor. The prolonged psychological anguish this young girl turns over in her psyche cannot be deemed by an objective person to be more or less painful than another facing the anguish of a terminal illness. Internal conflict is entirely subjective and a personal experience that cannot be standardized, measured, or compared. Universalism argues that a set of rules or norms are applicable to all human beings and cultures equally [14]. Therefore, across the various evolving global cultures, there should be an effort to promote and protect the sanctity of life. Understanding how suicide serves as an escape from an unbearable affliction, regardless of our objective judgment of the affliction, will improve our ability as clinicians to assess risk, explore other avenues of action, and mobilize hope.

At the end of his piece, Camus rejects suicide as an answer to the absurd or meaninglessness of life by embracing passion, freedom, and revolt despite how mundane or pointless life can seem at times. Even when suicide appears to be the only logical decision in an otherwise hopeless situation, while we should acknowledge the anguish and chosen solution, we are ultimately tasked with guiding an individual to see their unique potential and present alternatives that promote life.

References

1. Andrews, E. (2016). What is seppuku? History.com. www.history.com/news/what-is-seppuku
2. Bhugra, D. (2005). Sati: a type of nonpsychiatric suicide. *Crisis, 26*(2), 73–77.
3. Bilefsky, D. (2006). How to avoid honor killing in Turkey? Honor suicide. *The New York Times*, www.nytimes.com/2006/07/16/world/europe/16turkey.html
4. Blaise, L. (2017). Self-immolation, catalyst of the Arab spring, is now a grim trend. *The New York Times*, www.nytimes.com/2017/07/09/world/africa/self-immolation-catalyst-of-the-arab-spring-is-now-a-grim-trend.html
5. Bondy, B., Buettner, A., & Zill, P. (2006). Genetics of suicide. *Molecular Psychiatry, 11*(4), 336–351.
6. Brent, D. A., & Mann, J. J. (2005). Family genetic studies, suicide, and suicidal behavior. In *American Journal of Medical Genetics Part C: Seminars in Medical Genetics* (Vol. 133, pp. 13–24). Hoboken: Wiley.
7. Camus, A. (1942). *The myth of sisyphus*. Paris: Gallimard.
8. Carballo, J. J., Akamnonu, C. P., & Oquendo, M. A. (2008). Neurobiology of suicidal behavior. An integration of biological and clinical findings. *Archives of Suicide Research, 12*(2), 93–110.
9. Cassell, E. J. (1991). *The nature of suffering and the goals of medicine*. New York: Oxford University Press.
10. Cassell, E. J. (1982). The nature of suffering and the goals of medicine. *The New England Journal of Medicine, 306*, 639–645.
11. Cheikh, I. B., Rousseau, C., & Mekki-Berrada, A. (2011). Suicide as protest against social suffering in the Arab world. *The British Journal of Psychiatry, 198*(6), 494–495.
12. Desai, N. G., Sengupta, S., & Kumar, D. (2012). Ethical issues in suicide. In A. Shrivastava (Ed.), *Suicide from a global perspective* (p. 183). New York: Nova Science Publishers Inc..
13. Durkheim, E. (1951). *Suicide: A study in sociology (JA Spaulding & G. Simpson, Trans.)*. Glencoe: Free Press. (Original work published 1897).
14. Evanoff, R. J. (2004). Universalist, relativist, and constructivist approaches to intercultural ethics. *International Journal of Intercultural Relations, 28*(5), 439–458.
15. Fisher, M. (2011). In Tunisia, act of one fruit vendor sparks wave of revolution through Arab world. *The Washington Post*, WP Company. www.washingtonpost.com/world/in-tunisia-act-of-one-fruit-vendor-sparks-wave-of-revolution-through-arab-world/2011/03/16/AFjfsueB_story.html
16. Jafri, A. H. (2008). *Honour killing: dilemma, ritual, understanding*. Oxford: Oxford University Press.
17. Jaeschke, R., Siwek, M., & Dudek, D. (2011). Neurobiology of suicidal behaviour. *Psychiatria Polska, 45*(4), 573–588.
18. Kleinman, A., & Benson, P. (2006). Anthropology in the clinic: the problem of cultural competency and how to fix it. *PLoS Medicine, 3*(10), e294.
19. Liu, S. S. (2005). Suicide as protest. Fueling Unrest, 1.
20. Mann, J. J. (2003). Neurobiology of suicidal behavior. *Nature Reviews. Neuroscience, 4*(10), 819–828.
21. Mann, J. J., Brent, D. A., & Arango, V. (2001). The neurobiology and genetics of suicide and attempted suicide: a focus on the serotonergic system. *Neuropsychopharmacology, 24*(5), 467–477.
22. Mann, J. J., & Currier, D. M. (2010). Stress, genetics and epigenetic effects on the neurobiology of suicidal behavior and depression. *European Psychiatry, 25*(5), 268–271.
23. Nock, M. K., Borges, G., & Ono, Y. (2012a). Global perspectives on suicidal behavior. In M. Nock, M. K. Nock, G. Borges, & Y. Ono (Eds.), *Suicide: global perspectives from the WHO world mental health surveys*. Cambridge: Cambridge University Press.
24. Nock, M. K., Borges, G., Bromet, E. J., Cha, C. B., Kessler, R. C., & Lee, S. (2012b). The epidemiology of suicide and suicidal behavior. In M. Nock, M. K. Nock, G. Borges, & Y. Ono

(Eds.), *Suicide: global perspectives from the WHO world mental health surveys*. Cambridge: Cambridge University Press.
25. Osterman, L. L., & Brown, R. P. (2011). Culture of honor and violence against the self. *Personality and Social Psychology Bulletin, 37*(12), 1611–1623.
26. Petroni, S., Patel, V., & Patton, G. (2015). Why is suicide the leading killer of older adolescent girls? *Lancet, 386*(10008), 2031–2032.
27. Pierre, J. M. (2015). Culturally sanctioned suicide: euthanasia, seppuku, and terrorist martyrdom. *World Journal of Psychiatry, 5*(1), 4.
28. The Rajasthan Sati (Prevention) Act, 1987 (No. 40 of 1987), 26 November 1987. Annu Rev Popul Law. 1987;14:477–82. PubMed PMID: 12346744.
29. Richmond, J., Yakunina, E., & Werth, J. L., Jr. (2012). Complexities in assisted suicide and euthanasia. In A. Shrivastava (Ed.), *Suicide from a global perspective* (p. 183). New York: Nova Science Publishers Inc.
30. Roy, A., Rylander, G., & Sarchiapone, M. (1997). Genetics of suicide: family studies and molecular genetics. *Annals of the New York Academy of Sciences, 836*(1), 135–157.
31. Sanburn, J. (2011). A brief history of self-immolation. Time, Time Inc. content.time.com/time/world/article/0,8599,2043123,00.html
32. Shea, S. C. (1999). *The practical art of suicide assessment: a guide for mental health professionals and substance abuse counselors*. Wiley.
33. Schmutte, T. J., & Wilkinson, S. T. (2020). Suicide in older adults with and without known mental illness: results from the national violent death reporting system, 2003–2016. *American Journal of Preventive Medicine, 58*(4), 584–590.
34. Stack, S. (2004). Emile Durkheim and altruistic suicide. *Archives of Suicide Research, 8*(1), 9–22.
35. Stewart, A., & Smith, D. (2012). Suicide and gender. In A. Shrivastava (Ed.), *Suicide from a global perspective* (p. 183). New York: Nova Science Publishers Inc.
36. Toong, Z. J. (2008). Overthrown by the press: the US media's role in the fall of Diem. *Australasian Journal of American Studies, 27*(1), 56–72.
37. TNN. (2019). In Rajasthan's sati village, RoopKanwar still burns bright: Jaipur news – times of India. *The Times of India*.
38. Vijayakumar, L., Pearson, M., & Kumar, S. (2014). Suicide prevention trials. In G. Thornicroft & V. Patel (Eds.), *Global mental health trials*. Oxford: Oxford University Press.
39. Vijayakumar, L. (2005). Suicide and mental disorders in Asia. *International Review of Psychiatry, 17*(2), 109–114.
40. Watkins, P. L., & Whaley, D. (2000). Gender role stressors and women's health.
41. World Health Organization. (2019). *Suicide Data*. Retrieved from https://www.who.int/mental_health/prevention/suicide/suicideprevent/en/

Part III

Social Determinants and Global Mental Health

Rethinking Idioms of Distress and Resilience in Anthropology and Global Mental Health

10

Emily Mendenhall and Andrew Wooyoung Kim

Introduction

How we interpret concepts from suffering to survival has been historically debated in the field of anthropology, transcultural psychiatry, and global mental health [24, 28, 35, 36, 59, 70]. Mostly, these debates have centered on the notion that such concepts are cross-culturally reproducible. Anthropologists have put together an impressive body of work that reveals how and why suffering is experienced, expressed, and embodied differently from place to place and emphasized that it is not a universal construct. Some have gone so far as to challenge the notion that an international measurement of such suffering is realistic [29, 70], despite the fact that many of us use psychometric scales that have been "validated" among the communities with which we work. While these tools and the larger research agenda of global mental health are necessary to assess and produce culturally relevant understandings of psychological disease, health, and well-being across the world, we must critically reconsider the inherent cultural biases that alter our measurement of key concepts like suffering, resilience, and lived experience in hopes of designing more effective tools and producing more accurate and holistic knowledge of global mental health.

Anthropologists have long been concerned with how culture and experience shape the ways in which people interpret and express social and psychological suffering [12, 27, 31–33]. Yet, the impact of culture on the experience and expression of mental illness continues to be debated [21, 36]. Since the early 1980s, idioms of distress, first articulated by Mark Nichter [54, 55], have become a central construct

E. Mendenhall (✉)
School of Foreign Service, Georgetown University, Washington, DC, USA
e-mail: em1061@georgetown.edu

A. W. Kim
Center for Global Health, Massachusetts General Hospital, Boston, MA, USA
e-mail: awkim@mgh.harvard.edu

© Springer Nature Switzerland AG 2021
A. R. Dyer et al. (eds.), *Global Mental Health Ethics*,
https://doi.org/10.1007/978-3-030-66296-7_10

employed among anthropologists who aspire to understand the languages that individuals of certain sociocultural groups use to express suffering, pain, or illness. These idioms or modes of expression are "typically unquestioned normativity" [16, p. 211] that reveals culturally located norms, values, and practices that inform not only experiences with distress but also methods and patterns of care-seeking and healing [14, 22, 80]. Despite interest and inclusion in the glossary of the most current Diagnostic and Statistical Manual (DSM-5) in psychiatry, these idioms are rarely assessed in biomedicine. This is in part because such idioms convey more than a medical diagnosis, often pointing to "interpersonal, social, political, economic, and spiritual sources of distress" [54, p. 402].

Despite decades of inquiry into idioms of distress and a longer history of studies on social suffering and morbidity, very few anthropologists have investigated the sociocultural dynamics that shape and promote positive health and well-being [5, 6, 15, 68] and the core concepts and expressions that reflect these experiences, often referred to as "resilience." Resilience has been long defined by doing well amid adversity, with a focus on how individual traits may facilitate positive adaptation. Anthropological contributions have pushed thinking about resilience toward a more nuanced perception of what social and cultural complexities impact and how people and communities are resilient. Some have focused on the various processes through which social, cultural, and political factors foster resilience and vulnerability alike [9, 38, 39, 52, 56, 57, 74, 82]. Such work has been exemplified in scholarship among indigenous people and the collective identities that foster unique, locally rooted strength through time and space. For instance, Laurence Kirmayer et al. [26] argue that "collective and cultural terms" (85) are fundamental, such as the "Inuit concept of *niriunniq*, an Inuktitut word that can be glossed as hope. Faced with adversity, people talk of hope and wait for it to reveal itself. For many, it is an elusive experience, but its potency as a life-giving force is never questioned" (88). In her work among indigenous communities in the Arctic, Lisa Wexler [79] argues that "cultural ideas of self situate people as part of something larger" and "offer people a way to understand their problems and difficulties as part of a collective experience that has been overcome by people like them" (86). This is exemplified by Sara Lewis's [38] work with Tibetan Buddhists, where the practice of *lojong*, or mind training, can create the possibility to mitigate suffering by cultivating compassion for others (often in the same situation) and reflecting on emptiness – a term referring to resilience or "an active process – an approach for meeting life's inevitable problems with openness, humor, and compassion" [1]. Thus, many anthropologists consider resilience to be a concept or experience found within suffering, not in spite of it [29, 38, 39, 73, 79, 82].

In this chapter, we revisit central arguments we and others have made on idioms of distress and idioms of resilience (see [23, 46, 48]) across various cultural contexts and propose an extension of the idioms of distress framework as an effective approach to examine the culturally significant ways of exhibiting resilience in a given cultural context. First, we begin by introducing the idiom of distress "thinking too much" to address some of the key features and framing of the idiom. Then, we discuss the utility of idioms of resilience by revisiting our work on the idiom of resilience "acceptance." Finally, we discuss the advantages of using this framework from anthropology for thinking about global mental health and the drawbacks of moving within and between such thinking in anthropology and biomedicine when considering how to deliver high-quality, locally relevant mental health care in diverse contexts.

Idiom of Distress: The Case of Thinking Too Much

Scholarly interest in the idiom of distress "thinking too much" or "thinking a lot" exemplifies the ways in which such idioms hold global and local relevance because the idiom reveals both broad cross-cultural usage [16, 18, 22, 35, 62, 80] and localization of social, psychological, and somatic symptoms [19, 77]. Some of the earliest work on "thinking too much" in Zimbabwe, known as *kufungisisa* in Shona, exemplified this tension. On the one hand, *kufungisisa* revealed that the idiom communicated how people related distress with a supernatural cause or social stressor [61, 62]. On the other hand, Patel and colleagues argued that "thinking too much" in Zimbabwe demonstrated significant overlap with depression and anxiety, thereby signaling that it could inform biomedical diagnoses [60]. Their argument was met with criticism by those who argued that psychiatric utilization of cultural concepts often reifies culture, perceiving it as a static measure [70], when instead it is a fluid and interactive construct shaped by history, politics, and society [21, 25]. From this tension, we gain insight into how a globally relevant concept is situated into a cultural milieu, given meaning, and becomes relevant for both clinical and anthropological practice.

Many anthropologists believe that idioms like "thinking too much" are important because they communicate implicit critique of structural inequalities such as racism, sexism, and displacement [8, 45, 54, 63, 80]. For instance, Nicaraguan grandmothers used "thinking too much" (*pensando mucho*) to communicate distress associated with families fragmented by migration [80] that manifests somatically in the head and neck [81]. Similarly, the extensive work on trauma and recovery among Cambodian refugees embeds the experience of "thinking a lot" within a web of social, somatic, and psychological responses that eventually manifest in a form of panic and physical shock [16–18]. Despite the similarities in the idiom conveyed (thinking), the ways in which these idioms of distress were experienced differed significantly, revealing how "thinking too much" may take on different meaning from place-to-place and across landscapes of social inequality and also convey various social, cultural, political, and somatic factors. This is what Hinton et al. [19] have called a process of "localization" where the construct incorporates local social, psychological, and somatic experiences.

On the other hand, "thinking too much" is one of the most commonly catalogued idioms, represented globally in ethnographic studies and included as one of the cultural concepts of distress in the DSM-5 [16, 22]. This may be why many scholars have posed that "thinking too much" conveys biomedical useful symptoms to identify psychiatric disorders [3, 16, 22, 35, 60] and argue for the utility of using the cultural idiom in mental health interventions as markers of pathology [35, 72]. For example, research on idioms of distress among Cambodian refugees reveals that *khyâl* closely relates to anxiety and panic [17] and *kut caraeun* (or "thinking a lot") is an important indicator of post-traumatic stress disorder [18]. Similarly, *kufungisisa* closely relates to anxiety and depression among the Shona [60]. In Rwanda, *agahinda gakabije* encompasses symptoms of depression [4] and the idiom matched a diagnosis of depression [3]. In Kenya, "thinking too much" has been associated with depression [13, 49, 50] and identified as an independent distress diagnosis in community settings [44]. Yet, Paul Bolton [3] has argued that matching such idioms with psychopathology is not enough: in order to achieve validity, a local idiom of distress must be compared with a real-time psychiatric diagnosis to demonstrate how idioms may align with clinical diagnoses. In part, he argues that "legitimizing" such symptoms may empower patients and provide them greater access to available resources, such as counseling or social support, and improve diagnoses of mental illness in culturally diverse settings [3].

But matching cultural idioms with psychopathology also runs the risk of medicalizing cultural idioms to fit within a biomedical frame intelligible to clinical medicine, which may have unforeseen consequences, such as misinterpretations or failure to address the problem of greatest concern to the patient [35]. This speaks in part to what Derek Summerfield [71] has called "psychological imperialism," where acute trauma is co-opted in humanitarian or development contexts in order to provide quick technological fixes or counseling. For instance, Nichter [54] has argued that the pharmaceutical industry seeking profit might reframe an experience of suffering to reflect a psychiatric or medical problem. Abramowitz [1] has illuminated this phenomenon through the problem of the "Open Mole," an idiom of distress in Liberia that became an indicator for post-traumatic stress disorder through a process driven by humanitarian agencies. The Open Mole example shows how external actors may fundamentally shift how an idiom is utilized within a community and thereby transform how people interpret and internalize such idioms. Such an approach is misleading not only because it renders cultural idioms of distress to be static entities but also because it undermines the value of cultural idioms as embodiments of political, social, and somatic experiences.

The majority of research on "thinking too much" in Kenya focuses on how the idiom relates to pathology and specifically depression [13, 41, 43, 44, 49, 50, 53]. Many others associate "thinking too much" explicitly with social and psychological suffering, differentiating it from pathology. For instance, one study found traditional health practitioners who encounter patients with low mood in their Kenyan practices often give patients diagnoses of "thinking too much" or "stressed" rather than depression or another biomedical term [44]. Ice and Yogo (2005) found that the Luo ethnic community uses the term *jachir* to describe "thinking too much" when expressing stress. Pike and Williams (2006) found Turkana pastoralist women incorporate the mind-body interactions of thinking "so much your head hurts" and "your heart beats fast" (732). South Sudanese refugees in Kenya prioritized "thinking too much" as their most concerning psychosocial problem [2]. Similarly, a cross-cultural study of "thinking too much" among communities recovering from conflict in sub-Saharan Africa revealed that loss, sadness, and social withdrawal were key features, which required social remedies such as family support or traditional/faith healers as opposed to medical intervention [77].

The first author has argued that *kufikiria sana* (thinking too much in KiSwahili) plays a central role in the ethnopsychology of people seeking care at a public district hospital in urban Kenya by revealing some overlaps with pathology (depression, mostly) [13, 41, 43, 44, 49, 50, 53] as well as clear links to social and psychological suffering [2, 20, 44, 64]. Mendenhall, Bosire, and colleagues [47] found that *kufikiria sana* or "thinking too much" also relayed with emic narratives of *huzuni* to describe the increasing severity of grief [37]. But the most important finding was that "thinking too much" transverses emic and etic idioms of distress, weaving together concepts of *huzuni*, stress, and depression. These scholars argued that (1) an ethnopsychology of idioms of distress in Kenya highlights the role of social and political factors in driving people to express and experience cultural idioms of distress; (2) English terms stress and depression have been adopted into Kiswahili discourse and potentially taken on new meaning in the urban Kenyan context; (3) the role of rumination in how people express distress, with increasing severity, is closely linked to the concept of "thinking too much"; and (4) somatization is central to how people think about psychological suffering, locating social or political stress and distress in the heart and mind-brain.

In this way, thinking too much can provide a useful way to think about social and political drivers of psychological distress, integration of traditional/local and biomedical/global terms, rumination with increasing intensities, and somatization. In this case, *kufikiria sana* is both common idiom of distress and sign or symptom of increasing intensity of thinking within this ethnopsychology. As such, idioms of distress, while providing significant cultural and social meaning in their own right, may also reflect signs and symptoms of other idioms, from traditional idioms of distress to more biomedical terms. Using the same framework, we next examine the concept of resilience to understand its culturally specific meanings across contexts.

Theorizing Idioms of Resilience

Scholarship on resilience has emerged as a multidisciplinary research trend that explores the factors that contribute to positive psychological adaptation in the face of adverse social conditions across the life course [11, 39, 69]. Some of the earliest research on resilience pursued within fields like social psychology and neurobiology largely focused on the individual-level traits and characteristics that shape one's ability to successfully cope with adversity and lives in adverse social conditions. More recently, resilience research has adopted a socioecological and processual approach, examining how varying contexts shape positive outcomes despite adversity at the level of individuals, families, societies, and cultures [40, 58, 76]. Anthropological studies on stress, coping, and health repeatedly highlight the relational, societal, and structural dynamics that undergird both suffering and healing [10, 39, 42, 45, 52], and the field is ideally suited to advance resilience research.

Nevertheless, only a small handful of anthropologists has explicitly studied the processes that underlie psychological resilience (e.g., [9, 22, 23, 38, 39, 52, 56, 74, 82]). Attending to the full spectrum of subjective experiences of health and well-being not only helps us identify the social factors that facilitate "resilience" but also understand the complex cultural and sociopolitical dynamics that situate and structure disparities among individuals' responses to adversity.

An anthropological lens extends process-oriented and socioecological approaches further to trace how individuals and communities cultivate resilience by drawing on cultural and collective resources and meanings while facing constant interaction with adversity [30]. Here, the anthropological approach incorporates an understanding of life trajectories – from the physical realities of consistently facing adversity, to the social, economic, and cultural factors that foster strength, hope, and joy amid difficult times that may serve to protect one's health [58]. For example, Zraly and colleagues [82] illustrate that motherhood acts as a powerful social role that bolsters resilience among Rwandan genocide-rape survivors through reducing the stigma of genocide-rape, fostering positive emotions and reasons to live, and practicing maternal desire-mediated distress tolerance. Furthermore, anthropological scholarship contributes attention to political-economic forces as part of the intersectional forms of oppression individuals or communities face. For example, Aimee Cox [7] tactfully traces how Black women experiencing homelessness contest marginalizing stereotypes and exercise creative and nonnormative solutions to simultaneously combat poverty, antiblack racism, and sexism in their lives. Additionally, in her study of Afghan adults and children, Catherine Panter-Brick poignantly articulates how cultural values like living an "honorable life" (*izzat* in Dari and Pashto) bolstered resilience through developing a sense of order and meaning to life, though adherence to such values in the face of material poverty and educational insecurity was ultimately futile, forcing individuals to experience "entrapment" – the intense social frustrations brought about by failure to attain cultural milestones [9].

A second major contribution from the anthropology of resilience illuminates how collective and cultural ways-of-being shape how people are resilient [51, 74], moving beyond predominant resilience research that is "western-based with an emphasis on individual and relational factors" [75, p. 218]. The formation of meaning-making processes that structure resilience is specific to the social histories and cultural systems through which expressions of resilience emerge. For example, Foxen [11] describes how the K'iche' Mayan community in Guatemala draws on collective memories of successful community resistance against violent land claims and government militarization to heal from historic trauma and stay resilient to future political oppression. Ultimately, it is important to recognize that what fosters resilience among one individual, community, or population cannot be directly applied to another. Significantly, cultural examinations of resilience rectify how seemingly negative or maladaptive reactions to adversity may in fact be processes of resilience at play. Lewis [38] describes how Tibetan exiles enact the cultural practice of mind-training (*lojong*) and create more "flexible minds" to accommodate change, distress, and negative emotions. While it may seem that Tibetan exiles are merely coping and acquiescent to the extraordinary violence and suffering in their lives, learning to train one's mind to better deal with adversity fulfills religiously motivated goals of repaying one's karmic debt and ultimately achieving Buddhist cultural values of happiness.

We define resilience by a socially meaningful and culturally resonant means of experiencing and expressing positive adaption and well-being amid adverse situations – whether chronic or acute – achieved by drawing on personal, cultural, social, political, and economic resources (see [23, 46]). They might include forms of positive coping, thriving, and locally situated support systems. Idioms of resilience highlight the culturally salient processes that individuals use to cope with the complexities they face being-in-the-world. These culturally salient expressions of resilience can also serve as social markers to be used to uncover processes that may be otherwise unrecognized or undervalued by the clinician or researcher [40].

As previously discussed, the idiom of distress heuristic has been an effective tool to identify the wide variety of multidomain sources and manifestations of distress that are both culturally salient and socially patterned within a given cultural context. Idioms of distress not only are limited to linguistic utterances but also have included a wider array of semiotic expression such as clinically relevant behavior patterns (e.g., healthcare seeking and medication-taking behaviors), particular forms of cultural practice, and coping mechanisms (e.g., smoking and drinking) [54]. Similar to the diverse communicative nature of the idioms of distress heuristic, we recognize that resilience is also a multidomain phenomenon and can manifest through a wide variety of cultural expressions through language and behavior.

Idioms of resilience may also enrich cross-cultural clinical practice and health promotion efforts by identifying culturally salient resources and processes that structure and reinforce healing and recovery but may not be visible to clinical observation. Idioms of resilience may index certain perspectives of disease or health practices that are individually and culturally understood to promote healing and well-being but are inherently contradictory to biomedical models of disease. For example, supernatural expressions of health and illness are typically seen as barriers to healthcare-seeking by humanitarian practitioners in rural Haiti [34], but Kaiser [22] shows that concepts like sent spirits may be protective for well-being and should not be displaced for a more culturally sensitive approach to global mental health.

Idioms of resilience contributes to new theories, methods, research, and practice that cross-cut fields. Such an approach can serve the theoretical and methodological interests of multiple disciplines and provide an innovative way to understand points of intervention related to how individuals uncover ideas, reasons, and motivations to seek certain types of care within a pluralistic healthcare system. For instance, an idiom of resilience can serve as a methodological tool to develop culturally specific assessments of determinants and dimensions of resilience (see [65, 78] for examples of using idioms of distress to construct culturally specific mental health scales). We also hope the idiom of resilience concept will encourage deeper engagement and critical evaluation of the concept of resilience. In the following section, we describe our study of cancer patients in South Africa as one example of how idioms of resilience can be useful for broader discourses in anthropology, transcultural psychiatry, medicine, and public health (for other examples of idioms of resilience and well-being, see [6, 68]).

The Idiom of Acceptance as Process of Resilience

In our work in South Africa, we found that *ukwamukela,* the notion of "acceptance" of one's disease diagnosis (in this case, cancer), serves as an idiom of resilience (see [23]). We argued that acceptance is a *process* of resilience, which is necessarily shaped by the collective and relational factors that produce resilience in spite of the extraordinary social suffering. The embodied experience of accepting one's "fate," typically in relation to a disease diagnosis, injury, or social stress, facilitated a positive way of coping with the challenges people diagnosed with cancer face in Soweto. Despite intense treatment and, in many cases, a somewhat late diagnosis of cancer, many interlocutors conveyed a tepid view of their cancer and other medical conditions, recognizing how family priorities and social relations not only took precedence to individual vulnerability, disease, and social problems but also curbed negative emotions and feelings, facilitated adherence to clinical treatment, and helped normalize their condition. The themes that emerged from our study help support the shift away from a trait-based conceptualization and individual-level expression of resilience; the idiom of acceptance conveys a cognitive process rooted in ideas of the collective about putting social and religious community above the self.

We also found that the existence and impact of social support from individuals like family members, friends, church members, and in particular, a higher being (God) facilitated people's ability to avoid "holding in" stress by "letting go" of these concerns and, eventually, *accept* their circumstance. This process of acceptance was not only associated with people's cancer diagnosis but also other social traumas such as a car crash, family troubles, financial problems, other medical conditions, and so on. Receiving medical care played a similar salutogenic role as social support by allowing people to let go of their embodied social stress. The fact that many participants described releasing distress and worry as a form of prevention from disease explained how closely people interpreted the experience of internalizing social stress with materialization of problems in the brain and heart. Thus, understanding the process of cognition through which people perceive acceptance and the release of negative emotion as a form of disease prevention may be beneficial for clinical practice. Notwithstanding, the roles of social relationships, religious belonging, strong family bonds, and other communities of care in facilitating cancer patients to ultimately accept disease diagnosis could be relevant for clinicians and public health practitioners to promote medical adherence and reduce stigma.

While the acceptance of something like cancer may seem like an expression of fatalism, and thus, surrendering to hardship, the utility of acceptance as a tool for resilience is illuminated by situating it in a larger explanatory model and cultural context. Those who did not accept their present state of adversity were thought to develop a suite of stress-related diseases like depression and "high blood" (a cultural idiom for high blood pressure and/or hypertension). Individuals who accepted their cancer diagnosis or injury appeared to have fewer physical and psychological symptoms, such as "thinking too much," and thus appeared more "resilient" to the deleterious embodied impacts of internalizing distress associated with a new diagnosis and the experience of cancer. This finding reminds us that when researchers view resilience in relation to the cultural context that the resilient individual is situated in, the meanings and outcomes of "resilient" behavior may be different from what we assume (see [38]).

Thinking Forward

Before we close, we reflect on the utilities and applications of idioms of distress and idioms of resilience, their quantification, and translations across contexts. First, reorienting how we think about suffering and resilience is an imperative next step for anthropology and particularly applied, psychological, and medical anthropology. When thinking about resilience, we must keep culture-in-mind [66], as the power of how people envision themselves within the world around them plays an important role in how they perceive and respond to challenges from their social world. We suggest a rethink of medical anthropology's emphasis on the concept of *suffering* alongside the concept of *resilience* by cultivating a lens that moves within and between what fosters sickness and wellness. Jeff Snodgrass et al. [67] have described this approach as evaluating "emotional balance" between emotional frailty and emotional resilience/balance; this method and meditation focus on how people experience and navigate their emotional worlds in real time (as opposed to ex-factor remembrance). In this work, they focus more on the relative frequency in which people experience emotions—engaging agnostically with biomedical or local nosologies—and drawing from emotional realities. Such an approach should integrate the nuanced scholarship around resilience that focuses upon how resilience thrives through (as opposed to in spite) of suffering (see [79]).

Second, we need to reconsider the utility of quantifying the concept of resilience and translating it across contexts. This was the focus of a recent article [78] that focused on developing culturally rooted measures of distress through integration of ethnographic and empirical measures. Weaver and Kaiser state, "this ethnographic focus is important for preserving the variation in distress experiences, for making apparent to readers what specific aspects of distress are (or are not) measured by the scales being developed, and for increasing transparency" (p. 3). This statement further affirms the fact that local knowledge is imperative for designing such scales and for interpreting them (although this is no surprise to anthropologists studying resilience). Yet, such scales may tip the balance of focus within the context of biomedical thinking and evaluation of psychiatric distress. On the one hand, it may be that scales capturing resilience fail to do so in part because of the apathy toward the concept in biomedicine. On the other hand, ethnographically rooted scales – and perhaps those designed through participatory methods – may be meaningful because they require collective and cultural terms for strength, hope, survival, and other aspects of the social fabric that so often are excluded from the focus on distress or suffering. Similarly, Clare Herrick [15] has argued, "when our conceptualization of suffering extends beyond the individual as vulnerable victim to think through the contexts in which victimhood may be more problematically or ambiguously configured […] we become drawn to an array of different spaces of health production, erosion and negotiation where suffering is experienced and produced" (531). As such, resilience itself may be a community-level or political-level construct that becomes meaningless when conscribed to a scale-like format.

In conclusion, how people think about suffering and resilience – and what fosters both concepts from one place to the next – is culturally scripted and socially reproduced. We have considered how both distress and resilience are communicated across contexts. Returning to the question of scale, locally derived and collectively determined factors that may mediate "emotional balance" are imperative to understand a fair representation of "resilience" amid a preoccupation with "suffering". Taking stock of these meanings and the making of tools to evaluate how people feel and experience diverse emotions is imperative for understanding what drives good mental health and what causes the most distress. Communicating culturally relevant understandings of psychological disease, health, and well-being across the world, especially when care-seeking, will continue to be a critical challenge for global mental health.

References

1. Abramowitz, S. A. (2010). Trauma and humanitarian translation in Liberia: The tale of Open Mole. *Culture, Medicine and Psychiatry, 34*, 353–379. https://doi.org/10.1007/s11013-010-9172-0.
2. Adaku, A., Okello, J., Lowry, B., Kane, J. C., Alderman, S., Musisi, S., & Tol, W. A. (2016). Mental health and psychosocial support for South Sudanese refugees in northern Uganda: A needs and resource assessment. *Conflict and Health, 10*, 18. https://doi.org/10.1186/s13031-016-0085-6.
3. Bolton, P. (2001). Cross-cultural validity and reliability testing of a standard psychiatric assessment instrument without a gold standard. *The Journal of Nervous and Mental Disease, 189*, 238–242.
4. Bolton, P., Bass, J., Verdeli, H., Clougherty, K. F., & Ndogoni, L. (2003). Group interpersonal psychotherapy for depression in rural Uganda: Randomized controlled trial. *JAMA, 289*, 3117–3124.
5. Butt, L. (2002). The suffering stranger: Medical anthropology and international morality. *Medical Anthropology, 21*(1), 1–24.
6. Cassaniti, J. (2019). Keeping it together: Idioms of success and distress: In northern Thai Buddhist mindlessness. *Transcultural Psychiatry, 56*(4), 697–719.
7. Cox, A. M. (2015). *Shapeshifters: Black girls and the choreography of citizenship*. Durham, NC: Duke University Press.
8. Duncan, W. L. (2015). Transnational disorders: Returned migrants at Oaxaca's psychiatric hospital. *Medical Anthropology Quarterly, 29*, 24–41.
9. Eggerman, M., & Panter-Brick, C. (2010). Suffering, hope, and entrapment: Resilience and cultural values in Afghanistan. *Social Science & Medicine, 71*, 71–83. https://doi.org/10.1016/j.socscimed.2010.03.023.
10. Farmer, P. (2001). *Infections and inequalities: The modern plagues*. Berkeley: University of California.

11. Foxen, P. (2010). Local narratives of distress and resilience: Lessons in psychosocial well-being among the K'iche'Maya in postwar Guatemala. *The Journal of Latin American and Caribbean Anthropology, 15*(1), 66–89.
12. Good, B. (1997). Studying mental illness in context: Local, global, or universal? *Ethos, 25*, 230–248.
13. Grant, E., Murray, S. A., Grant, A., & Brown, J. (2003a). A good death in rural Kenya? Listening to Meru patients and their families talk about care needs at the end of life. *Journal of Palliative Care, 19*, 159–167. https://doi.org/10.1016/S1636-6522(04)97849-X.
14. Guarnaccia, P. (1992). Ataque de nervios in Puerto Rico: Culture-bound syndrome or popular illness? *Medical Anthropology, 15*, 1–14.
15. Herrick, C. (2017). When places come first: Suffering, archetypal space and the problematic production of global health. *Transactions of the Institute of British Geographers, 42*(4), 530–543. https://doi.org/10.1111/tran.12186.
16. Hinton, D. E., & Lewis-Fernández, R. (2010). Idioms of distress among trauma survivors: Subtypes and clinical utility. *Culture, Medicine and Psychiatry, 34*, 209–218. https://doi.org/10.1007/s11013-010-9175-x.
17. Hinton, D. E., Pich, V., Marques, L., Nickerson, A., & Pollack, M. H. (2010). Khyâl attacks: A key idiom of distress among traumatized Cambodia refugees. *Culture, Medicine and Psychiatry, 34*, 244–278.
18. Hinton, D. E., Reis, R., & de Jong, J. (2015). The "thinking a lot" idiom of distress and PTSD: An examination of their relationship among traumatized Cambodian refugees using the "thinking a lot" questionnaire. *Medical Anthropology Quarterly, 29*, 357–380. https://doi.org/10.1111/maq.12204.
19. Hinton, D. E., Reis, R., & de Jong, J. T. (2016). A transcultural model of the centrality of "thinking a lot" in psychopathologies across the globe and the process of localization: A Cambodian refugee example. *Culture, Medicine and Psychiatry, 40*, 570–619.
20. Ice, G. H., & Yogo, J. (2005). Measuring stress among luo elders: Development of the luo perceived stress scale. *Field Methods, 17*(4), 394–411.
21. Jenkins, J. (2015). *Extraordinary conditions: Culture and experience in mental illness*. Berkeley: University of California Press.
22. Kaiser, B. N., Haroz, E. E., Kohrt, B. A., Bolton, P. A., Bass, J. K., & Hinton, D. E. (2015). "Thinking too much": A systematic review of a common idiom of distress. *Social Science & Medicine, 147*, 170–183. https://doi.org/10.1016/j.socscimed.2015.10.044.
23. Kim, A. W., Kaiser, B., Bosire, E., Shahbazian, K., & Mendenhall, E. (2019). Idioms of resilience among cancer patients in urban South Africa: An anthropological heuristic for the study of culture and resilience. *Transcultural Psychiatry, 56*(4), 720–747.
24. Kirmayer, L. J. (2006). Culture and psychotherapy in a creolizing world. *Transcultural Psychiatry, 43*, 163–168. https://doi.org/10.1177/1363461506064846.
25. Kirmayer, L. J. (2012). Rethinking cultural competence. *Transcultural Psychiatry, 49*, 149–164. https://doi.org/10.1177/1363461512444673.
26. Kirmayer, L. J., Dandeneau, S., Marshall, E., Phillips, M. K., & Williamson, K. J. (2011). Rethinking resilience from indigenous perspectives. *Canadian Journal of Psychiatry, 56*, 84–91. https://doi.org/10.1177/070674371105600203.
27. Kirmayer, L. J., Gone, J., & Moses, J. (2014). Rethinking historical trauma. *Transcultural Psychiatry, 51*, 299–319.
28. Kirmayer, L. J., Lemelson, R., & Barad, M. (2007). *Understanding trauma: Integrating biological, clinical, and cultural perspectives*. Cambridge: Cambridge University Press.
29. Kirmayer, L., & Pedersen, D. (2014). Toward a new architecture for global mental health. *Transcultural Psychiatry, 51*, 759–776. https://doi.org/10.1177/1363461514557202.
30. Kirmayer, L. J., Sehdev, M., Whitley, R., Dandeneau, S. F., & Isaac, C. (2013). Community resilience: Models, metaphors and measures. *International Journal of Indigenous Health, 5*(1), 62–117.
31. Kirmayer, L. J., & Young, A. (1998). Culture and somatization: Clinical, epidemiological, and ethnographic perspectives. *Psychosomatic Medicine, 60*, 420–430.

32. Kleinman, A. (1980). *Patients and healers in the context of culture: An exploration of the borderland between anthropology, medicine, and psychiatry*. Berkeley: University of California Press.
33. Kleinman, A., & Good, B. (1985). *Culture and depression: Studies in the anthropology and cross-cultural psychiatry of affect and disorder*. Berkeley: University of California Press.
34. Khoury, N. M., Kaiser, B. N., Keys, H. M., Brewster, A. R. T., & Kohrt, B. A. (2012). Explanatory models and mental health treatment: Is vodou an obstacle to psychiatric treatment in rural Haiti? *Culture, Medicine and Psychiatry, 36*(3), 514–534.
35. Kohrt, B. a., Rasmussen, A., Kaiser, B. N., Haroz, E. E., Maharjan, S. M., Mutamba, B. B., De Jong, J. T. V. M., & Hinton, D. E. (2014a). Cultural concepts of distress and psychiatric disorders: Literature review and research recommendations for global mental health epidemiology. *International Journal of Epidemiology, 43*, 365–406. https://doi.org/10.1093/ije/dyt227.
36. Kohrt, B. A., & Mendenhall, E. (2015). *Global mental health: Anthropological perspectives*. Walnut Creek, CA: Left Coast Press.
37. Kumar, M., Ongeri, L., Mathai, M., & Mbwayo, A. (2015). Translation of EPDS questionnaire into Kiswahili: Understanding the cross-cultural and translation issues in mental health research. *Journal of Pregnancy Child Health, 2*, 1–5. https://doi.org/10.417 2/2376-127X.1000134.
38. Lewis, S. (2018). Resilience, agency, and everyday Lojong in the Tibetan diaspora. *Contemporary Buddhism, 19*(2), 342–361. https://doi.org/10.1080/14639947.2018.1480153.
39. Lewis, S. E. (2013). Trauma and the making of flexible minds in the Tibetan exile community. *Ethos, 41*, 313–336. https://doi.org/10.1111/etho.12024.
40. Luthar, S. S. (2015). Resilience in development: A synthesis of research across five decades. In D. Cicchetti & D. J. Cohen (Eds.), *Developmental psychopathology: Risk, disorder, and adaptation* (pp. 739–795). Hoboken: Wiley.
41. Mamah, D., Striley, C., Ndetei, D., Mbwayo, A., Mutiso, V., Khasakhala, L., & Cottler, L. (2013). Knowledge of psychiatric terms and concepts among Kenyan youth: Analysis of focus group discussions. *Transcultural Psychiatry, 50*, 515–531.
42. Manderson, L., & Smith-Morris, C. (2010). *Chronic conditions, fluid states: Chronicity and the anthropology of illness*. New Brunswick: Rutgers University Press.
43. Marangu, E., Sands, N., Rolley, J., Ndetei, D., & Mansouri, F. (2014). Mental healthcare in Kenya: Exploring optimal conditions for capacity building. *African Journal of Primary Health Care & Family Medicine, 6*, 5.
44. Mbwayo, A., Ndetei, D., Mutiso, V., & Khasakhala, L. (2013). Traditional healers and provision of mental health services in cosmopolitan informal settlements in Nairobi, Kenya. *The African Journal of Psychiatry, 16*, 134–140.
45. Mendenhall, E. (2012). *Syndemic suffering: Social distress, depression, and diabetes among mexican immigrant women*. New York: Routledge.
46. Mendenhall, E., & Kim, A. W. (2019). How to fail a scale: Reflections on a failed attempt to assess resilience. *Culture, Medicine and Psychiatry, 43*(2), 315–325.
47. Mendenhall, E., Rinehart, R., Musyimi, C., Bosire, E., Ndetei, D., & Mutiso, V. (2019). An ethnopsychology of idioms of distress in urban kenya. *Transcultural Psychiatry, 56*(4), 620–642.
48. Mendenhall, E., Rinehart, R., Musyimi, C. W., Bosire, E., Ndetei, D. M., & Mutiso, V. I. (2018). An ethnopsychology of idioms of distress in Urban Kenya. *Transcultural Psychiatry, 56*(4), 620–642.
49. Muga, F., & Jenkins, R. (2008a). Training, attitudes and practice of district health workers in Kenya. *Social Psychiatry and Psychiatric Epidemiology, 43*, 477–482.
50. Muga, F. A., & Jenkins, R. (2008b). Public perceptions, explanatory models and service utilisation regarding mental illness and mental health care in Kenya. *Social Psychiatry and Psychiatric Epidemiology, 43*, 469–476. https://doi.org/10.1007/s00127-008-0334-0.
51. Mullings, L. (2005). Resistance and resilience: The sojourner syndrome and the social context of reproduction in central Harlem. *Transforming Anthropology, 13*, 79–91.
52. Mullings, L., & Wali, A. (2001). *Stress and resilience: The social context of reproduction in central Harlem*. New York: Springer. https://doi.org/10.1007/978-1-4615-1369-8.

53. Musyimi, C. W., Mutiso, V. N., Nandoya, E. S., & Ndetei, D. M. (2016). Forming a joint dialogue among faith healers, traditional healers and formal health workers in mental health in a Kenyan setting: Towards common grounds. *Journal of Ethnobiology and Ethnomedicine, 12*, 4. https://doi.org/10.1186/s13002-015-0075-6.
54. Nichter, M. (2010). Idioms of distress revisited. *Culture, Medicine and Psychiatry, 34*, 401–416. https://doi.org/10.1007/s11013-010-9179-6.
55. Nichter, M. (1981). Idioms of distress: Alternatives in the expression of psychosocial distress: A case study from south India. *Culture, Medicine and Psychiatry, 5*, 379–408.
56. Obrist, B., & Büchi, S. (2008). Stress as an idiom for resilience: Health and migration among sub-Saharan Africans in Switzerland. *Anthropology & Medicine, 15*, 251–261.
57. Panter-Brick, C. (2014). Health, risk, and resilience: Interdisciplinary concepts and applications. *Annual Review of Anthropology, 43*, 431–448. https://doi.org/10.1146/annurev-anthro-102313-025944.
58. Panter-Brick, C., & Eggerman, M. (2012). Understanding culture, resilience, and mental health: The production of hope. In *The social ecology of resilience* (pp. 369–386). New York: Springer.
59. Patel, V. (2014). Why mental health matters to global health. *Transcultural Psychiatry, 51*, 777–789.
60. Patel, V., Abas, M., Broadhead, J., Todd, C., & Reeler, A. (2001a). Depression in developing countries: Lessons from Zimbabwe. *BMJ, 322*, 482–484.
61. Patel, V., Gwanzura, F., Simunyu, E., Lloyd, K., & Mann, A. (1995a). The phenomenology and explanatory models of common mental disorder: A study in primary care in Harare, Zimbabwe. *Psychological Medicine, 25*, 1191–1200.
62. Patel, V., Simunyu, E., & Gwanzura, F. (1995). Kufungisisa (thinking too much): A Shona idiom for non-psychotic mental illness. *The Central African Journal of Medicine, 41*, 209–215.
63. Pedersen, D., Kienzler, H., & Gamarra, J. (2010). Llaki and Ñakary: Idioms of distress and suffering among the highland Quechua in the Peruvian Andes. *Culture, Medicine and Psychiatry, 34*, 279–300.
64. Pike, I. L., & Williams, S. R. (2006). Incorporating psychosocial health into biocultural models: Preliminary findings from Turkana women of Kenya. *American Journal of Human Biology, 18*, 729–740.
65. Rasmussen, A., Katoni, B., Keller, A. S., & Wilkinson, J. (2011). Posttraumatic idioms of distress among Darfur refugees: Hozun and Majnun. *Transcultural Psychiatry, 48*(4), 392–415.
66. Shore, B. (1998). *Culture in mind: Cognition, culture, and the problem of meaning*. Oxford: Oxford University Press.
67. Snodgrass, J. G., Lacy, M. G., & Upadhyay, C. (2017). Developing culturally sensitive affect scales for global mental health research and practice: Emotional balance, not named syndromes, in Indian Adivasi subjective well-being. *Social Science & Medicine, 187*, 174–183. https://doi.org/10.1016/j.socscimed.2017.06.037.
68. Snodgrass, J. G., Dengah, H. F., Polzer, E., & Else, R. (2018). Intensive online videogame involvement: A new global idiom of wellness and distress. *Transcultural Psychiatry, 56*(4), 748–774.
69. Southwick, S. M., Bonanno, G. A., Masten, A. S., Panter-Brick, C., & Yehuda, R. (2014). Resilience definitions, theory, and challenges: Interdisciplinary perspectives. *European Journal of Psychotraumatology, 5*(1), 25338.
70. Summerfield, D. (2008). How scientifically valid is the knowledge base of global mental health? *BMJ, 336*, 992–994.
71. Summerfield, D. (1999). A critique of seven assumptions behind psychological trauma programmes in war-affected areas. *Social Science & Medicine, 48*, 1449–1462.
72. Sweetland, A. C., Belkin, G. S., & Verdeli, H. (2014). Measuring depression and anxiety in Sub-Saharan Africa. *Depression and Anxiety, 31*, 223–232.
73. Trout, L., Wexler, L., & Moses, J. (2018). Beyond two worlds: Identity narratives and the aspirational futures of Alaska Native youth. *Transcultural Psychiatry, 55*(6), 800–820.
74. Ulturgasheva, O., Rasmus, S., & Morrow, P. (2015). Collapsing the distance: Indigenous-youth engagement in a circumpolar study of youth resilience. *Arctic Anthropology, 52*, 60–70.

75. Ungar, M. (2008). Resilience across Cultures. *British Journal of Social Work, 38*, 218–235. https://doi.org/10.1093/bjsw/bcl343.
76. Ungar, M. (2011). The social ecology of resilience: Addressing contextual and cultural ambiguity of a nascent construct. *The American Journal of Orthopsychiatry, 81*(1), 1.
77. Ventevogel, P., Jordans, M., Reis, R., & de Jong, J. (2013). Madness or sadness? Local concepts of mental illness in four conflict-affected African communities. *Conflict and Health, 7*, 3. https://doi.org/10.1186/1752-1505-7-3.
78. Weaver, L. J., & Kaiser, B. N. (2015). Developing and testing locally derived mental health scales examples from North India and Haiti. *Field Methods, 27*, 1150130.
79. Wexler, L. (2013). Looking across three generations of Alaska Natives to explore how culture fosters indigenous resilience. *Transcultural Psychiatry, 51*, 73–92.
80. Yarris, K. (2014). Pensando mucho ("Thinking Too Much"): Embodied distress among grandmothers in Nicaraguan transnational families. *Culture, Medicine and Psychiatry, 3*, 473–498.
81. Yarris, K. E. (2011). The pain of 'thinking too much': dolor de Cerebro and the embodiment of social hardship among Nicaraguan women. *Ethos, 39*, 226–248. https://doi.org/10.1111/j.1548-1352.2011.01186.x.THE.
82. Zraly, M., & Nyirazinyoye, L. (2010). Don't let the suffering make you fade away: An ethnographic study of resilience among survivors of genocide-rape in southern Rwanda. *Social Science & Medicine, 70*, 1656–1664.

Epidemiologic Linkages Between Childhood Trauma, Health, and Health Care

11

Megan Quinn

Introduction

Adverse Childhood Experiences (ACEs), such as neglect, physical, emotional, or sexual abuse, and household dysfunction, have been shown to be sources of extreme stress during childhood, which can have long-term consequences on health and well-being throughout the life course [42]. In the United States, the landmark ACE Study by Vincent Felitti and Robert Anda identified that trauma during childhood had a tremendous impact on adult health [16]. ACE survey methodology has become one of the standard tools for measuring the prevalence and correlates of childhood trauma, neglect, and household dysfunction. The ACE questions are typically asked along with other health-related questions and are asked to adults regarding experiences that occurred before the age of 18. The Violence Against Children Survey (VACS) is another standard tool for measuring violence against children. VACS asks questions to adolescents and adults of age 13–24 and provides nationally representative information for various countries on violence against children. The World Health Organization (WHO) ACE international questionnaire (ACE-IQ) was developed with the aim of measuring ACEs in all countries [42]. The ACE-IQ highlights multiple types of abuse, neglect, violence between parents or caregivers, household dysfunction, community, and war/collective violence, with the goal of understanding a comprehensive picture of the trauma that an individual may be exposed to before the age of 18, inclusive of all geographies.

Despite these tools, many countries lack extensive research on violence against children, ACEs, and comprehensive data on exposure to childhood trauma. Globally, the impact of different forms of trauma on the mental and physical health of adults has not been clearly established, but by understanding exposure to various forms of

M. Quinn (✉)
Department of Biostatistics and Epidemiology, College of Public Health, East Tennessee State University, Johnson City, TN, USA
e-mail: quinnm@etsu.edu

© Springer Nature Switzerland AG 2021
A. R. Dyer et al. (eds.), *Global Mental Health Ethics*,
https://doi.org/10.1007/978-3-030-66296-7_11

violence and dysfunction, future initiatives to reduce this adversity can be developed to address mental health needs in the global community.

We do know that ACEs are common and highly interrelated, and the occurrence of one should evoke the search for others. A dose-response relationship exists between a person's ACE score, the total of ACEs that occurred before the age of 18, and subsequent problems, such that as one's ACE score increases, so does the risk of problems across the lifespan [16]. In particular, United States-based ACE research has noted the strong, graded relationship between exposure to childhood adversity and a range of negative adult outcomes including smoking, severe obesity, depression, suicide attempts, alcoholism, and drug abuse [16]. ACEs have been shown to represent a conduit to lifelong behavioral, health, and social problems [2].

The original ACE study included 10 dichotomous items measuring child abuse, neglect, and family dysfunction; however, subsequent research involving urban youth in the United States identified an even broader domain of common adverse experiences, with evidence of polyvictimization that included exposure to violence, personal victimization, bullying, discrimination, and economic hardship [10]. At the socioeconomic level, child physical abuse has been associated with a lower likelihood of marriage and decreased education level and income, while parental intimate partner violence is associated with reduced income, and community violence exposure is associated with high odds of unemployment [10]. Conversely, adulthood socioeconomic factors including marriage, divorce and separation, income, educational attainment, and insurance status all mediate the association between ACEs and adult health risks [2]. Figure 11.1 illustrates ACEs, their impact, and long-term consequences of unaddressed ACEs.

Therefore, beyond the cumulative effect of adversity, furthering our understanding of the influence of individual types of ACEs, the interplay between ACEs and the social determinants of health, and the costs of childhood trauma is imperative. Furthermore, the connection between exposure to trauma during childhood and how that exposure serves as a foundation for how the mind and body develop throughout the lifespan is not fully understood.

Following the original ACE study, Robert Anda was quoted saying, "what's predictable is preventable," meaning that since we know that childhood trauma and exposure to toxic stress during childhood can cause negative effects in adulthood, we should be able to prevent and/or mitigate childhood trauma to deter negative adult physical and mental health outcomes [16]. In order to do that though, we must have a firm understanding of the contributors to childhood trauma, how childhood trauma can disrupt or influence mind-body connections and drive negative health, and how health care, mental health, and public health need to work together to address trauma and promote resilience for individuals and communities.

Adverse Childhood Experience* ACE Categories (Birth to 18)	Impact of Trauma and Health Risk Behaviors to Ease the Pain	Long-Term Consequences of Unaddressed Trauma (ACEs)	
Abuse of Child	*Neurobiologic Effects of Trauma*	*Disease and Disability*	
■ Emotional abuse	■ Disrupted neuro-development	■ Ischemic heart disease	
■ Physical abuse		■ Cancer	
■ Contact Sexual abuse	■ Difficulty controlling anger-rage	■ Chronic lung disease	
Trauma in Child's Household Environment	■ Hallucinations	■ Chronic emphysema	
	■ Depression - other MH Disorders	■ Asthma	
■ Alcohol and/or Drug User		■ Liver disease	
■ Chronically depressed, emotionally disturbed or suicidal household member	■ Panic reactions	■ Skeletal fractures	
	■ Anxiety	■ Poor self rated health	
	■ Multiple (6+) somatic problems	■ Sexually transmitted disease	
■ Mother treated violently	■ Sleep problems	■ HIV/AIDS	
	■ Impaired memory	*Serious Social Problems*	
■ Imprisoned household member	■ Flashbacks	■ Homelessness	
	■ Dissociation	■ Prostitution	
■ Not raised by both biological parents (Loss of parent - best by death unless suicide, - Worse by abandonment)	***Health Risk Behaviors***	■ Delinquency, violence, criminal	
	■ Smoking	■ Inability to sustain employment	
	■ Severe obesity		
	■ Physical inactivity	■ Re-victimization: rape, DV, bullying	**ACE>4**
Neglect of Child	■ Suicide attempts		AIOH x 7
■ Physical neglect	■ Alcoholism	■ Compromised ability to parent	Sex<15 x2
■ Emotional neglect	■ Drug abuse		Cancer x2
	■ 50+ sex partners	■ Negative alteratins in self perceptions and relationships with others	Emphysema x 4
* Above types of ACEs are the "heavy end" of abuse. *1 type = ACE score of 1	■ Repetition of original trauma		
	■ Self Injury	■ Altered systems of meaning	**ACE>6**
	■ Eating disorders		suicide attempt x30
	■ Perpetrate interpersonal violence	■ Intergenerational trauma	
		■ Long-term use of multiple human service systems	

Fig. 11.1 ACEs, impact, and long-term consequences [16]

Social Epidemiology and Epigenetics: Factors Influencing Childhood Trauma

Following the original ACE study, an ACE pyramid depicting how ACEs can impact an individual throughout the lifespan was created and distributed (Fig. 11.2). The figure also indicated scientific gaps that needed to be better understood—factors that could either protect from negative adult consequences or promote further negative effects throughout the life course.

However, the updated ACE pyramid illustrates a more comprehensive picture of childhood trauma and the contextual factors, including the social determinants of health, intergenerational, and historical trauma that the child is born into [6]. The life a child is born into lays the foundation for many health outcomes and can contribute to or deter from trauma during childhood. Figure 11.3 illustrates how those factors are the building blocks and how they influence ACEs.

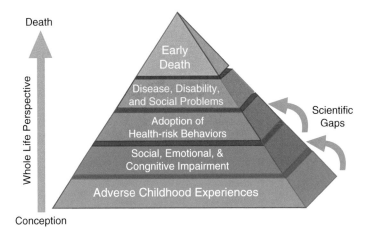

Fig. 11.2 ACE Pyramid [5]

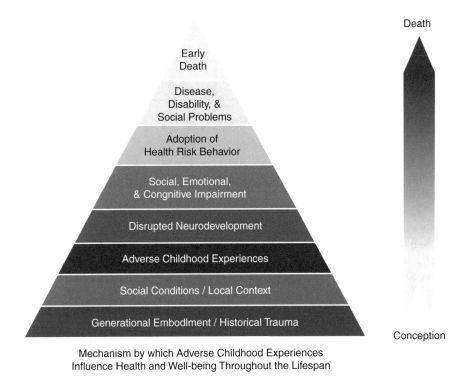

Mechanism by which Adverse Childhood Experiences
Influence Health and Well-being Throughout the Lifespan

Fig. 11.3 CDC ACE Pyramid [6]

Social Determinants of Health

Figure 11.3 depicts the social conditions/local context as the level on the pyramid before ACEs. These conditions and context include the social determinants of health, which were outlined in detail in the 2003 World Health Organization report, Social Determinants of Health: The Solid Facts, edited by Professor Richard Wilkinson and Sir Michael Marmot. The report indicated that a person's lifestyle and their living and working conditions influenced health and that genes alone did not determine an individual's health status [40]. Social determinants of health are defined as conditions in the environment where a person is born, lives, works, learns, grows, etc. that contribute to a variety of health, quality of life, and risk factors [20]. For example, social determinants of health such as access to health care, literacy, and social support can play a large role in an individual's overall well-being and quality of life. Furthermore, when social determinants of health are less than ideal, this can provide an environment for ACEs to flourish. For example, social determinants like parent education and poverty can contribute to increased ACEs associated with household dysfunction such as parental divorce, witnessing interpersonal violence in the home, parent/caregiver abuse of alcohol or substances, or parent/caregiver incarceration.

While public health regularly uses social determinants of health in research, programs, and interventions, health care has not historically intervened on issues related to social determinants of health. Community mental health resources may account for social determinants of health, but not all mental health services would address issues related to social determinants consistently. For example, if a client did not have transportation to an appointment, most healthcare providers, whether predominately physical or mental health providers, would not intervene to create opportunities to alleviate the transportation issue for the client. Furthermore, in many places, health care is either difficult to access due to proximity to the local health center or can be overburdened by a large number of patients and a lack of trained, skilled workers, thus increasing the burden on those who are already marginalized.

Intergenerational and Historical Trauma

Generational embodiment and historical trauma are recognized as the first level of the pyramid, and neither can be overlooked when discussing childhood trauma and epidemiologic linkages of trauma. The transfer of individual traits, abilities, behavior, and outcomes from parents to their children is known as intergenerational transmission. Evidence shows that maternal illness or adverse childhood experiences (ACEs) are transmitted through different generations and result in negative early childhood development that includes impaired personal-social, communication, motor, and problem-solving skills. Adverse experiences can be measured by the ACE score, and an individual's high ACE score points toward also having parents or children with high ACEs [3].

Maternal and perinatal exposure to ACEs demonstrates a strong correlation with child mental health including anxiety and depression [17]. Recently, research has shown that males may be at greater risk than females to negative events that occur to their mother during pregnancy [26]. In addition, maternal ACEs are more strongly associated with child behavior complications than paternal ACEs. Parents' ACEs and children's behavioral problem index scores, aggravation, and emotional distress also show a positive association [34]. Furthermore, children who live in high alcohol density areas have also shown high ACE scores, with ACEs related to sexual assault, child neglect and abuse, and domestic violence [35].

The psychological and biological mechanism is mainly responsible for intergenerational risks [17]. During pregnancy, maternal early life stress is transmitted to offspring via Hypothalamic Pituitary Adrenal (HPA) axis. Prenatal and postnatal social support is crucial to infant ACEs and moderated by HPA axis function and newborn cortisol reactivity. The HPA axis's social sensitivity and the importance of social relationships have been documented in the research [37]. Various other studies have been performed to examine intergenerational transmission of trauma. A prospective study focusing on black, low-income women was performed in Philadelphia and found that mothers who experienced violence or physical abuse as a child were more likely to use infant spanking [8]. Similarly, a retrospective cohort study of two-year-old children, collected from a primary healthcare setting, illustrated an 18% increase in suspected developmental disorders [17]. Likewise, a community-based cross-sectional telephone survey demonstrated intergenerational negative health outcomes such as less physical activity, obesity, asthma, sedentary life, unhealthy food choices (high soda consumption, low vegetable, and fruit consumption), lack of accessibility, and availability of health care or dental care, which were related to trauma [27].

Identification of behavioral problems and children at higher risk for trauma could help practitioners to prevent downstream results of health issues such as mental illness, interactions with the justice system, low academic performance, and substance abuse [34]. A proper understanding of ACEs, poor adult mental health, and intergenerational transmission could prevent leading causes of negative childhood and adult health outcomes. Historical trauma, the cumulative emotional and psychological adversities experienced by a group across generations, can directly influence intergenerational trauma and cannot be overlooked when developing trauma-informed programming or discussing global mental health. Recognizing historical trauma, finding common language to discuss historical trauma, and using culture and community connection can help to heal historical traumas.

Epigenetics

Historical and intergenerational trauma, along with an individual's social and environmental experience, leads to epigenetic modifications [29]. The interactions between a person's genome and environmental factors could result in an altered phenotype due to methylation, histone modifications, and acetylation, which modify the gene accessibility for transcription [4]. ACEs are linked to gene methylation, a mechanism in which a methyl group or small chemical groups attach to stress responding genes and suppress their activity. The molecular changes related to continuous stress-inducing circumstances could result in physiological or psychological disorders. Moreover, the hormonal, immune, and neurotransmitter activity also changes in response to methylation [4, 18]. The biological changes due to methylation result in chronic conditions such as cancer, heart disease, obesity, diabetes, depression, and autoimmune diseases [4, 15].

Various studies have been performed to show the correlation between ACEs and disabilities and also to increased psychotropic drug consumption in adults. One study showed that a low level of maternal care in rodents was strongly related to glucocorticoid receptor (GR) gene changes and leads to an increase in methylation of the promoter region. A similar study was performed in a group of healthy human subjects, demonstrating changes in NR3C1 (GR) gene in leukocyte DNA [4]. Decreased methylation of the stress-regulator gene (FKBP5) and modified HPA (Hypothermic-Pituitary-Adrenal) axis activity have also been observed [4, 29, 33]. Another study shows that child abuse is related to modified C_pG methylation, which alters the regulation of SLC6A4 (Serotonin Transporter) gene [39]. Moreover, stress-related hormonal changes such as low cortisol level and elevated inflammation in maltreated children are also linked to pathophysiological and psychiatric changes [4]. Stress markers, mitochondrial DNA, and telomere length illustrate biological links among ACEs and poor health consequences, providing a further understanding of intergenerational trauma transmission. Stress molecular markers play a significant role in moderating adverse childhood events and associated health risks as well as understanding the role of resilience and the development of effective interventions [32].

Governmental policies, medicine, community partnerships, and epigenetic research provide a starting point to develop early intervention for childhood trauma. Thus, a proper understanding of the epigenetic mechanism and gene-environmental interactions is required to prevent childhood trauma or stress consequences, and also across generation transmission [33].

Life Course Epidemiology, Trauma, and Health

It is not often that an indirect nonchemical and nonbiological exposure occurring during infancy can have a profound impact throughout the life course, potentially leading to a number of maladaptive behaviors, revictimization, and negative health outcomes. However, research has shown that infants who are exposed to interpersonal violence in the home remember and respond to that exposure to violence, potentially modifying the size, structure, and function of their brain [23]. Exposure to interpersonal violence in the home and other adverse childhood experiences before the age of 18 can continue to impact individuals throughout the life course. Psychologists, sociologists, and anthropologists have promoted a life course approach to health, development, and aging; however, public health and epidemiology, specifically, have integrated this approach into their discussion and methodology more so over the last 20 years [12, 24, 25]. It is vital to look at trauma and health from a life course perspective for a myriad of reasons, most importantly for the mind body connection that exists and can persist in negative ways with underlying chronic stress or unaddressed trauma.

Mind Body Connections of Trauma and Health

The ACE study provided one of the most profound demonstrations of the impact of trauma on health outcomes and established the foundation for understanding the mind body connection of how childhood experiences can be imprinted in the brain and cause negative physiological and psychological effects later in life. Although humans are a resilient species, traumatic experiences leave marks on our minds, emotions, biology, and immune systems [29]. These marks can be large, affecting a history or culture, or more intimate, affecting our families and potentially being passed down through generations [29]. Trauma and its after effects can cause the brain to release stress hormones at the slightest perception of danger. In turn, this can cause survivors of trauma to become hypervigilant, disconnected, avoidant, or angry, regularly feeling like they might be "broken" or "damaged" [30, 38].

What we now know is that reactions to trauma are not bad behavior; so to say, they are normal reactions to abnormal situations. Trauma elicits physiological reactions, which include an increase in the production of stress hormones, altering the brain's alert system, and modifying the brain mechanisms that sort information and its relevance [38]. While stress and trauma are related concepts and experiences at basic biological and psychosocial levels, it is worth noting that the terms are not interchangeable [13]. Stress involves the complex interactions of mind and body mediated through the endocrine and immune systems. Trauma refers to experiences, such as experiencing or witnessing an event that is overwhelming and thus changes the person in profound ways. Because stress and trauma are not synonymous, and because everyone who experiences stressful situations does not become traumatized, the Inter-Agency Standing Committee on Mental Health and Psychosocial Support recommends not using the word trauma when stress is meant [13, 21].

From a basic evolutionary perspective, the body has selected mechanisms to survive stressful experiences. For example, the fight or flight mechanism of the autonomic nervous system has historically enabled humans to survive dangerous encounters with predators. The body automatically increases heart rate and blood pressure, converts stored glycogen in the liver to energy glucose, which is adaptive in the short-term, and keeps you alive long enough to pass your genes to another generation, but repeated stresses, with the exaggerated cortisol response leading to the adverse health outcomes, such as hypertension, diabetes, hypercholesterolemia, asthma, decreased immune function, increased infections, and depression [13]. As noted by Bessel van der Kolk [38], the body keeps the score. The brain, mind, and body are all connected, and if untreated, trauma can cause real changes in the brain, potentially altering the overall health of individuals and societies over time.

Costs of Trauma

It is difficult to fully understand the costs of trauma. This is in part due to the fact that having an accurate measure of the size and scope of trauma at a local, regional, national, and international level is hard to gauge, given that the trauma reported is the tip of the iceberg and not an accurate portrayal of all cases of trauma. Trauma is likely to be highly underestimated in many places throughout the world as abuse is often not reported or tracked on a systems level and household dysfunction may not be reported or tracked at all. The costs of trauma are often estimated in two ways: economic costs and disability adjusted life years (DALYs).

Economic Costs

Peterson et al. [31], based on 2010 data, estimated the economic costs associated with child maltreatment was $428 billion dollars over the course of the lifespan [33]. This is a staggering figure, and it only estimates those cases of child maltreatment that were substantiated and does not account for ACEs that are not related to all types of abuse, domestic violence, parent/guardian substance abuse, mental illness, or incarceration. A similar study in the United Kingdom predicted an average lifetime cost of £89,390 for nonfatal child maltreatment by a primary caregiver, with costs ranging from £44, 896 to £145,508 [9].

Recently, in the United States, the economic costs of trauma have been estimated by determining medical costs and worker absenteeism from health issues that can be contributed to trauma. Alaska estimated that their annual medical cost for adult Medicaid, smoking, diabetes, binge drinking, arthritis, and obesity linked to ACEs was $775,649,000 [1]. A similar study in Tennessee determined that in 2017, an estimated $5.2 billion in direct medical costs and lost productivity from employees missing work could be attributed to ACEs [36]. Needless to say, ACEs are financially expensive if left untreated. Additional estimates on a global scale need to be assessed to better understand the economic burden associated with ACEs.

Disability Adjusted Life Years (DALYs)

DALYs provide a measure of overall disease burden, estimating the number of years lost due to poor health, disability, or early death [43]. Globally, mental illnesses account for the greatest disability that receives the least amount of resources and attention [14]. The outcomes associated with trauma, such as depression or mental disorders, are used to determine the DALYs associated with those trauma-associated outcomes. Mental disorders accounted for 12% of the estimated disability and depression accounted for 4.3% of disability according to the 2004 Global Burden of Disease Report [41]. Furthermore, depression is the leading cause of years of life lived with disability due to disease [41]. ACEs and other life traumas are well known to be associated with negative mental health outcomes, but they are also known to be associated with negative physical health outcomes and increase risk for many of the other major contributors to the disease burden such as HIV/AIDS, ischemic heart disease, stroke, and diabetes.

Cuijpers et al. [11] found that in the Netherlands, the burden of disease related to ACEs was greater than any other common mental disorders combined. That said, globally ACEs likely contribute more DALYs than current estimates predict. Finally, as we better understand ACEs and how to measure ACEs in culturally appropriate methods at a local level, we will likely see the costs of trauma as it relates to DALY rise exponentially.

Case Examples and Personal Experience

Munsieville, South Africa, ACE and Trauma-Informed Care Project

Over the past few years, I have been working on an ACE and trauma-informed care (TIC) project in Munsieville, South Africa, to determine how to best measure ACEs, understand the prevalence and types of trauma in this underserved community, and determine how to build capacity for addressing trauma. Thus far, the project has included three parts: (1) focus groups with community members to discuss the WHO's ACE-IQ and modifications to culturally adapt the survey, (2) a community wide survey using the adapted ACE-IQ, and (3) dissemination of the findings of the community wide survey and discussing next steps through focus groups and key informant interviews.

In a location where historical trauma is evident and recent from Apartheid, which meant that all citizens were not provided with equal rights until after 1994, there is a need for community healing and resilience building. While the effects of Apartheid are still felt today, the consequences of Apartheid from an epigenetic standpoint have not been explored and are not understood. The community anecdotally reported large amounts of child sexual and physical abuse, neglect and abandonment, domestic violence, and community violence. The community also reported a desire to heal, learn from one another, and create a better environment for the next generation. All of these factors showed the need and readiness of the community to understand ACEs and intervene on trauma-related issues.

While in Munsieville, for the community-wide survey on ACEs, a couple of interesting events occurred. On arrival, the nongovernment organization (NGO) we were working with mentioned that they had a recent case of child abuse and neglect with infant twins. The mother was suspected to have postpartum depression and was being hospitalized. One of the twins had recently left the hospital due to some respiratory complications from his mother's attempt to drown him. In less than 8 weeks of life, the twins had been born into a family in poverty who had recently immigrated from Malawi, had a parent suffering from a mental health issue, received little to no attention, food, or love, were unwanted by their mother, and had suffered major physical abuse. The foundation on the ACE pyramid was not setting these children up for success, and we could not help but wonder how life would pan out for these two children, one male and one female.

We learned about the twins the day before we started the community wide survey, so this somewhat set the tone for our work, and we realized the level of trauma in this community might be more than initially suspected. When completing the survey with our first participant, we learned that this individual's father treated her as if she was a servant in the household and used her for chores, cooking, and sex— sexually, physically, and emotionally abusing her for years. In an attempt to get out of her negative home environment, she ended up dating a series of people who treated her in similar ways to her father and became pregnant. Several years and a couple children later, she was living on her own and learning how to navigate life. During our administration of the survey with her, she cried, stating that she had never told anyone about these events, no one had ever asked, and so she never said anything. She also mentioned she knew she sometimes yelled or hit her children and that might be because of her negative childhood. She cried as she shared her story and cried harder as she shared that she does not feel like she is a good parent because of her upbringing. We referred her to a social worker with the NGO for follow-up care.

I had several initial reactions to the first participant's survey on day one of a 7–10 day project. Initially, I thought, maybe that was healing for her and now she knows there is help she can use. Second, I thought the community is right; there are many instances of child abuse, domestic abuse, and community violence. Lastly, I thought, wow, that survey took over an hour to complete and we might be doing more harm than good... I wondered how the project would turn out. Survey administration progressed much quicker after the first day of the survey, and we were able to survey all areas of the community and refer any individuals who needed additional support to a social worker for follow-up care.

When I came back to the community to complete key informant interviews to disseminate the survey findings and learn what community members wanted to do to address trauma, one stakeholder, a governmental youth development worker, that I spoke with, when asked the question, "if you had one thing you could do in Munsieville to address childhood and family trauma, what would it be?" responded with an equally necessary question, "how do you discuss trauma and issues related to community level violence without addressing some of the economic issues that contributed to trauma and violence?" When I asked some follow-up questions to gain more insight, he proceeded to tell me about the second and third economies that existed in his community, and likely do in most communities, due to a lack of employment opportunities. The second economy where crimes like robbery and hijacking provide a method to buy and sell goods and the third economy where drugs and sex are sold to make money typically have been shown to increase levels of violence, neglect, and abuse, and the Munsieville community was no different. The stakeholder also commented that unless there are opportunities for people to make money and rise out of poverty, the second and third economies would continue to exist, thrive, and contribute to trauma.

Despite the intentional work to comprehensively understand adverse experiences and the role of trauma in the lives of those in Munsieville, we have only scratched the surface on the work that needs to be done. A key finding from disseminating the results to the community was the need for a physical location that could serve as a one-stop shop for those dealing with trauma. A center would allow people to report abuse, receive social support and treatment, have a safe space to stay, and have their basic needs met during the crisis. However, in order to build a center, substantial amounts of background work are required, funds need to be raised and/or allocated, and a method is required to "prove" that this concept will work to be able to receive additional funds, through grants, to sustain the project. Furthermore, more research is essential to better understand ACEs in adults and current trauma in children to further measure these traumas, their effects, and understand how to best intervene in a culturally appropriate way. We know there is unaddressed trauma in the community, and we know there are interventions available that have worked in other communities, but proof of concept in this community may not be fully established and funding agencies may not be willing to allocate funds. So, ethically how do we not treat the trauma in this community and how can we overlook a problem we know exists? If the community suffered from a natural disaster causing physical injuries to over 20% of the community, those health effects would be addressed; but since this is a human made disaster through Apartheid, poverty, and lack of mental health resources, the community has to wait until all of the research has been done to prove this work is needed, which seems to be quite a dilemma.

Langtang Valley, Nepal, and the 2015 Earthquake

Recent historical trauma of the earthquake and subsequent landslide in 2015 in the Langtang Valley of Nepal, coupled with the historical trauma of the Tibetan population in this community, has left an entire community in need of healing from trauma. No one in the Langtang Valley was not affected by loss due to the earthquake and its after effects. While the community was able to come together to determine a memorial and how certain funds should be spent, there have not been opportunities to fully treat individuals for mental health issues related to the trauma of the earthquake in a culturally competent manner that is acceptable to local community members. This was obvious when I was in Nepal in late March and early April 2019 working with the Flagstaff International Relief Effort (FIRE). The purpose of our work in Nepal was to learn about the needs of the community, how to support FIRE's existing projects and expand their work, and determine if there were opportunities to establish partnerships between two United States universities who were interesting in working with FIRE. The work was not specifically focused on the earthquake or trauma; however, it was obvious through our community conversations that there was unaddressed trauma in the community.

We worked with FIRE to complete a series of focus groups with community members to understand their health needs, health issues in the community, and what resources were available in the community. Through these conversations, we learned that many people in the community were living in poverty, dependent on fluctuating income from tourism, and that the effects of the earthquake were still felt throughout the community, physically, mentally, and emotionally. We learned that while the community initially worked together in the aftermath of the earthquake and landslide, as donations started to come into the community individuals who were community leaders were allocating those funds to their family and friends first instead of on a need-based system. As you might expect, this caused some difficulties in the community and many individuals had to rebuild their lives with little to no support. This was surprising to find out given my initial reactions when I arrived in Langtang Valley. From an outsider's perspective, my initial reactions were that the community worked together, donated land and built a memorial for those who died in the natural disaster, and planned to add additional cultural information stops along the trekking route that traveled through the various towns in the area. All positive things that made it seem like a close-knit, remote community that worked together for the good of the whole. However, as we gained more knowledge and understanding of the community and the effects of the natural disaster, we learned that things were not always fair or equal and that the community has had to work to rebuild in multiple ways to get to where they are now and there is still more work to do—structurally, culturally, and emotionally.

Our time in the community also helped us to learn that most adults suffered from some kind of physical ailment—joint pain, back pain, headaches, and gastritis—or mental health ailments, such as worrying or feeling hopeless. Many of the children in the community were only home during school breaks, as most children were sent to the capital, Kathmandu, to boarding school. The child's ability to go to school and the school conditions varied greatly by the ability for the parents/guardians to pay or to obtain school sponsorship from an outside entity. Several of the children we met lost an immediate family member in the natural disaster or had immediate family members leave the area to set up a better life elsewhere following the earthquake and landslide. One of the children lost her mother and a younger sibling, three others had their mother move to another country, and one of those three broke of his legs both due to the weather events and aftershocks following the initial earthquake.

Based on our conversations and observations in the community, it did not seem like anyone genuinely processed the natural disaster. People did what they needed to do to survive, helped others as they could, and then went right back to life the way it was before, almost as if things never happened. However, for an area with a small population that is spread out along the mountain trekking trail, they lost 20–30% of their population from the earthquake, due to either death or relocation. As mentioned, many of the children are not always in the community, but now when they come home from boarding school, one of their parents and/or siblings is no longer there and those facts do not seem to be discussed. Furthermore, I could not help but wonder if some of the physical and mental health conditions reported during the focus groups and the way people acted following the earthquake were potentially related unaddressed trauma from earlier in life or residual trauma from the earthquake.

I also wondered what long-term effects might prevail from the earthquake, especially for those children who lost a parent/guardian or sibling. The young girl who lost her mother was already experiencing some stomachaches and having difficulty expressing her emotions, and she had a solid support system. While the stomachaches could be related to food or water-borne diseases and the difficulty expressing her emotions might be related to her developmental age, it is hard not to think that they might be related to the unaddressed trauma of losing her mother in a natural disaster. I expect that people in the Langtang Valley would fare better if they talked about their loss instead of trying to forget those individuals. Eric Lindemann's study of the Cocoanut Grove fire in Boston, USA, supports this idea and found that short-term individual counseling following disasters can be beneficial [28]. Likely though, the community of Langtang Valley would benefit from a more community-based approach that included community health workers (CHWs) trained in psychosocial support and care, much like the models used following a variety of natural disasters that occurred globally in the early 2000s [22]. This approach would provide an opportunity to train local individuals to provide supports, with oversight from a mental health professional, which would assist in sustainability and cultural competency. Unfortunately, I do not think these resources are available and those in the Langtang Valley would likely not know if they were available or how to advocate for those services, given that so much of their daily lives are focused on meeting basic needs for survival. Great improvements have been made to integrate mental health into disaster response over the past 20 years. However, gaps in care, resource allocation, and prioritizing mental health still persist.

Understanding ACEs and Building a Trauma-Informed System of Care in Appalachia

The Appalachian region is no stranger to adversities and hardships. This region is also no stranger to a strong work ethic and grassroots efforts to help their fellow community members. In my work in the northeast Tennessee area of the Appalachian region, I have learned about the intergenerational cycles of adversity and how those hardships have impacted economic status, education, and health. I have also had the opportunity to participate in community-based efforts to address these issues across various sectors, such as education, economic development, and health. This dichotomy is important to note, in both the Appalachian region and other regions when working to address trauma. In northeast Tennessee, much like many other places, the strength and perseverance people exhibit to survive and provide a better life for their family is impressive. The amount of barriers that must be overcome to not only survive but also thrive is equally impressive. Two experiences in this region provided me with the opportunity to witness this dichotomy first hand.

Dr. Katie Baker and I collaborated on a maternal caregiver-teenage daughter (from now on referred to as mother-daughter) ACE project based on Katie's expertise in mother-daughter health communication and our mutual interest to work with underserved populations. We wanted to gain a better understanding on mothers' self-report of their own ACEs, mothers' report of daughters' ACEs, and daughters' self-report of their own ACEs and to identify what, if any, influence ACEs had on how maternal caregivers and daughters communicated about health issues. The project included individual interviews for mothers and daughters, along with the administration of an ACE questionnaire. We were certain we would gain interesting insights into the types of ACEs reported and how mothers and daughters communicate about health issues. However, we did not expect that the interviews would elicit such raw information from mothers about their own upbringing and maternal influences played a role in how they interacted with their daughter and their concerns for their daughter's well-being. Katie and a graduate research assistant completed all of the interviews in the northeast Tennessee region. As I read transcripts to complete qualitative analysis, there were interviews where I felt like I was in the room, hearing that mother talk through the ACEs that occurred in her life and how she wanted to prevent those same ACEs from happening to her daughter. From my review of the transcripts, it seemed that simply asking mothers about their ACEs was helpful in providing terminology and an understanding of how ACEs might contribute to current parenting practices. One mother discussed the sexual abuse that she experienced as a child and how she wanted to make sure that her daughters did not experience the same thing. She recognized that she adopted certain parenting practices out of fear that her daughters would experience sexual abuse in childhood. Another mother discussed her mother's lack of communication on health-related issues and how that influenced how she discussed these issues with her daughter. We heard about childhood neglect and abuse, parental drug and alcohol use, parental mental illness, and domestic violence. We heard about the struggles to parent while dealing with their own ACEs, while living in poverty, and in today's society to connect with a teenager while competing with external influences. We learned of the many barriers that women in the Appalachian region face to overcome their upbringing. We completed the project with a better understanding of what types of ACEs were occurring and the role those ACEs likely play in mother daughter communication. What we still did not know was how these mothers and daughters could receive support from their community to help understand and address these issues. This is where a system of care for trauma-informed care comes into the picture.

Around the same time Katie and I were learning about ACEs in mothers and daughters, Dr. Andi Clements and Becky Haas were building a system of care to address ACEs in the northeast Tennessee region. Andi and Becky started providing the Substance Abuse and Mental Health Services Administration's (SAMHSA) trauma-informed care trainings throughout the region, inviting others to receive the training and, where appropriate, to become trainers themselves. They also started meeting regularly with community members to share information on what services were available in the region and how those services could be trauma informed. Andi and Becky were early adopters of the SAMHSA National Center for Trauma-Informed Care's advice to engage your local community and build a system of care for trauma-informed care. Their grassroots effort was well received throughout the community and provided time and space for school systems, libraries, nonprofit organizations, healthcare providers, police departments, and local businesses to discuss ACEs and trauma-informed approaches. Organizations learned from each other and quickly identified ways to best support local families, even though there were limited resources available for these efforts. Andi and Becky made sure to track the number of people who received trauma-informed care training, assessed attendees' ideas about trauma-informed care before and after the training, and document all of their steps to build a system of care. These efforts resulted in thousands of individuals receiving training and completing assessments, over a 100 individuals or organizations in the original system of care, at least three additional community specific systems of care in the region, and a toolkit for how communities can create their own system of care for trauma-informed care [19]. The impact made in the northeast Tennessee region to address ACEs through Andi and Becky's grassroots efforts can easily be noticed. Whether it is increased attendance and graduation rates at the local alternative high school, trauma informed, patient centered care at the children's hospital, or the police department recognizing how to best respond to situations to mitigate ACEs—Andi and Becky's efforts, trainings, and passion are woven throughout. As a member of the system of care, I had the opportunity to watch the group grow and develop strategies to address ACEs. I also had the opportunity to become a trauma-informed care trainer through Andi and Becky's train-the-trainer course, which has allowed me to not only complete research on ACEs and trauma but also provide communities with an understanding of trauma and tools to address trauma. This grassroots effort is a prime example of how the Appalachian region is persistent and works hard to help their community. These efforts have received regional, national, and international attention—illustrating just how far hard work and engaging with your local community can go to understand and address ACEs and trauma and how much other communities are craving tools to address these issues in their own backyard.

Analysis in an Ethical Framework

We know that childhood trauma is common in societies throughout the world, yet measures have not fully been put in place to prevent or mitigate this trauma. Trauma has physical, mental, and societal health consequences, and continuing to overlook the prevalence of trauma and its effects on individuals and communities throughout the life course will result in a lack of economic and social development globally. From a public health perspective, the field aims to prevent and control disease and factors that contribute to poor health outcomes. If childhood trauma or trauma in general was viewed as an outbreak to an infectious disease or better yet, a global pandemic of infectious disease, public health practitioners globally would respond to trauma as an emergency and major public health threat. Trauma and its effects are an emergency and a major public health threat, but how do we prevent and control something that is not fully understood and multidimensional in nature requires various treatment modalities based on the individual experience?

Responding to and mitigating trauma is extremely difficult due to the lack of an understood and clearly defined case definition for trauma or even more specifically, for ACEs. We know that as the number of ACEs increases, the number of negative health outcomes increases, but that is not necessarily true for each individual as everyone has their own lived experience, which may recognize an event as traumatic. Furthermore, there are a number of protective factors related to exposure to trauma, such as having a responsive caregiver or a healthy role model, and every individual has their own resilience factors that can mitigate the effects of trauma. As an epidemiologist, I can typically rely on case definitions, specifically for infectious disease. For example, a confirmed case of measles is defined by an acute febrile rash illness with one of the following: isolation of measles virus from a clinical specimen, detection of measles-virus specific nucleic acid from a clinical specimen using polymerase chain reaction, IgG seroconversion or a significant rise in measles immunoglobulin G antibody using any evaluated and validated method, a positive serologic test for measles immunoglobulin M antibody, or direct epidemiologic linkage to a case confirmed by one of the above methods [7]. While that is a highly involved definition, if a case does not meet those criteria, then it is not a confirmed case of measles. Unfortunately, we do not fully have this luxury when defining and diagnosing trauma since trauma is not quite as straightforward. Mental health practitioners may work with a client for quite some time before the client reveals that trauma occurred during childhood and many individuals around the world may not have the access to a mental health practitioner to diagnose and treat trauma.

That said, do we urge health officials to encourage health practitioners to screen for trauma, and if trauma is screened for, do communities around the world have the capacity to treat that trauma? Ethically, we cannot and should not screen for something for which we do not have treatment options. Imagine screening for breast or cervical cancer and finding multiple cases but not having affordable or effective treatment available in that community. Then, ethically, the screening is harmful and not helpful. I have concerns that this could be the case in screening for trauma. Health entities such as local health departments or ministries of health have to build capacity for community mental health practitioners before screening for trauma. I imagine that if trauma is screened for in a culturally sensitive manner at a local level, the prevalence of trauma at a global level will be overwhelming.

However, with what is known about trauma, I do not know if we actually need to screen for trauma. I think that we can almost assume that everyone has experienced trauma of some kind in their lives. Then, we come to the dilemma of what to actually do about the trauma that individuals have experienced. I have more questions than I have answers about this, but I do know that we cannot continue to overlook trauma and its effects on individuals and societies. We have to work across disciplines to develop unique, cost-effective strategies to prevent and mitigate trauma at an individual and societal level.

Conclusions

Childhood traumas are common throughout the world and consist of physical, emotional, and sexual abuse along with household dysfunction factors such as parent/guardian substance abuse, incarceration, or mental illness, witnessing interpersonal violence, and neglect. In natural disaster or conflict situations, these traumas may extend to loss of family members, displacement, and destruction or loss of property. The connection between trauma and the mind and body is clear, and trauma is associated with health risk behavior and costly negative physical and mental health outcomes throughout the lifespan. Trauma is an important public health problem throughout the world and we must find effective methods to prevent and mitigate trauma at an individual and societal level in order to have healthy, economically stable communities.

References

1. Alaska Department of Health and Social Services. (2019). *Economic costs of adverse childhood experiences: The price of not intervening before trauma occurs*. Retrieved from: http://dhss.alaska.gov/abada/ace-ak/Documents/ACEsEconomicCosts-AK.pdf
2. Anda, R. F., Felitti, V. J., Bremner, J. D., Walker, J. D., Whitfield, C. H., Perry, B. D., Dube, S. R., & Giles, W. H. (2006). The enduring effects of abuse and related adverse experiences in childhood. *European Archives of Psychiatry and Clinical Neuroscience, 256*(3), 174–186.
3. Anda, R. F., Dong, M., Brown, D. W., Felitti, V. J., Giles, W. H., Perry, G. S., Valerie, E. J., & Dube, S. R. (2009). The relationship of adverse childhood experiences to a history of premature death of family members. *BMC Public Health, 9*(1), 106.
4. Brockie, T. N., Heinzelmann, M., & Gill, J. (2013). A framework to examine the role of epigenetics in health disparities among Native Americans. *Nursing Research & Practice, 2013*, 410395.
5. Centers for Disease Control and Prevention (CDC). (2012). *Adverse childhood experiences (ACE) study: ACE pyramid*. National Center for Chronic Disease Prevention and Health Promotion. Retrieved from http://www.cdc.gov/ace/
6. Centers for Disease Control and Prevention (CDC). (2019). *Adverse childhood experiences study, the ACE pyramid*. Retrieved from: https://www.cdc.gov/violenceprevention/childabuseandneglect/acestudy/ace-graphics.html
7. Centers for Disease Control and Prevention (CDC). (2019). *Measles/Rubeola 2013 case definition*. Retrieved from: https://wwwn.cdc.gov/nndss/conditions/measles/case-definition/2013/
8. Chung, E. K., Mathew, L., Rothkopf, A. C., Elo, I. T., Coyne, J. C., & Culhane, J. F. (2009). Parenting attitudes and infant spanking: The influence of childhood experiences. *Pediatrics, 124*(2), e278–e286.
9. Conti, G., Morris, S., Melnychuk, M., & Pizzo, E. (2017). *The economic costs of child maltreatment in the UK*. London: NSPCC.
10. Cronholm, P. F., Forke, C. M., Wade, R., Bair-Merritt, M. H., Davis, M., Harkins-Schwarz, M., Pachter, L. M., & Fein, J. A. (2015). Adverse childhood experiences: Expanding the concept of adversity. *American Journal of Preventive Medicine, 49*(3), 354–361.
11. Cuijpers, P., Smit, F., Unger, F., Stikkelbroek, Y., ten Have, M., & de Graaf, R. (2011). The disease burden of childhood adversities in adults: A population-based study. *Child Abuse & Neglect, 35*(11), 937–945.
12. Davey Smith, G., Gunnell, D., & Ben-Shlomo, Y. (2001). *Life-course approaches to socioeconomic differentials in cause-specific adult mortality. Poverty, inequality and health: An international perspective*. New York: Oxford University Press.
13. Dyer, A. (2014). Mind-body adaptations to adverse experiences. Retrieved from: https://allendyer.files.wordpress.com/2014/12/mind-body-adaptations.pdf
14. Dyer, A., & Bhadra, S. (2014). *Global disasters war, conflict, and complex emergencies: Caring for special populations*. Retrieved from: https://allendyer.files.wordpress.com/2014/12/2012-dyer-bhadra-global-disasters.pdf
15. Ehlert, U. (2013). Enduring psychobiological effects of childhood adversity. *Psychoneuroendocrinology, 38*(9), 1850–1857.

16. Felitti, V. J., Anda, R. F., Nordenberg, D., & Williamson, D. F. (1998). Adverse childhood experiences and health outcomes in adults: The Ace study. *Journal of Family and Consumer Sciences, 90*(3), 31.
17. Folger, A. T., Eismann, E. A., Stephenson, N. B., Shapiro, R. A., Macaluso, M., Brownrigg, M. E., & Gillespie, R. J. (2018). Parental adverse childhood experiences and offspring development at 2 years of age. *Pediatrics, 141*(4), e20172826.
18. Gershon, N. B., & High, P. C. (2015). Epigenetics and child abuse: Modern-day darwinism— the miraculous ability of the human genome to adapt, and then adapt again. *American Journal of Medical Genetics. Part C, Seminars in Medical Genetics, 169*(4), 353–360.
19. Haas, B. & Clements, A. D. (2019). Building a Trauma Informed System of Care. Retrieved from: https://www.tn.gov/content/dam/tn/dcs/documents/health/aces/building-strongbrains-tn/Building%20a%20Trauma%20Informed%20System%20of%20Care%20Toolkit.pdf
20. Healthy People. Social determinants of health. (2019). Retrieved from: https://www.healthy-people.gov/2020/topics-objectives/topic/social-determinants-of-health
21. Inter-Agency Standing Committee on Mental Health and Psychosocial Support. (2011). Retrieved from: https://interagencystandingcommittee.org/system/files/legacy_files/MHPSS%20Protection%20Actors.pdf
22. Kasi, S., Bhadra, S., & Dyer, A. (2007). A decade of disasters: Lessons from the Indian experience. *Southern Medical Journal, 100*(9), 929–931.
23. Kendall-Tackett, K. (2019). *Brain trauma.* Retrieved from: https://www.gannett-cdn.com/experiments/usatoday/responsive/graphics/2019/01/012519-brain-trauma/index.html
24. Kuh, D., Ben-Shlomo, Y., Lynch, J., Hallqvist, J., & Power, C. (2003). Life course epidemiology. *Journal of Epidemiology and Community Health, 57*(10), 778.
25. Kuh, D., & Shlomo, Y. B. (Eds.). (2004). *A life course approach to chronic disease epidemiology.* Oxford: Oxford University Press.
26. Lê-Scherban, F., Wang, X., Boyle-Steed, K. H., & Pachter, L. M. (2018). Intergenerational associations of parent adverse childhood experiences and child health outcomes. *Pediatrics, 141*(6), e20174274.
27. Letourneau, N., Dewey, D., Kaplan, B. J., Ntanda, H., Novick, J., Thomas, J. C., Deane, A. J., Leung, B., Pon, K., Giesbrecht, G. F., & APrON Study Team. (2019). Intergenerational transmission of adverse childhood experiences via maternal depression and anxiety and moderation by child sex. *Journal of Developmental Origins of Health and Disease, 10*(1), 88–99.
28. Lindemann, E. (1944). Symptomatology and management of acute grief. *The American Journal of Psychiatry, 101*(2), 141–148.
29. McEwen, B. S. (2017). *Neurobiological and systemic effects of chronic stress* (p. 1). Thousand Oaks: Chronic Stress.
30. National Child Traumatic Stress Network. (2019). Retrieved from: https://www.nctsn.org/what-is-child-trauma/about-child-trauma
31. Peterson, C., Florence, C., & Klevens, J. (2018). The economic burden of child maltreatment in the United States, 2015. *Child Abuse & Neglect, 86*, 178–183.
32. Ridout, K. K., Khan, M., & Ridout, S. J. (2018). Adverse childhood experiences run deep: Toxic early life stress, telomeres, and mitochondrial dna copy number, the biological markers of cumulative stress. *BioEssays, 40*(9), 1800077.
33. Rubin, L. P. (2016). Maternal and pediatric health and disease: Integrating biopsychosocial models and epigenetics. *Pediatric Research, 79*(1–2), 127.
34. Schickedanz, A., Halfon, N., Sastry, N., & Chung, P. J. (2018). Parents' adverse childhood experiences and their children's behavioral health problems. *Pediatrics, 142*(2), e20180023.
35. Schofield, T. J., Donnellan, M. B., Merrick, M. T., Ports, K. A., Klevens, J., & Leeb, R. (2018). Intergenerational continuity in adverse childhood experiences and rural community environments. *American Journal of Public Health, 108*(9), 1148–1152.
36. The Sycamore Institute. (2019). *The economic cost of ACEs in Tennessee.* Retrieved from: https://www.sycamoreinstitutetn.org/wp-content/uploads/2019/02/2019.02.01-FINAL-The-Economic-Cost-of-ACEs-in-Tennessee.pdf

37. Thomas, J. C., Letourneau, N., Campbell, T. S., Giesbrecht, G. F., & Apron Study Team. (2018). Social buffering of the maternal and infant HPA axes: Mediation and moderation in the intergenerational transmission of adverse childhood experiences. *Development and Psychopathology, 30*(3), 921–939.
38. Van der Kolk, B. A. (2015). *The body keeps the score: Brain, mind, and body in the healing of trauma*. New York: Penguin Books.
39. Vijayendran, M., Beach, S., Plume, J. M., Brody, G., & Philibert, R. (2012). Effects of genotype and child abuse on DNA methylation and gene expression at the serotonin transporter. *Frontiers in Psychiatry, 13*(3), 55.
40. World Health Organization. (2003). *Social determinants of health: The solid facts*. Retrieved from: http://www.euro.who.int/__data/assets/pdf_file/0005/98438/e81384.pdf
41. World Health Organization. (2004). *Global burden of disease 2004 update*. Retrieved from: https://www.who.int/healthinfo/global_burden_disease/GBD_report_2004update_full.pdf?ua=1
42. World Health Organization. (2019). *Adverse childhood experiences international questionnaire*. Retrieved from: https://www.who.int/violence_injury_prevention/violence/activities/adverse_childhood_experiences/en/
43. World Health Organization. (2019). *Metrics: Disability-adjusted life year (DALY)*. Retrieved from: https://www.who.int/healthinfo/global_burden_disease/metrics_daly/en/

Part IV

Interventions and Public Health Programs

Coping With Addictive Opioid Markets 12

Amir A. Afkhami and Javad John Fatollahi

Introduction

Opioid dependence is a significant contributor to the global disease burden. Over the past generation, both the range of opiates and markets for the drugs have expanded to unprecedented levels. On the supply side, opioid drug markets have seen record levels of production and manufacture. On the demand side, nonmedical use of opioids and their synthetic analogues have reached epidemic proportions in parts of the world. Opioid dependence is a chronic disorder that prompts users to persist in using the drug despite the negative downstream effects of its consumption including imprisonment, exposure to infectious diseases, and possible fatal overdose. Social, political, geographical factors are important determinants of opiate dependence rates, morbidity, and mortality in a population. Drugs also play an important role in eroding stability and governance, particularly in low- and middle-income nations, through conflict, criminality, and corruption fueled by the profits of the opiate trade. Globally, there is increasing realization that combating opioid dependence is an essential component of a healthy and stable society. Despite this recognition, most individuals struggling with addiction do not receive appropriate care. The prevailing stigma across cultures and the criminalization of the disorder have largely shifted the opioid-dependent population into prisons instead of clinics, which has worsened the impact of opioid misuse.

A. A. Afkhami (✉) · J. J. Fatollahi
Department of Psychiatry and Behavioral Sciences, The George Washington University, Washington, DC, USA
e-mail: aafkhami@mfa.gwu.edu; jfatollahi@gwu.edu

© Springer Nature Switzerland AG 2021
A. R. Dyer et al. (eds.), *Global Mental Health Ethics*,
https://doi.org/10.1007/978-3-030-66296-7_12

Population Health and the Opiate Drug Market

Economic/Social/Legal Impacts

The economic burden of opioids was estimated to have cost the US $55.7 billion in 2007. Lost workplace productivity contributed $25.6 billion, healthcare costs contributed $25 billion, and criminal justice costs accounted for the remaining $5.1 billion [3]. In 2013, the CDC estimated that the cost had risen to $78.5 billion per year [11], and in 2015, The White House Council of Economic Advisers estimated that the cost of the opioid epidemic exceeded $500 billion, largely because of lost productivity from premature death [17]. Since the start of the war on drugs campaign led by the US federal government in the early 1970s, the number of addicts incarcerated in American prisons has increased exponentially. Other countries that have adopted similar strict interdiction and criminalization drug policies have also witnessed a dramatic increase in their prison populations. Besides an increase in incarcerations, opioid dependence has been shown to correlate with a higher proportion of criminal activity outside of crimes specific to drug use and possession. Typically the more the addict uses, the more crime they are likely to commit. The cause for this is likely twofold; increased risk-taking behaviors coupled with the strength of addiction which causes addicts to be motivated to procure their next dose by any means necessary.

Global Burden of Opioid Use

The contribution of opioid use to premature mortality varies across the globe, with North America, Eastern Europe, and Southern Sub-Saharan Africa being the regions most affected by this growing epidemic. Nearly two-thirds of the deaths attributed to drug use disorders in 2017 were due to opioids [8]. In 1990, there were an estimated 10.4 million people globally who were opioid-dependent. That number skyrocketed to 15.5 million people in 2010, resulting in 9.2 million disability-adjusted life years (DALYs) lost to opioid-related ill health and premature mortality (approximately 7 million years lived with disability (YLD) and 2 million years of life lost (YLL)) [5]. There is also a geographic variation in the contribution of YLD versus YLL due to opioid dependence. For example, in the majority of regions, burden was mainly due to YLD, but in North America, Eastern Europe, and Southern Sub-Saharan Africa, there was a higher burden (>50%) due to YLL [6]. By 2016, there were an estimated 34.3 million past-year users of opioids which corresponded to roughly 0.7 percent of the global population (aged 15–64 year). The prevalence of past-year opioid users in 2016 was especially high in regions like North America (4.2 percent) and Oceania (2.2 percent) [12].

The rise of synthetic opioids is also a cause for concern in today's drug climate. Fentanyl, which was first synthesized in 1959, was approved initially for use as an anesthetic in the USA in 1972. With a potency of 50–100 times that of morphine, it is produced using inexpensive and readily available chemical precursors. This surge in potency, coupled with Fentanyl's ease in traversing across the blood-brain barrier, narrows the therapeutic window of the drug, with small dosage increases resulting in fatal respiratory depression [17]. The rate of overdose deaths in the USA due to synthetic opioids, like fentanyl, increased from 1 per 100,000 people in 2013 to 9 per 100,000 in 2017. This was approximately double the corresponding 2017 rates for heroin (4.9 per 100,000) or prescription opioids (4.4 per 100,000) giving rise to the concern that inexpensive, readily accessible, and mass-produced synthetic opioids were changing the morbidity and mortality patterns of opioid dependence in the USA [14].

Associated Medical Comorbidities

One of the major downstream consequences of opioid dependence is the surge of blood-borne infectious diseases associated with their use, including higher rates of Acquired Immune Deficiency Syndrome (AIDS) caused by the human immunodeficiency virus (HIV), viral hepatitis, infective endocarditis, and other skin and soft tissue diseases. This creates a converging public health concern that requires a coordinated effort by both infectious disease specialists and substance use disorder providers to address. Most of these infections are spread via intravenous injection through the sharing of needles [19]. According to WHO data, injecting drug use is reported in 136 countries, of which 93 reported HIV infection among those who are injecting [4]. Injecting drug use as a global risk factor for HIV accounted for 2.1 million DALYs and as a global risk factor for hepatitis C accounted for 0.5 million DALYs in 2010. In 2017, there was an estimated 11 million people worldwide who inject drugs and more than half of them live with Hepatitis C and close to one in eight live with HIV [8].

According to the US National Institute of Drug Abuse (NIDA), roughly 30–60% of individuals with a diagnosis of substance use disorder met the criteria for post-traumatic stress disorder (PTSD) as well. The most prominent example of this dual diagnosis phenomenon can be found among American veterans of the Vietnam War. A study found that 75% of combat Vietnam veterans with diagnosed PTSD also met criteria for a substance use disorder (mainly due to heroin addiction). These same veterans also faced a higher risk of fatal overdose when compared to the general population. Similarly, American veterans of the Iraq/Afghanistan War shared an increased prevalence of opioid dependency. But unlike their predecessors, these soldiers were becoming addicted to prescription opioids. A veterans affairs healthcare study showed that roughly 11% of veterans who served in operations in Iraq and Afghanistan were diagnosed with a substance use disorder and 22% of the veterans diagnosed with PTSD had a comorbid substance use disorder.

Addiction in Humanitarian Settings

While growing addiction rates and its burden on the developing world have been cause for concern, the prevalence of opioid dependence in humanitarian settings (zones of conflict, natural disasters, and displaced populations) is just as glaring. In these settings, addiction has been linked to issues ranging from organized crime, to gender violence, to the unfortunate neglect of small children. Like soldiers returning from war, refugees have shown a similar trend in increasing addiction rates. Refugees are at a higher risk for dependence when compared to the general population due to higher levels of stress, unemployment, and difficulties adapting to a new environment. Lack of access to treatment services along with cultural, economic, and language barriers can increase the risk of developing a drug habit or create barriers to accessing appropriate addiction treatment. Dependence can develop in the country of origin, while in transit, or in the setting of temporary or permanent residence. Risk factors in these settings include male gender, exposure to combat, and coexisting mental health problems. The Assimilation/Acculturation Model postulates that refugees tend to adopt the social norms of their new environment, including harmful behaviors such as substance misuse. The Acculturative Stress Model, on the other hand, theorizes that difficulties in managing new cultural and societal norms result in drug use as a coping mechanism [13]. The Syrian refugee crisis has brought a resurgence of interest in this topic. There are approximately 6.6 million Syrian refugees that have fled their country and another 6.1 million that have been displaced from their homes with in Syria. Of those, 12 million people, 90% of them live outside of camps in makeshift shelters, which are often overcrowded. What is even more disheartening is that roughly 50% of all registered Syrian refugees are under the age of 18 meaning millions have spent their formative years experiencing high levels of poverty, malnutrition, and conflict [20]. While opioid dependence is considered a public health issue in humanitarian settings, it is an area that has been overlooked given the lack of relevant literature on the matter. The challenges of collecting data in emergency settings and stigma are major barriers to empirical studies that can shed light on supporting a correlation between humanitarian emergencies and increased addiction rates. However, the Acculturative Stress Model and the know significant traumas of conflict, deprivation, and displacement make it very plausible that illicit opioid use in these regions may increase as more individuals seek to self-medicate and treat mental/physical pain or to alleviate the stress of adapting to a new lifestyle and environment. There are also instances where during or following a national emergency, supply of medications used for the treatment of opioid use disorders (like methadone and buprenorphine) can abruptly be discontinued. The Ukrainian revolution in 2014 was a prime example as to how discontinuation of medication-assisted treatment (MAT) can cause sudden withdrawal and return to illicit opioid use among dependent users. Even more cause for concern is the dangerous shift in how opioids are being consumed. Afghanistan, for example, has had a shift from its traditional smoking of opium to more high-risk use via intravenous injection of heroin. This shift can be attributed to a combination of outdated drug policies and a war that destabilized an already fragile nation. This instability led to a lack of proper border control, which in turn increased trafficking and access to drugs. Libya, a country that had back-to-back civil wars in less than a decade, experienced a similar shift of increasing intravenous opioid use, which was also coupled with an HIV epidemic that nearly crippled the entire country's health system [13].

Impact on National Security and Stability

The transnational trade and domestic trade in illicit opioids are significant threats to public health, law enforcement, and overall stability throughout the world. The actors involved in the production and trade of this illegal commodity include civilian farmers and manufacturers; criminal groups such as drug trafficking organizations and mafias; belligerent actors, such as terrorist, insurgent, and paramilitary groups; and corrupt government and law enforcement officials. Mexican transnational criminal organizations, including the Sinaloa Cartel and Jalisco New Generation Cartel, are the principal suppliers, traffickers, and distributors of opioid drugs in the USA. They work closely with US-based actors to distribute the drugs on a local level [16]. National and neighborhood-based street gangs and prison gangs continue to dominate the market for the street sales and distribution of illicit drugs in their respective territories. The profit from this trade fuels the criminality, violence, and disruptions to the social fabric across both rural and urban communities in the USA. The adulteration of heroin with fentanyl and the increased purity of opioids by cartels to maximize profits have been the primary drivers of rising overdose deaths in the USA in the last 4 years.

Terrorist or insurgent actors involved in the global illicit opioid market represent a particularly significant threat to nations and regional stability since these groups often seek to disrupt or eliminate the existing sovereign governing structures of a state. In Afghanistan, the world's largest opium producer, most of the poppy cultivation tends to take place in areas and villages controlled by insurgent and other non-state actors, compared with just 26 percent for non-poppy villages. Insurgent groups such as the Taliban enforce a variety of taxes on the production and sale of the agricultural product, earning them tens of millions yearly, which fuels the armed conflict in the country. Moreover, poppy-producing villages controlled by insurgents have worst access to med medical and educational facilities, especially for girls and women. The United Nations estimates that in villages not under state control only 13 percent of women have access to culturally sanctioned female providers, resulting in higher maternal and child mortality and morbidity figures [1].

Case Examples

The Portuguese Case

Background
The location of Portugal on the southwest border of Europe makes it the perfect gateway for drug trafficking. Despite this, the lifetime prevalence of illicit drug use in the country has been historically low. However, in the 1990s there was a significant increase of intravenous (IV) drug users within the country, which increased the rates of infectious diseases like HIV, AIDS, Hepatitis B, and Hepatitis C. By the turn of the century, Portugal had the highest rate of

drug-related AIDS and the second highest rate of HIV among IV drug users in the European Union [2]. Drug-related deaths also peaked within the country and drug users were slowly becoming marginalized and socially excluded. Drug-related offenders made up 44% of the Portuguese prison population, and overcrowding was becoming an issue [15]. It was around this time that law enforcement and health sectors within the country started viewing criminalization of drug use more as a problem than a real solution.

Model Intervention

Efforts at harm reduction could be seen in Lisbon as early as the 1990s, when Odette Ferreira, an experienced pharmacist and pioneering HIV researcher, started an unofficial needle exchange program to address the growing HIV epidemic. Ferreira, whose fieriness made up for her small stature, began giving away clean syringes in the middle of Europe's biggest open-air drug market, in the Casal Ventoso neighbourhood of Lisbon. She also collected donations of clothing, soap, razors, condoms, fruit, and sandwiches, and distributed them to users. Her efforts were met with death threats from drug dealers and legal threats from politicians. Not one to back down easily, she eventually convinced the Portuguese Association of Pharmacies into running the country's—and arguably the world's—first national needle exchange program [9].

Along with harm reduction programs, the Portuguese government eventually appointed an expert commission that proposed decriminalization of all illicit drugs for personal use as its first national drug strategy. Their goal was to provide a more evidence-based approach to drug use and decriminalization aimed to create a more humane legal framework [7]. Decriminalization of illicit drugs ultimately went into full effect in Portugal on July 1, 2001. Prior to this reform, drug possession or cultivation was punishable by up to 1 year of imprisonment, but with decriminalization, these minor drug offenders were now being funneled through the drug treatment system rather than the criminal justice system [15].

Results

While decriminalization caused a slight increase in apparent drug use within Portugal, its effects on the criminal justice system, drug treatment, mortality, and infectious disease were considerably profound. The number of people arrested for criminal drug offences reduced from over 14,000 offenders in 2000 to an average of 5000 per year after decriminalization went into effect. The number of drug-related offenders in the Portuguese prison population decreased from 44% in 1999 to 21% in 2008. As the number of incarcerated drug users decreased, so did the rate of drug use within prisons. Between 1998 and 2008, the overall number of drug users in treatment expanded from 23,654 to 38,532 [18]. The proportion of drug-related deaths due to opioids decreased from 95% in 1999 to 59% in 2008 [15]. From 2000 to 2008, the number of new HIV cases decreased among drug users from 907 to 267 and the number of new AIDS cases decreased from 506 to 108 [18].

The Iranian Case

Background

For much of the twentieth century, the Iranian government's strategy for curbing the country's growing problem with opiate misuse was one of interdiction, by stopping the flow of opium products, banning, and destroying the poppy crop, and increasingly draconian criminal justice laws against trafficking and possessing narcotics. When, in the late 1960s, it became clear that this approach was not working due to a rising heroin epidemic, Iranian authorities adopted policies that focused more on prevention and treatment, with promising results. The Iranian government allowed the resumption of opium cultivation and use, increased access to overdose management, detoxification services, and pilot MAT programs. But the country returned to strict zero-tolerance narcotics laws after the 1979 revolution that overthrew the secular monarchy. Iran's new Islamic government saw drug use not as a medical or public health issue but as a moral shortcoming, believing that addiction and abuse could be addressed through religiously sanctioned punitive measures. Penalties for addicts included fining, imprisonment, and physical punishment; drug dealers and smugglers were often considered to be "at war with God" were either imprisoned or executed. But by the late 1980s, the rising number of incarcerated addicts had become a burden on the prison system, and a boot camp approach, led by the Ministry of Justice but administered by The Ministry of Welfare and Social Security, was adopted to address the increasing opioid-dependent population. Tehran began sending thousands of addicts to these camps, where they were supposed to abruptly detoxify without medical assistance and atone for their sins through forced labor and minimal social work approach to supporting the process. As expected, many relapsed after release from the camps.

These draconian measures were matched with similarly aggressive operations to prevent the flow of opiates across the border from Afghanistan. By the late 1980s, an estimated 50 percent of Afghan opiate production was passing through Iranian territory, and the Iranian markets were flooded with Afghan opium, heroin, and morphine. Starting in the early 1990s, Tehran constructed more than 260 kilometers of static defenses—including concrete dams that blocked mountain passes, anti-vehicle berms, trenches, minefields, forts, and mountain towers— at a cost of over $80 million. By the late 1990s, more than 100,000 police officers, army troops, and Revolutionary Guardsmen were committed to antinarcotic operations. Yet both the social policies and the border fortifications were fruitless. Although the Iranian authorities seized nearly eight times the amount of narcotics in 1999 than they had in 1990, they could not keep up with the expansion of Afghan opium production, which rose in those years from approximately 1500 metric tons to roughly 4500. Iran also found that the number of intravenous drug users was growing. Ironically, the prisons and camps where addicts were expected to kick their habits became epicenters of drug use, in which people learned how to inject heroin and shared primitive infection-prone needles. The rise in malignant drug use brought with it more deaths, more cases of addiction, and most embarrassingly for Iran's leaders, a full-blown HIV/AIDS epidemic.

Model Intervention

These setbacks prompted a turnaround in Iran's approach to fighting narcotics in 1994 when the Iranian government began focusing on primary prevention programs against opiate misuse for the first time since the revolution. By 2002, over 50 percent of the country's drug-control budget was dedicated to preventive public health campaigns, such as advertisement and education. In 1996, the Iranian government amended its criminal justice codes on opiate misuse, acknowledging the legality of medical and nonmedical interventions for treating opiate dependence. This opened the way for outpatient treatment centers and abstinence-based residential centers to start operating in Tehran and the provinces. The Islamic Republic also began to allow nongovernmental organizations to launch their own prevention and treatment efforts. The government began to implicitly support needle exchange programs, going so far as to encourage the distribution of clean needles in the Iranian prison system. Gradually, the road was paved for methadone maintenance treatment centers and clinics that dispensed locally produced opium pills, in a bid to turn injection drug users into medicated patients.

Results

In making this shift, Iran sought not only to halt the growing HIV/AIDS epidemic but also to reduce the demand for illicit narcotics and to reintegrate drug users back into the economy. These new measures began to show results: The number of new HIV cases among intravenous drug users dropped from a high of 3111 in 2004–1585 in 2010. This trend was particularly notable among Iran's prison population, which witnessed a drop in HIV prevalence from a high of 7.92 percent in 1998 to a low of 1.51 percent in 2007. Additionally, in areas where the country set up harm reduction programs, improvements were observed in addicts' life expectancies and psychological well-being, coupled with an overall reduction in the illicit consumption of opiates.

Analysis

These cases clearly show that strict zero-tolerance criminalization of opiate misuse and interdiction of drug trafficking without a wraparound population health approach not only fail at significantly shifting the opiate drug market, but also can actually worsen health, social, and economic indicators. Effective interventions to change the opiate drug market need to include upstream prevention approaches and a downstream treatment approaches to opiate misuse that improves the overall health outcomes and socioeconomic well-being of the affected population. To succeed, this process requires broad-based coalitions and partnerships across both the healthcare sector, government agencies, including judiciary and criminal justice systems, and communities grappling with opiate addiction. Given the evidence internationally that the incarceration of opiate consumers and sellers is not an effective remedy for opiate use disorder, treatment should be prioritized over incarceration while making sure that those who are imprisoned receive adequate treatment and care after release, including access to public benefits that will allow them to reintegrate into the social fabric.

Primary Prevention: Education/Public Health Campaigns

Primary prevention should begin by addressing the stigma associated with opiate use disorder by educating stakeholders in the community that opiate addiction is a medical illness, not a moral weakness. In the Iranian case, this involved educating clerics and government officials on the biological underpinnings of opioid dependence, allowing the ratifications to the criminal justice laws that were necessary to establish drug treatment programs in the country.

Misapprehensions surrounding harm reduction and medication-assisted treatment of addiction remain a stubborn problem in both low- and high-income countries as evidenced by the position of the US Secretary of Health and Human Services in 2017 that such interventions do little to "move the dial" against opiate use disorders. Educating stakeholders on harm reduction is an important factor in the establishment, expansion, and utilization of programs that focus on reducing the deleterious downstream health and social outcomes of opiate misuse. In the Iranian case, the establishment and widespread use of prison needle exchange programs and its impact on reducing the rate of HIV/AIDS in the Iranian prison system show that investments in harm reduction education pay significant dividends. Such interventions maximize the health of users that are not ready for treatment or face barriers to obtaining care.

Increased community knowledge of risk of opioids, overdose, and overdose prevention strategies through advertisement and education campaigns can have an impact on the both morbidity and mortality associated with opioid misuse in a population.

Secondary Prevention: Focusing on at Risk Populations

This intervention involves screening and more intensive education of the subset of the population more vulnerable to opiate misuse due to increased biological, psychological, or social risk factors. This can include individuals with mental illness, prior substance misuse, and the incarcerated or homeless population. Individuals who screen positive should then receive an in-depth assessment. Self-report questionnaires like the Screener and Opioid Assessment for Patients in Pain (SOAPP) and Opioid Risk Tool (ORT) help assess for the risk of opioid misuse. Preventing initial exposure to opioids should be considered whenever possible and is particularly warranted for minor surgical procedures in which non-opioid modalities can provide effective postsurgical analgesia. Patients with preexisting psychiatric comorbidities or those with family histories of opioid dependence would also benefit from opioid-sparing analgesic strategies. For the acute care surgical patient, the use of multimodal analgesic regimens, including the use of long-acting local anesthetics, has become an approach for expediting movement away from opioid-centric prescribing practices for postsurgical pain management.

Tertiary Prevention: Interventions

Widespread Naloxone Distribution
Broadly expand access to and training for administering naloxone to prevent overdose deaths. Studies show that in communities where overdose education and naloxone distribution were implemented, there was a 27–46 percent decrease in opioid overdose deaths. High implementation of training and naloxone distribution does not increase rates of riskier opioid use as emergency department visits, and hospitalizations after overdose were equivocal in both high and low implementation communities [21].

Needle and Syringe Programs
Allow injection drug users to access clean hypodermic needles at little to no cost or via exchange of used needles. This harm reduction model intervention can help decrease the spread of communicable blood borne infections and by extension reduce the disease burden of addiction on the individual user and their community. A 2004 World Health Organization study showed that needle and syringe programs markedly decreased the rates of HIV transmission among IV drug users without increasing IV drug use rates at the individual or societal level [23].

Medication-Assisted Treatment (MAT)
The use of FDA-approved medications, in combination with counseling and behavioral therapies, to treat opioid use disorders and prevents overdoses. There are currently 3 FDA-approved medications for treating opioid use disorder: methadone, naltrexone, and buprenorphine. Studies show that a combination of medication and therapy can successfully treat and sustain recovery. Medications work by blocking the euphoric effects of opioids, relieve cravings, and normalizing body functions without the negative effects of opioids [22].

Monitoring and Evaluation Frameworks for MAT for Opioid Dependence

MAT programs for opiate dependence have historically been strictly regulated by political authorities. These top-down regulations and guidelines have unintentionally disincentivized individual programs from monitoring outcomes and implementing innovations that respond to changing local needs. Without outcome evaluations, programs risk not meeting their stated goals, and fail to respond to shifting social, medical, and opiate market conditions over time. Objective measures of outcomes can be taken in the following way: (I) medical/psychiatric: laboratory analyses, physical examination results, or hospitalizations; (II) relapse: random urinalysis evaluations, record of hospitalizations for overdose, or complications of opiate misuse; (III) employment: verification via pay stub or third party; (IV) crime: arrest records, probation/parole violations. Patient retention and length of time in treatment are also good proxy measures of the ability of a program to engage a patient in rehabilitation. This process can be facilitated through the use of a number of reliable performance tools including the Methadone Treatment Quality Assurance System (MTQAS), Addiction Severity Index, Treatment Services Review, Family Burden Interview/Short Form (SF) Schedule.

Ethical Considerations

Patients should be free to choose whether to participate in treatment as prescribed by the ethical principle of autonomy unless a person can no longer care for themselves or poses an imminent risk to self or others as a result of their opiate dependence. It is preferable to offer individuals the option of having their opioid dependence treated in a clinical setting as an alternative to incarceration if they are convicted of crimes related to their opioid use. These diversion programs have shown to have high rates of success in treating addicts and low rates of criminal recidivism once treated [10]. Prisoners should not be denied adequate health care associated with their history of addiction because of their imprisonment. Treatment options available to the non-incarcerated population should be available in prisons, and increased efforts at prevention and harm reduction, such as needle exchange programs, should be implemented in prison systems which have higher rates of blood-borne pathogenic transmission due to intravenous opiate consumption compared to the non-incarcerated population. Opioid withdrawal agonist maintenance and naltrexone treatment should be available in prison settings, and prisoners should not be forced to accept any particular treatment. Patients should have the right to privacy and confidentiality while receiving treatment and when possible, central registration of patients receiving methadone or buprenorphine maintenance treatment should be avoided to reduce the chance of breaching privacy.

Conclusion

Evidence-based methods that focus on preventing and treating opiate misuse and addiction have been shown to be far more effective in reducing demand, mortality, and morbidity associated with addictive markets as compared to punitive tactics, such as criminalization, interdiction, and incarceration. The more progressive aspects of the Iranian and Portuguese experience demonstrate that a more ethical, public-health-oriented, harm reduction approach to opiate misuse holds the best hope of decreasing the impact of addiction on the individual and populations throughout the world. Yet, effective evidence-based gold standard medical treatments for addiction remain out of reach for most who need it, driven mostly by the prevalence of stigma and sociocultural prejudices in most policy-making bodies and governments. Coping with addictive opiate markets, therefore, demands a renewed effort to raise global public awareness on proven biomedical treatments for addiction and preventive approaches to curb this growing public health crisis.

References

1. Afghanistan opium survey 2018: Challenges to sustainable development, peace and security. (2019). Retrieved from https://www.unodc.org/documents/crop-monitoring/Afghanistan/Afghanistan_opium_survey_2018_socioeconomic_report.pdf
2. Annual report on the state of the drugs problem in the European Union. (2000). Retrieved from http://www.emcdda.europa.eu/system/files/publications/151/ar00_en_69639.pdf
3. Birnbaum, H. G., White, A. G., Schiller, M., Waldman, T., Cleveland, J. M., & Roland, C. L. (2011). Societal costs of prescription opioid abuse, dependence, and misuse in the United States. *Pain Medicine, 12*(4), 657–667. https://doi.org/10.1111/j.1526-4637.2011.01075.x.
4. Data and statistics. (2019). Retrieved from http://www.euro.who.int/en/health-topics/disease-prevention/illicit-drugs/data-and-statistics
5. Degenhardt, L., Charlson, F., Mathers, B., Hall, W. D., Flaxman, A. D., Johns, N., & Vos, T. (2014). The global epidemiology and burden of opioid dependence: Results from the global burden of disease 2010 study. *Addiction, 109*(8), 1320–1333. https://doi.org/10.1111/add.12551.
6. Degenhardt, L., Whiteford, H. A., Ferrari, A. J., Baxter, A. J., Charlson, F. J., Hall, W. D., et al. (2013). Global burden of disease attributable to illicit drug use and dependence: Findings from the Global Burden of Disease Study 2010. *Lancet, 382*(9904), 1564–1574. https://doi.org/10.1016/s0140-6736(13)61530-5.
7. Estratégia Nacional de Luta Contra a Droga: Relatório da Comissão para a Estratégia Nacional de Combate à Droga. (1998). Retrieved from http://www.sicad.pt/BK/Publicacoes/Lists/SICAD_PUBLICACOES/Attachments/48/ENcomissao.pdf
8. Executive summary. (2019). Retrieved from https://wdr.unodc.org/wdr2019/prelaunch/WDR19_Booklet_1_EXECUTIVE_SUMMARY.pdf
9. Ferreira, S. (2017). *Portugal's radical drugs policy is working. Why hasn't the world copied it?*. Retrieved from https://www.theguardian.com/news/2017/dec/05/portugals-radical-drugs-policy-is-working-why-hasnt-the-world-copied-it
10. Fielding, J. E., Tye, G., Ogawa, P. L., Imam, I. J., & Long, A. M. (2002). Los Angeles County drug court programs: Initial results. *Journal of Substance Abuse Treatment, 23*(3), 217–224. https://doi.org/10.1016/s0740-5472(02)00262-3.
11. Florence, C. S., Zhou, C., Luo, F., & Xu, L. (2016). The economic burden of prescription opioid overdose, abuse, and dependence in the United States, 2013. *Medical Care, 54*(10), 901–906. https://doi.org/10.1097/mlr.0000000000000625.
12. Global overview of drug demand and supply. (2018). Retrieved from https://www.unodc.org/wdr2018/prelaunch/WDR18_Booklet_2_GLOBAL.pdf
13. Hanna, F. (2017). Alcohol and substance use in humanitarian and post-conflict situations. *Eastern Mediterranean Health Journal, 23*(3), 231–235. https://doi.org/10.26719/2017.23.3.231.
14. Hedegaard, H., Miniño, A. M., & Warner, M. (2018). *Drug overdose deaths in the United States, 1999–2017.* Hyattsville: National Center for Health Statistics, Centers for Disease Control and Prevention. Data Brief No. 329.
15. Hughes, C. E., & Stevens, A. (2010). What can we learn from the Portuguese decriminalization of illicit drugs? *British Journal of Criminology, 50*(6), 999–1022. https://doi.org/10.1093/bjc/azq038.

16. National drug threat assessment. (2018). Retrieved from https://www.dea.gov/sites/default/files/2018-11/DIR-032-18%202018%20NDTA%20final%20low%20resolution.pdf

17. Pardo, B., Taylor, J., Caulkins, J., Kilmer, B., Reuter, P., & Stein, B. (2019). *The future of fentanyl and other synthetic opioids*. Santa Monica: RAND.

18. Relatório annual 2008: a situação do país em matéria de drogas e toxicodependências, vol. I – Informação estatística. 2009. Lisbon Portugal: Instituto da Droga e da Toxicodependência

19. Schwetz, T. A., Calder, T., Rosenthal, E., Kattakuzhy, S., & Fauci, A. S. (2019). Opioids and infectious diseases: A converging public health crisis. *The Journal of Infectious Diseases, 220*(3), 346–349. https://doi.org/10.1093/infdis/jiz133.

20. Syrian refugee crisis: Aid, statistics and news: USA for UNHCR. (n.d.). Retrieved from https://www.unrefugees.org/emergencies/syria/

21. Walley, A. Y., Xuan, Z., Hackman, H. H., Quinn, E., Doe-Simkins, M., Sorensen-Alawad, A., et al. (2013). Opioid overdose rates and implementation of overdose education and nasal naloxone distribution in Massachusetts: Interrupted time series analysis. *BMJ, 346*, f174. https://doi.org/10.1136/bmj.f174.

22. Walsh, L. (2019). *Medication and counseling treatment*. Retrieved from https://www.samhsa.gov/medication-assisted-treatment/treatment#medications-used-in-mat

23. Wodak, A., & Cooney, A. (2004). *Effectiveness of sterile needle and syringe programming in reducing HIV/AIDS among injecting drug users*. Geneva: World Health Organization. Retrieved from https://www.who.int/hiv/pub/prev_care/effectivenesssterileneedle.pdf.

Resilience and Ethics in Post-conflict Settings: *Kwihangana*, Living After Genocide Rape, and Intergenerational Resilience in Post-genocide Rwanda

Maggie Zraly and Marie Grâce Kagoyire

Resilience and Gender-Based Violence in Humanitarian Settings

Resilience is a concept of growing importance in global mental health. It emerged in the 1970s in the field of developmental psychopathology to help explain how people could achieve adaptive outcomes despite exposure to adversity. In contemporary global mental health literature, *resilience* is generally defined as the capacity of individuals, communities, and groups to adapt and cope in the presence of adversity, risk, and/or traumatic experience as well as with future negative events. It is particularly relevant in emergency contexts where, despite multiple forms of adversity, conflict, and violence, affected populations tend to develop relatively low rates of long-term mental disorders [28]. Increasingly, efforts by global mental health researchers and practitioners in humanitarian and post-conflict settings aim to focus on protecting and promoting mental health and well-being, which calls for a rigorous understanding of human resilience in order to develop salutogenic approaches that stand in distinction to treating pathology.

Support for strengthening resilience among disaster- and conflict-affected people has become recognized as a critical component of good practice for provision of mental health and psychosocial support (MHPSS) in humanitarian settings [9]. Individual resilience in the face of political violence is supported by internal and external resources such as hope, optimism, determination, religious/spiritual beliefs, and connection to community as well as interacting biological, psychological, and social systems [35]. *Collective resilience* in the context of political

M. Zraly (✉)
Mental Health and Psychosocial Support (MHPSS) Collective, Copenhagen, Denmark

M. G. Kagoyire
Historical Trauma and Transformation, Stellenbosch University, Stellenbosch, South Africa

© Springer Nature Switzerland AG 2021
A. R. Dyer et al. (eds.), *Global Mental Health Ethics*,
https://doi.org/10.1007/978-3-030-66296-7_13

violence has been theorized to be a context-dependent process that counteracts social trauma and aims to create relationships that heal the wounds of trauma, heal the losses of war, and reconstruct a sense of belonging and identity [6]. Practice recommendations based on this theoretical ground call for providing safe space after an initial phase of post-disaster stabilization for people to come together, enabling them to share their stories and develop pathways to re-establish communities [4].

However, the uniqueness of each humanitarian setting and the diversity of cultures and socio-historic contexts make it challenging to specify prescriptions for resilience promotion. The complexity of this problem has to do with the ways that culture and context play a defining role in both in what constitutes resilience itself and the dynamics of violence. During humanitarian emergencies, some of the most complicated challenges involve the protection of individuals, families, and communities from multiple forms of gender-based violence (GBV), defined as *any harmful act that is perpetrated against a person's will and that is based on socially ascribed (i.e., gender) differences, including physical, sexual, or mental harm or suffering, threats of such acts, coercion, and other deprivations of liberty* [10]. Conflict-related sexual violence, one type of GBV, violates individuals, cultural systems, and social bonds which creates widespread fear, shame, and demoralization among the people under assault making it harder to recover and rebuild. Sexual and other forms of gender-based violence are known risk factors for mental health and psychosocial well-being in conflict settings. While there is some evidence that strengthening community-based supports is a promising approach to improve well-being and prevent or treat mental disorders among survivors of GBV in post-conflict and recovery settings, more attention and focus is needed to develop effective resilience promotion strategies [38].

Brief Ethnohistory of Rwanda

Since the onset of European colonization (1899–1962), people in Rwanda have experienced waves of catastrophic political violence, including massacres, war crimes, crimes against humanity, and genocide. Although aspects of this history are contested, there is global agreement that one of the most abject events in human history was the 100 days of systematic genocide of Tutsis and political moderate Hutus by the Hutu extremist led by Rwandan army and local Rwandan *Interahamwe*[1] militias in 1994. During what has come to be known as the 1994 Rwandan genocide against the Tutsi, an estimated 800,000 to over 1 million Rwandan people were killed, including 70% of the minority Tutsi population. As many as 10,000 people were killed per day, and sexual violence was used as a weapon of genocide against upward of 250,000 mostly Tutsi women and girls [2]. Women and girls aged 2 to over 70 years old were targeted for rape, gang rape, sexual torture, and

---

[1] *Interahamwe* means those who stand/work/fight/attack together and refers to the Hutu paramilitary organization that participated in the mass killings of Tutsis during 1994 genocide.

forced "marriage" [23]. The United Nations Security Council, led by the United States at the time, voted to withdraw UN troops from Rwanda, avoided acknowledging what was happening as genocide, and did not organize a response to halt the killing.

Rwandan people, the *Banyarwanda*, have for centuries shared a common language, history, and cultural world with meaningful, rich, and enduring interpersonal and generational relationships across social groups. Pre-colonial Rwandan society was largely organized by ethnically flexible clans, patron-client relationships, and gender systems with power structures that were more or less influenced by state politics according to proximity to the geographic reach of a central monarchy [22]. In the early twentieth century, Belgian colonizers crystallized a sense of ethnic distinction and institutionalized ethnic inequality through creating a system of indirect rule by the Tutsi monarchy and identity cards that encoded the categories of Tutsi, Hutu, and Twa as "ethnicity." Ethnic group classification by the Belgians was assigned in a bureaucratic way according to degree of wealth expressed through cattle ownership. With Rwanda's independence (1959–1961) came a revolution of the Hutu majority that resulted in the formation of a Hutu-dominated republic that brought discrimination against, massacres of, and exile of Tutsis into neighboring countries.

Following episodes of political violence, such as in 1959, 1963, and 1973, more and more Rwandans took refuges outside Rwanda's borders, and they eventually formed the Rwandan Patriotic Front (RPF), a political group who launched a war in 1990 to seize control of the country [30]. While a peace agreement (the Arusha Peace Accords) was being negotiated between the RPF and Rwandan government to end the war, a plane with Rwandan President Juvénal Habyarimana and Burundian President Cyprien Ntaryamira was shot down on April 6, 1994, killing everyone aboard. Immediately claiming that the RPF had assassinated the President, the Interahamwe militias supported by the former army and *gendarmerie*[2] set up road blocks in the capital city of Kigali that same day and launched a country-wide genocidal campaign against the Tutsi ethnic group. The RPF ended the war and genocide 3 months later by defeating the civilian and military authorities responsible for the genocide and taking control and leadership of the country.

During and after the genocide, about two million civilians, a number of whom participated in the genocide and some of their family members, fled to neighboring countries, such as the Democratic Republic of Congo (DRC) (then Zaire) and Tanzania, where they became refugees primarily in camps. Leaders, enforcers, and perpetrators of the genocide used the same escape routes from Rwanda, forcing some Tutsi women to move and stay with them as sexual slaves [23], and in many places genocide militia leaders seized control of camps. Regional histories of the late 1990s during the first Congo war, the mass return of Rwandan refugees from

---

[2] Gendarmerie was used by the then former government. It has been replaced by the police in post-genocide Rwanda.

DRC and Tanzania to Rwanda, and the insurgency and counter-insurgency in northwest Rwanda are particularly contested and "sensitive," and the numbers of victims are not yet well-known [17, 39]. During these same years, Rwandan genocide rape survivors who were living in and returning to Rwanda had disproportionately high rates of HIV/AIDS, persistent psychiatric suffering and mental health problems, threats of stigma and social marginalization, and danger due to being direct targets and witnesses of genocide crimes [18, 47].

Post-genocide Rwandan Context

In post-genocide Rwanda, Rwandan "home-grown" solutions to Rwandan problems are valued, as is pride in having successfully prevented genocide from reoccurring and in rebuilding a society aimed toward national unity and reconciliation. For example, the Rwandan institution of *gacaca* (justice on the grass) was re-imagined and deployed as an experimental, community-based, transitional justice system to process backlog of over 100,000 suspects of genocide-related crimes that would have taken over 200 years to try within a conventional national court system. Likewise, *ingando*[3] (temporary military encampments for soldiers) was recreated as liminal spaces of intense learning and transformation for a wide variety of Rwandan groups to become incorporated as good citizens in the new post-genocide social order. Others intentionally conceived of "traditional," "local," and "participatory" national unity and reconciliation activities that operate as tools for social transformation include *itorero* schools, *ubudehe* "mutual assistance" schemes, and *ubusabane* "public conviviality meetings" [31].

Similarly, *Kwibuka* (to remember/to memorialize) is the now annual public period of commemorating the 1994 genocide against the Tutsi in Rwanda. *Kwibuka* is a national, and international, social backdrop to more traditional mourning rituals (*icyunamo*) for lost loved ones that can involve locating mass graves, unearthing people's bodies, washing skeletal remains, entering the remains in coffins, and holding traditional all-night vigils with visitors around a fire for ideally at least seven nights. During Kwibuka, there are also pilgrimages by survivors and their supporters to remembrance ceremonies at genocide memorial sites and graveyards. The aim of the annual memorialization, which lasts for 100 days to mark the period of the genocide, is to remember the genocide victims, heal the wounds of the past, and enable Rwandans to reflect on the causes and the consequences of past divisions, all in order to prevent the recurrence of the collective violence [20]. Kwibuka socially acknowledges of the situation and suffering of genocide survivors[4] and also works toward reinforcing a sense of shared national and cultural identity among all as "Rwandans."

Most Rwandans hope for and appreciate social acknowledgment of their pain and suffering during the genocide and war, but participation in some transitional

---

[3] Ingando in post-genocide society refers to solidarity or reeducation or reintegration camps established in 1999 [22]. Ingando (in singular) refers to Rwanda's peace/civic education program, taken from the Kinyarwanda verb *kugandika*, which is about halting normal activities in order to reflect on and find solutions to national challenges [21].

[4] Anyone who was directly targeted during the genocide and survived.

justice and national reconciliation mechanisms have been re-traumatizing and otherwise dangerous for many genocide survivors, including women and girls who were raped. Platforms like gacaca and Kwibuka offered opportunities for giving public testimony about what happened during the genocide, yet many women and girls who survived genocide rape and who dared to speak out about their experiences have been harassed before, during, and after giving testimony and faced threats of traumatic experience, stigma from the community, ill-health, social isolation, and insecurity [3]. And, while gacaca was remarkable in opening up space for genocide rape survivors to take up community leadership positions as *inyangamugayo* (judges in the community-based courts), research findings suggest that doing so was related to women and girl survivors needing or taking more time alone to themselves for emotional self-care or self-protection [43].

Western Conceptions of Resilience vs. Local Variation in Accounts of Resilience

In 2005, I (the first author) conducted an ethnographic study of resilience among Rwandan women who survived genocide rape.[5] Early in the fieldwork in southern Rwanda, I realized how specific the concept of resilience was to Western/US culture at that time. No one I talked to in the first few months, except for two Rwandan psychologists, was familiar with or seemed to be interested in the idea of resilience. I attempted to explain it with academic and technical definitions, which were abstract and fuzzy, or more colloquial expressions like "being able to bounce back from adversity." Slowly, through working with multiple interpreters and translators during participant observation and informal interviews, I identified three Rwandan psychosocial concepts that together seemed to open a lens on resilience in relation to genocide rape among members of genocide survivor associations: *kwihangana* (to withstand, to bear, to be patient), *kwongera kubaho* (to live again), and *gukomeza k'ubuzima* (to continue life/living). These concepts unlocked a rich world of dozens of practices, processes, and resources involving self, emotion, and sociality that Rwandan genocide rape survivors used to live life despite exquisite traumatic experience and extreme adversity [45].

Kwihangana was particularly salient to wider everyday Rwandan social life, especially in its imperative form, *Ihangane*. It can generally be considered an expression of care or interest in one's emotional well-being. People commonly said "Ihangane" in an encouraging way to me and others across a broad spectrum of situations, ranging from mundane frustrations and slights, like having someone cut in front of you in line while waiting for help to get access to a basic service like electricity or medical care, to intense tragedies and losses like the death of a family member. Interestingly, shortly after my research, kwihangana also emerged as an important finding in a separate public health study in northern Rwanda on resilience among children and families at risk for psychosocial difficulties due to HIV/AIDS. In that context,

[5] This research was supported by the National Science Foundation under Grant No. 0514519.

kwihangana, translated as perseverance or withstanding despite hardship, was identified as one of five key sources of resilience along with self-esteem/self-confidence
(*kwigirira ikizere*), family unity/trust (*kwizerana*), good parenting (*kurera neza*), and
collective/communal support (*ubufasha abaturage batanga*). It was also singled out
as a potentially widespread Rwandan cultural value [1].

In a more recent study of the politics of patience in Rwanda, Løvgren [15] argues
that kwihangana is not passive nor is it constituted by suffering, but it is an active
bearing with or being patient with something that becomes most relevant when that
something is suffering. Based on her research with graduates from a rehabilitation
center for loitering and "delinquent" male youth on Iwawa Island in Rwanda,
Løvgren describes an empirical framing of being patient as an agentive emotional
processing of violence that attempts to control its effects. This resonates with
Rwandan genocide-survivors accounts of kwihangana (see Box 13.1).

Preliminary research by the second author with Rwandan women survivors of rape
who have children born of rape, and who are supported by a local non-governmental

---

Box 13.1 Rwandan Genocide rape Survivor Narratives of Kwihangana,
Translated as to Withstand

Can you imagine somebody who sees your naked body and aims to harm your
life so much that you are unable to work and earn a living like before? Being
unable to find something [food] for yourself like you used to be able to is
worse. Still, we try to withstand, as we can do nothing else. It is possible to
withstand. – *Adelyn, age 57*

When I say to make myself strong, there is a time, I mean, as we talk about
it, I feel palpitations, and then, but I keep quiet and think that everything is
possible. You create in yourself something to be strong and you withstand. –
Eloise, age 58

To strengthen yourself, of course, it's you feel that you don't let the suffering make you fade away; otherwise, you could die. You hurry up and go
through it. You do not linger in that pain. But, as it goes, to withstand causes
you to feel that you brought force inside yourself … That's withstanding; it is
like this of course. – *Noelle, age 43*

Kwihangana simply means to withstand something you have experienced
that has hurt your heart. You withstand it to avoid committing. You feel as if it
were the end of life, but you eventually realize you are not the only one who
has suffered because there are other people with whom you share problems.
This then makes you withstand and you no longer experience these feelings. –
Elaina, age 42

Withstanding when somebody is confronted with a problem. When one
fails to withstand when facing problems, he or she is likely to go mad.
Therefore, all they need is to be like any other mature person when facing a
problem that makes them feel pain. People may then ask themselves: how
should we go about this problem? Let us stand firm. People then stand firm
this way. – *Gabrielle, age 44*

organization called Kanyarwanda, points to their definition of kwihangana as to strengthen a/your vein (*gukomeza umutsi*)[6] or to keep going courageously despite enduring hardships (*kudacika intege*). Here, kwihangana involves committing oneself to leave the past behind in order to move on, or going beyond one's personal suffering to try to face the present and future. According to some of these women, kwihangana is also seen as an outcome of a back and forth process that consists of trying to understand, live with, accept, and find a way of managing/dealing with the consequences of an unbearable situation that happened in life while oriented toward a better future. In addition, both of us have gleaned from our long-term study that key intersections of resilience and kwihangana among survivors in the Rwanda post-genocide setting involved having people around who faced similar experiences and among whom a survivor may feel a sense of family and belonging, as well as having access to a platform or safe setting where a survivor can go meet like others, share her/his emotional distress, laugh with others, and learn from others' ways of dealing and coping with everyday stressors.

Resilience and kwihangana are not the same, nor can kwihangana be conceived of as a simple mechanism of positive coping with severe traumatic experience. Kwihangana has cultural meaning, value, and logic in relation to suffering in the Rwandan post-genocide context that resilience does not. Kwihangana connects self and emotion to everyday social interaction and to what it means to be a "good person" in a sociopolitical context where the stakes of not engaging in it can include risks of loss of dignity, bodily distress, mental illness, and death. In the Rwandan context, engaging in kwihangana appears to index a type of moral person who is a strong person in terms of being able to manage difficult or intense emotions and hardships. Yet, the relationships between kwihangana and resilience are important, as both are capacities for non-pathological, protective responses to violence and trauma that enable people to adapt and exceed expectations of the impacts of adversity.

Though kwihangana involves fundamental human capacities of the self and psyche, the psychosocial components of kwihangana may be the more important aspects to focus on for fostering and strengthening resilience. We explore collective dimensions of resilience in the next section and note that the case material on resilience and kwihangana that we present in this chapter focuses on Rwandan women survivors of genocide rape who had already accessed safe spaces – some they had created themselves and most that received some form of support from the Rwandan government and/or non-governmental organizations.

---

[6] In the study of Rwandan ethnomedicine, where it is theorized that flow is valued as health, strengthening veins would be a symbol of restoring well-being by perpetuating the process of flow [38].

Collective Resilience in Politically Sensitive Environments: Narrating Suffering vs. Unspeakability

In the aftermath of the genocide, the population of Rwanda was 70% female and thousands of new Rwandan women's associations formed in the void left by the disruption and destruction of families, friendships, and communities [29]. During the study of resilience referenced above, I (MZ) worked closely with three of these associations: a district-level branch of AVEGA, a national-level association of genocide widows; Tugane Umuhoza, a sub-group of AVEGA members living with HIV/AIDS; and Abasa, a district-level association of genocide rape survivors. Genocide

---

Box 13.2 Rwandan Genocide rape Survivor Narratives of Association Membership

One of the best things I like about AVEGA is the way we used to meet there to withstand together and discuss a number of our problems and thoughts. This was helpful because we were no longer isolated. – *Jolie, age 42*

When we are with others, that is when we feel happy because we chat about our problems and end up finding that we share the same problems. That's how the Abasa community, our association, grew strong. – *Liana, age 42*

When I joined Abasa, I had to say all I went through, no secrets. So those who didn't want to say it didn't become members because they didn't want to say it; they kept it secret. So we said it because there was no need keeping it a secret. Mostly because it [genocide rape] was done in public where people were watching. So there was no need to hide it anymore. – *Emmeline, age 40*

The reason why Abasa members can discuss it together; look, this is a hill. You are the same children, and you live in the same family. And all of your parents have died, and only girls remained, who were raped ... We also had another person, Violet, who was a hero. Violet could speak it [experiencing genocide rape] out. And we said: "why not say it if she can say it?" And we discussed it a lot. And when you are free to talk, it is impossible to know how it starts; you can't know how it started when you are talking freely with other people, to any one else who has the same problems as yours. We often sit and talk about it; we ask each other if we all are the same: "is it also the same for you?" This makes us unite in that way, because we have same problems. We didn't hide anything from each other because we realized that we had a same problem. – *Colette, age 34*

AVEGA people set up an association and invited widowed survivors to join. So we used to meet there and talk together so that everyone told about her experiences. We sometimes sat together, cried, and closed curtains. After feeling relieved, we went back home. – *Estelle, age 38*

I mean we generally share the same problems. When we were hiding in sorghum plantations [during the genocide], you could meet someone there who's gone through same ordeal as you, and she tells you what happened to people you knew, those who were killed after being raped, because that's what Interahamwe were busy doing. – *Adette, age 40*

rape survivors, genocide widows, and people living with HIV/AIDS all faced different forms of stigma in the post-genocide Rwandan context. Through association membership, women and girls who survived genocide rape adapted to the risk of social marginalization by connecting with like others. These relationships provided psychosocial support and enabled members to do the collective emotional and cultural work of sharing problems, making meaning, and normalizing extreme experience (see Box 13.2).

What I observed among women survivors' associations in Rwanda in the mid-2000s supports the conceptualization of collective resilience as a context-dependent process involving the re-making of relationships, belonging, and identity. Membership in these associations created a protected space where genocide rape survivors could speak their truth and bear witness to the often painful and courageous truths of others who shared similar experiences. However, this collective resilience through women's associations was juxtaposed with everyday social dynamics outside associations where it was not always safe to speak openly about experiences of the excruciating pain and anguish of the genocide rape they endured and its continuing impacts on their lives. In daily life, women and girls navigated multiple sources of threat and harassment by employing tactics of self-silencing and self-censoring, feigning naivety, and exchanging gossip to survive [44]. This highlights the live-saving nature and importance of associations like AVEGA and *Abasa* in the post-genocide context.

The theme of "unspeakability" in reference to experiences of political violence also arose in a most recent study of community resilience in northern Rwanda by Otake [26]. She found that Rwandan adults in these communities used the coping and protection strategy of selective silence and avoidance of speaking about sensitive past war experiences. Sharing of suffering narratives, when it happened, took place as part of sharing everyday life (*gusangira*), like in *ubusabane* (convivial public get-togethers). Sharing everyday life was related to helping each other, and talking for mutual understanding as ordinary aspects of "living together," among people of different identities, in post-genocide Rwandan community. Collective resilience to war experience in the northern Rwandan context did not take place through support groups or associations, and instead consisted of creating and maintaining relationships of mutual support in the ordinary processes of living [25]. This helps illustrate that even when experiences of political violence and trauma are not openly appreciated and acknowledged, collective resilience dynamics can still occur in muted ways.

Strengthening Resilience in Practice: Singular Focus on Humanitarian Mental Health and Well-Being vs. Simultaneously Addressing Peace-Building and Post-conflict Development

There is a small but growing evidence base for potentially scalable psychosocial interventions that activate individual, family, and community resilience humanitarian settings [11]. For example, practiced in Rwanda for the past 15 years, sociotherapy is an approach that the World Health Organization describes as using "the interactions between individuals and their social environment to facilitate the re-establishment of values, norms, and relationships and at the same time provide the opportunity for debate, the sharing of experiences and coping mechanisms" ([42]:33). Whether implemented in formal or informal group settings, sociotherapy provides safe space and dialogue to create peer support structures that enhance social networks and improve mental health and psychosocial well-being. Supporting and protecting safe space for people who have survived humanitarian disasters, like war and genocide, to meet and share their past experiences and current life issues is thought to be a key element in sociotherapy and some other community- and group-based interventions to strengthening resilience [7]. Findings from ongoing research in Rwanda suggest that by sharing their own wounds in a series of structured peer support group sessions, people start to find and commit themselves to living a new life in a positive way while setting common ground rules for achieving a more beneficial future together. As they increasingly practice these life orientations within their group, the practice ripples out to their families and communities as well [33].

Interestingly, improved psychosocial well-being among Rwandan survivors of genocide- and war-related traumatic events who participate in community-based sociotherapy may cascade to produce additional positive impacts for the generation who was born after the conflict. Findings on the intergenerational effects of socio-therapy among genocide rape survivors in Rwanda revealed that children seek to develop their own strategies of coping with the past in response to their parents' patterns of resilience and suffering [12]. For example, depression symptoms were common among mothers and children before the intervention, while after both had developed more feelings of self-confidence. Moreover, sociotherapy enabled women survivors to be less violent and more open, communicative, and caring toward their children, which conferred a sense of emotional release among the children themselves. This unburdening co-occurred with a variety of child outcomes, including participating in family decision-making, having less worries related to their mother's suffering, improving their school performance, and having hope for the future.

Box 13.3 Children with a Parent in Sociotherapy Speak of Ending Violence
Before, I used to think that when I will meet my mother's perpetrator, I should get revenge. But my mother always warned me that it is not good… As I said above, one day I threw stones at him [the perpetrator]. But our mother challenged us; she asked us what we think might have been her own reasons for not seeking revenge for that perpetrator? Then we stopped doing so. – *Adeline, age 21*

The way our parents got empowered gave me the strength to cope with what happened. They are the ones who should hold that grudge, because they know what they went through, they were the ones to suffer because of the history, instead of us having that grudge about things we do not know. Since our parents have no grudge, we should not have it. – *Adeline, age 21*

> So, when you read the stories, how parents lived day after day, you come to easily understand how things were during the genocide... The mothers have described well how the genocide was done. If you read how it started, you will prevent yourself from committing same acts. Through reading the stories, you may learn how it started and plan how to fight against anything that can bring back the genocide. On my side, I can have love and be of service to others [*kwitanga*]. – *Celie, age* 24

Furthermore, some youth expressed a lessening of feelings of wanting revenge or holding grudges due to receiving positive guidance from their mothers, reading the stories of their mother's suffering and resilience (or of death and rebirth), and witnessing the smiling of their mothers. Some youth even expressed feeling a commitment to preventing another genocide (see Box 13.3).

Women's self-help groups, like AVEGA and Abasa, and community-based sociotherapy are types of evidence-based resilience-focused psychosocial interventions that may promote transmission of resilience across generations. For example, Zraly et al. [46] had also previously reported a case of a Rwandan woman genocide rape survivor who engaged in a mode of resilience that she hoped bolstered her children's resilience, especially the resilience of her daughter who also had survived genocide rape as a child. Resilience activated through groups, communities, or networks may also work as a mechanism of trauma-informed restorative justice resulting in peace-building at family and community levels, as well as wider social change. If resilience can be transmitted intergenerationally from primary sufferers of the traumatic events, then it is possible that such resilience transmission could contribute to the prevention of mental health problems among future generations as well as a reduction in the likelihood of future political violence and the promotion of peace in communities. This means that it may be possible for interventions that strengthen resilience in humanitarian or recovery settings to achieve indirect impacts that exceed intended short-term MHPSS outcomes among participants. What is most critical to making these group/community interventions more successful is to contextualize them and empower local people to drive them within their own communities.

Ethical Frameworks for Interpreting Resilience in Post-conflict Contexts

According to the Humanitarian Charter in the Sphere Handbook for humanitarian responses, all people affected by disaster or conflict have a right to receive protection and assistance to ensure the basic conditions for life with dignity [36]. One form of protection in humanitarian settings consists of strengthening community psychosocial support and self-help, which creates a protective environment that allows the people affected to help each other toward psychosocial resilience and recovery. In alignment with the principles and rights outlined in the Humanitarian Charter, Inter-Agency Standing Committee (IASC) MHPSS Reference Group has issued guidelines on mental health and psychosocial interventions for emergency settings [9]. The core principles of the MHPSS in emergencies guidelines are to promote human rights and equity, maximize local participation, do no harm, build on available resources and capacities, integrate support systems (rather than stand-alone services for specific groups), and ensure multi-layered supports (i.e., basic services and security, community and family supports, focused non-specialized supports, and specialized services). The do no harm principle includes the imperative to use methods and approaches that are sensitive to and fit the context and culture.

Central to resilience-based approaches, the IASC guidelines recommend both to support local people's engagement with understanding adversity and shaping interventions and to take context and culture into account. This means building on existing strengths and resources within affected communities, recognizing especially the role that non-specialists and community members can play, and accounting for local perceptions and knowledge of psychosocial well-being and distress. While support for community self-help activities is generally considered resilience enhancing, it is critical to also determine the needs of diverse people across age, gender, and disability, in relation to specific protective and resilience-promoting factors in each particular humanitarian setting. In addition, the guidelines note that ethical sensitivity is needed in the provision of all forms of community support in order to ensure that any existing cultural, religious, and spiritual practices that could be amplified are in alignment with human rights. With regard to resilience and GBV in humanitarian settings, the goals of the related *IASC Guidelines for Integrating GBV Interventions in Humanitarian Action* (2015) include promoting resilience by strengthening community-based systems that enable survivors and those at risk of GBV to access appropriate care and support.

While the IASC guidelines critically highlight the ethical importance to consider culture and context in humanitarian MHPSS practice to do no harm at the field level, the discipline of medical anthropology takes this further [14] and elevates the imperative to grapple more deeply with theoretical, technical, and ethical issues, such as the following:

- Is resilience a universal process or is it different across cultures?
- What are the local cultural concepts of well-being and recovery that contribute to culturally specific patterns of resilience?
- How are local beliefs about resilience related to wider ethnomedical traditions as they pertain to mental health?
- What is essential to know about resilience in the particular contexts of humanitarian disaster and complex emergency settings in order to ensure safe, accessible, effective MHPSS interventions for diverse groups, including GBV survivors?

In addition, when it comes to ethics, medical anthropology highlights the concept of moral experience, defined as *what is "at stake" for people in the course of ordinary living in a local social world*. Moral experience outlines the stakes that occur throughout the flow of everyday interactions, including our responses to perceived threats, our hopes, and our coping with loss, pain, and suffering [13]. From this perspective, resilience among survivors of genocide and other complex humanitarian disasters illuminates itself as deeply imbued with moral dimensions implicit in survival, endurance, and adaptation to adversity that register through the navigation of threats and dangers in specific local worlds. As a process that is embedded and meaningful in local social networks and communities, resilience among people living through and recovering from the extraordinary conditions of war, genocide, and sexual violence is thought to involve realizing, or enacting, cultural values in ways that counter disintegration or shattering of the self and emotion and retain claims to moral personhood, or being a "good person," and these cultural values maybe more or less aligned with human rights. A focus on moral experience also empowers MHPSS in emergencies practitioners to determine what constitutes "good" resilience-focused psychosocial care at the field level [19].

For many survivors of political violence, moral experience includes hope for social acknowledgment of war- and genocide-related pain and suffering. The concept of social acknowledgment has been operationalized in the health sciences literature as a survivor/victim's experience of positive reactions from society that show appreciation for and acknowledge the survivor/victim's unique state and difficult situation [16]. It stands in counterpoint to what's been called the denial syndrome, a combination of selective perception, selective recollection, and selective interpretation that prevent the acknowledgment of unbearable information [32]. Social acknowledgment can be a powerful resilience resource or protective factor, while denial of experiences of political violence can undermine resilience. As an ethical frame, social acknowledgment of the pain and suffering from genocide, conflict-related sexual violence, and other forms of political violence taps into a shared sense of what it means to be human and promotes the humanitarian basis for survivors to assert rights to dignity, safety, and freedom from stigma and to claim space to express experiences of suffering and resilience. It also has key implications for ensuring that resilience-based MHPSS in humanitarian action is guided by both discouraging the selective denial of violence and suffering and a taking on the responsibility to bear the knowledge of violence and suffering in its most complex and horrific forms.

Humanitarian action is increasingly interconnected with development efforts through the humanitarian-development-peace nexus. The nexus offers a framework that reflects the understanding that humanitarian relief, development programs, and peace-building are not sequential processes; all are needed at the same time [27]. The implementation of a nexus approach could provide a substantial opportunity to enhance psychosocial resilience, including through long-term support to community-based resilience promotion programs and ensuring that resilience approaches are integral to both immediate responses and longer-term development and peace-building outcomes. However, the nexus is challenging to put into practice at the field level. If possible, there is an ethical duty to do all three at once: (1) support resilience of disaster- or conflict-affected people, (2) ensure those supports translate into longer-term recovery and mental health and well-being for all, and (3) contribute to preventing future violence and building sustainable justice and peace. From a MHPSS humanitarian point of view, it is paramount to ensure in settings where political violence is perpetrated against people by the state that taking on all three goals does not compromise the first – the delivery of accessible, high-quality psychosocial resilience support among disaster- and conflict-affected people (see [34]).

Recommendations

Global mental health is becoming more accustomed to and familiar with taking cultural difference seriously when it comes to establishing diagnostic categories and criteria for mental disorders. We recommend that the same consideration should be applied to "positive" mental health or salutogenic psychological and psychiatric phenomena like resilience [40]. We need more refined understandings of resilience and related human capacities that encompass a broader spectrum of human experience and cultural variation, and we need better understanding of the categories and underlying process for mental health itself, not just as the absence of disorder, across culture and context. We support Eggerman and Panter-Brick's [5] proposal to inform practice with an anthropological and social-ecological accounting of variations in resilience across peoples' conceptions of resilience, cultural values, culturally recognized life course and development milestones, and conceptions of suffering and hope. This approach values both emic views and social determinants of resilience, and it can illuminate subjectivities (senses of self and emotional experience), social experiences, and structural conditions that shape how the life trajectories of people situated in particular social worlds can arc toward or achieve good mental health and psychosocial outcomes after exposure to traumatic events or violence.

The evidence base for resilience promotion interventions, particularly in post-conflict humanitarian settings and LMIC with limited resources, is scant but growing. Supporting people's resilience is an essential part of MHPSS during and after complex humanitarian disasters involving political violence. Psychosocial resilience should be routinely supported as part of post-conflict mental health promotion efforts. To increase access to resilience-enhancing programs, scalable, community-based resilience-strengthening interventions that can be delivered by trained and supervised local, non-specialist facilitators need to be developed. Even though conceptions of resilience based on Western cultural assumptions can be used productively in cross-cultural mental health practice as a point of departure, tools and curricula developed for resilience promotion interventions should be systematically tested for cross-cultural relevance and effectiveness and amenability to cultural adaptation. Ideally, ethnographic inquiry into local individual and collective resilience patterns and resources should be identified, mapped, and analyzed from a do no harm, human rights, and moral experience lens to inform the design and prioritization of resilience-based interventions. We recommend concerted investment in the development and dissemination of resilience-focused interventions that are appropriate, safe, and effective for diverse populations, including survivors of GBV and conflict-related sexual violence, and we suggest that that such interventions be designed for results across the humanitarian-development-peace nexus.

For resilience-based approaches, it is important to consider how to create an environment that enables people to feel connected and to share their daily problems as well as past experiences with violence. In order to do no harm, existing coping and protection mechanisms and resilience should not be disrupted by humanitarian intervention. Resilience-focused interventions must maximize the engagement of local people and prioritize facilitating authentic local ownership. Individual survivors of complex humanitarian disasters can be supported to engage in opportunities for social reintegration and to decide for themselves when to speak, what to say about their experiences, and to whom. Collective resilience can be supported by identifying safe spaces to narrate or otherwise express suffering, making meaning of extreme experiences of violence and loss, and building toward possible futures of accountability and social justice for all. When working with conflict-related sexual violence survivors, safe spaces need to be survivor-centered to avoid survivors being silenced and stigmatized about their experiences and to actualize the right of survivors to decide when and how they share their experiences, and for what purposes [41].

Social acknowledgment supports resilience by increasing the social spaces where survivors can safely express their experiences of violence and suffering, reinforcing the positive moral personhood of survivors, and driving resources to address survivors' wounds. Social acknowledgment in the sense we have described it here never means forcing or coercing survivors to speak out about their story in any way. For practitioners and researchers in complex humanitarian disaster contexts, we recommend becoming increasingly responsive to all forms of disaster-/conflict-related violence and suffering and supporting individuals, communities, [I]NGOs, governments, and UN organizations to create and enact norms that publicly recognize what people have been through. This public recognition should also highlight the obligation of states to realize the rights to health and well-being among all survivors.

We recommend that evolving humanitarian-development-peace nexus approaches to resilience prioritize the right of protection and assistance to survivors in complex humanitarian settings with scaffolding for room to grow toward linkages with development and peace-building. Resilience work at the nexus needs to account for cultural or contextual specificities that can render some violent or traumatic experiences unspeakable, support safe spaces that allow for reckoning with these problems, ensure that community-based resilience efforts are aligned with human rights, and engage with efforts to promote social acknowledgment of what survivors of recent and historical traumas have endured. Increased attention should be given to fostering intergenerational resilience efforts that lead to better long-term mental health and peace-building outcomes. In fragile and conflict-affected settings, resilience action should inform the articulation of formal collective outcomes, which are concrete and measurable results that humanitarian, development, and other peace actors aspire to achieve jointly over a period of 3–5 years to reduce people's needs, risks, and vulnerabilities and increase their resilience (see [24]).

References

1. Betancourt, T. S., Meyers-Ohki, S., Stulac, S. N., Barrera, A. E., Mushashi, C., & Beardslee, W. R. (2011). Nothing can defeat combined hands (Abashyize hamwe ntakibananira): Protective processes and resilience in Rwandan children and families affected by HIV/AIDS. *Social Science & Medicine, 73*(5), 693–701. https://doi.org/10.1016/j.socscimed.2011.06.053.
2. Bijleveld, C., Morssinkhof, A., & Smeulers, A. (2009). Counting the countless. *International Criminal Justice Review, 19*(2), 208–224. https://doi.org/10.1177/1057567709335391.
3. Brounéus, K. (2008). *Rethinking reconciliation: Concepts, methods, and an empirical study of truth telling and psychological health in Rwanda.* (Unpublished doctoral dissertation). Institutionen för freds-och konfliktforskning, Uppsala
4. Diaz, J. O. P. (2013). Recovery: Re-establishing place and community resilience. *Global Journal of Community Psychology Practice, 4*(3), 1–10.
5. Eggerman, M., & Panter-Brick, C. (2010). Suffering, hope, and entrapment: Resilience and cultural values in Afghanistan. *Social Science & Medicine, 71*(1), 71–83. https://doi.org/10.1016/j.socscimed.2010.03.023.
6. Hernandez, P. (2002). Resilience in families and communities: Latin American contributions from the psychology of liberation. *The Family Journal, 10*(3), 334–343. https://doi.org/10.1177/10680702010003011.
7. Hogwood, J., Auerbach, C., Munderere, S., & Kambibi, E. (2014). Rebuilding the social fabric: Community counselling groups for Rwandan women with children born as a result of genocide rape. *Intervention, 12*(3), 393–404. https://doi.org/10.1097/WTF.0000000000000053.
8. Ingabire, C. M., Kagoyire, G., Karangwa, D., Ingabire, N., Habarugira, N., Jansen, A., & Richters, A. (2017). Trauma informed restorative justice through community based sociotherapy in Rwanda. *Intervention, 15*(3), 241–253. https://doi.org/10.1097/WTF.0000000000000163.
9. Inter-Agency Standing Committee (IASC). (2007). IASC Guidelines on mental health and psychosocial support in emergency settings. https://www.who.int/mental_health/emergencies/guidelines_iasc_mental_health_psychosocial_june_2007.pdf.
10. Inter-Agency Standing Committee. (2015). Guidelines for integrating gender-based violence interventions in humanitarian action: Reducing risk, promoting resilience and aiding recovery. https://interagencystandingcommittee.org/working-group/documents-public/iasc-guidelines-integrating-gender-based-violence-interventions.
11. International Federation of Red Cross and Red Crescent Societies (IFRC). (2014). Strengthening resilience: A global selection of psychosocial interventions. http://pscentre.org/resources/strengthening-resilience/.
12. Kagoyire, M., & Richters, A. (2018). "We are the memory representation of our parents": Intergenerational legacies of genocide among descendants of rape survivors in Rwanda. *Torture, 28*(3), 30–45. https://doi.org/10.7146/torture.v28i3.111183.
13. Kleinman, A. (1999). Moral experience and ethical reflection: Can ethnography reconcile them? A quandary for "the new bioethics". *Daedalus, 128*(4), 69–97.
14. Kohrt, B. A., Mendenhall, E., & Brown, P. J. (2018). Global mental health. In *The international encyclopedia of anthropology.* John Wiley & Sons, Ltd. New York.
15. Løvgren, R. (2019). *Politics of patience: Lessons on sovereignty and subjectivity from failed fieldwork in Rwanda.* (Unpublished doctoral disseration). Københavns Universitet, Copenhagen). https://curis.ku.dk/ws/files/218355795/Ph.d_adhandling_2019_L_vgren.pdf.
16. Maercker, A., & Müller, J. (2004). Social acknowledgment as a victim or survivor: A scale to measure a recovery factor of PTSD. *Journal of Traumatic Stress, 17*(4), 345–351. https://doi.org/10.1023/B:JOTS.0000038484.15488.3d.
17. Mushikiwabo calls for more UN Cooperation. (2010, 25 Oct). *The New Times.* https://www.newtimes.co.rw/section/read/25274.
18. Mukamana, D., & Brysiewicz, P. (2008). The lived experience of genocide rape survivors in Rwanda. *Journal of Nursing Scholarship, 40*(4), 379–384. https://doi.org/10.1111/j.1547-5069.2008.00253.x.

19. Myers, N., & Yarris, K. E. (2019). Extraordinary conditions: Global psychiatric care and the anthropology of moral experience. *Ethos, 47*(1), 3–12. https://doi.org/10.1111/etho.1222.
20. National Unity and Reconciliation Commission (NURC). (2016). *Unity and reconciliation process in Rwanda.* (Government of Rwanda). http://www.nurc.gov.rw/fileadmin/Documents/Others/Unity_and_Reconciliation__Process_in_Rwanda.pdf.
21. Ndushabandi, E. (2015). La gouvernance des mémoires au Rwanda au travers du dispositif « ingando »: Une analyse critique des représentations sociales. *Journal of African Peace and Conflict Studies, 2*(2), 37–61. https://doi.org/10.5038/2325-484X.2.2.2.
22. Newbury, D., & Newbury, C. (2000). Bringing the peasants back in: Agrarian themes in the construction and corrosion of statist historiography in Rwanda. *The American Historical Review, 105*(3), 832–877. https://doi.org/10.1086/ahr/105.3.832.
23. Nowrojee, B. (1996). Shattered lives: Sexual violence during the Rwandan genocide and its aftermath. *Human Rights Watch, 3169*, no. 164.
24. OCHA. (2018). *Collective outcomes.* Operationalizing the new ways of working. https://www.agendaforhumanity.org/sites/default/files/resources/2018/Apr/OCHA%20Collective%20Outcomes%20April%202018.pdf.
25. Otake, Y. (2018). Community resilience and long-term impacts of mental health and psychosocial support in northern Rwanda. *Medical Science, 6*(4), 94. https://doi.org/10.3390/medsci6040094.
26. Otake, Y. (2019). Suffering of silenced people in northern Rwanda. *Social Science & Medicine, 222*, 171–179. https://doi.org/10.1016/j.socscimed.2019.01.005.
27. Oxfam. (2019). The humanitarian-development-peace nexus: What does it mean for multi-mandated organizations?. https://reliefweb.int/sites/reliefweb.int/files/resources/dp-humanitarian-development-peace-nexus-260619-en_0.pdf.
28. Patel, V., Saxena, S., Lund, C., Thornicroft, G., Baingana, F., Bolton, P., Chisholm, D., Collins, P. Y., Cooper, J. L., Eaton, J., & Herrman, H. (2018). The Lancet Commission on global mental health and sustainable development. *Lancet, 392*(10157), 1553–1598. https://doi.org/10.1016/S0140-6736(18)31612-X.
29. Powley, E. (2003). *Strengthening governance: The role of women in Rwanda's transition.* Hunt Alternatives Fund. https://www.inclusivesecurity.org/wp-content/uploads/2012/08/10_strengthening_governance_the_role_of_women_in_rwanda_s_transition.pdf.
30. Prunier, G. (1995). *The Rwanda crisis: History of a genocide 1959–1994.* Kampala: Fountain.
31. Purdeková, A. (2011). *Rwanda's Ingando Camps: Liminality and the reproduction of power.* (Oxford Refugee Studies Centre Working Paper Series, no. 80). Refugee Studies Centre. https://purehost.bath.ac.uk/ws/portalfiles/portal/174005236/Purdekova_WP_Sep_20_2011.pdf.
32. Ramet, S. P. (2007). The denial syndrome and its consequences: Serbian political culture since 2000. *Communist and Post-Communist Studies, 40*(1), 41–58. https://doi.org/10.1016/j.postcomstud.2006.12.004.
33. Richters, A. (2015). Enhancing family and community resilience and wellbeing across the generations: The contribution of community-based sociotherapy in post-genocide Rwanda. *International Journal of Emergency Mental Health and Human Resilience, 17*(3), 661–662.
34. Slim, H. (2019, 23 Oct). Searching for the nexus: How to turn theory into practice. *The New Humanitarian.* https://www.thenewhumanitarian.org/opinion/2019/10/23/Triple-nexus-theory-practice.
35. Sousa, C. A., Haj-Yahia, M. M., Feldman, G., & Lee, J. (2013). Individual and collective dimensions of resilience within political violence. *Trauma, Violence, & Abuse, 14*(3), 235–254. https://doi.org/10.1177/1524838013493520.
36. Sphere Association. (2018). *The sphere handbook: Humanitarian charter and minimum standards in humanitarian response.* https://spherestandards.org/wp-content/uploads/Sphere-Handbook-2018-EN.pdf.
37. Taylor, C. (2002). The cultural face of terror in the Rwandan genocide of 1994. In A. Hinton (Ed.), *Annihilating difference: The anthropology of genocide* (pp. 137–178). University of California Press. Berkeley and Los Angeles, California.

38. Tol, W. A., Stavrou, V., Greene, M. C., Mergenthaler, C., Van Ommeren, M., & Moreno, C. G. (2013). Sexual and gender-based violence in areas of armed conflict: A systematic review of mental health and psychosocial support interventions. *Conflict and Health, 7*(1), 16. https://doi.org/10.1186/1752-1505-7-16.

39. UN Office of the High Commissioner for Human Rights (UNHCHR). (2010). *Report of the mapping exercise documenting the most serious violations of Human Rights and International Humanitarian Law Committed within the Territory of the Democratic Republic of the Congo between March 1993 and June 2003.* http://www.refworld.org/docid/4ca99bc22.html.

40. Ungar, M., & Theron, L. (2019). Resilience and mental health: How multisystemic processes contribute to positive outcomes. *Lancet Psychiatry.* https://doi.org/10.1016/S2215-0366(19)30434-1.

41. UNSCR. S/RES/2467 (2019) Security Council Distr.: General 23 April 2019. Resolution 2467 (2019) Adopted by the Security Council at its 8514th meeting, on 23 April 2019. 2019. http://unscr.com/en/resolutions/2467.

42. WHO. (2014). *Social determinants of mental health.* (World Health Organization). https://apps.who.int/iris/bitstream/handle/10665/112828/9789241506809_eng.pdf;jsessionid=62184BC33F343CD8E53344FAF6E1CC76?sequence=1.

43. Zraly, M. (2008). *Bearing: Resilience among genocide-rape survivors in Rwanda.* (Unpublished doctoral dissertation). Cleveland: Case Western Reserve University, https://etd.ohiolink.edu/!etd.send_file?accession=case1189191843&disposition=inline.

44. Zraly, M. (2010). Danger denied: Everyday life and everyday violence among Rwandan genocide-rape survivors. *Voices, 10*(1), 18–23. https://doi.org/10.1111/j.1548-7423.2010.00001.x.

45. Zraly, M., & Nyirazinyoye, L. (2010). Don't let the suffering make you fade away: An ethnographic study of resilience among survivors of genocide-rape in southern Rwanda. *Social Science & Medicine, 70*(10), 1656–1664. https://doi.org/10.1016/j.socscimed.2010.01.017.

46. Zraly, M., Rubin, S. E., & Mukamana, D. (2013). Motherhood and resilience among Rwandan genocide-rape survivors. *Ethos, 41*(4), 411–439. https://doi.org/10.1111/etho.12031.

47. Zraly, M., Rubin-Smith, J., & Betancourt, T. (2011). Primary mental health care for survivors of collective sexual violence in Rwanda. *Global Public Health, 6*(3), 257–270. https://doi.org/10.1080/17441692.2010.493165.

Ethical Challenges of Nonmaleficence in Mental Health Care for Forcibly Displaced Children and Adolescents

14

Edith Stein and Suzan J. Song

The Changing Ecology of Conflict and Displacement

In 2018, violent conflict and persecution forced about 37,000 people to flee their homes each day, and the total number of displaced people grew to 70.8 million globally; forcibly displaced children and adolescents make up around half of that total [88]. Many children who are unaccompanied or separated from their caregivers and families must navigate perilous migration journeys on their own. The ecology of conflict and displacement has dramatically changed over the past few decades. As opposed to nations being involved in a war, civil wars, non-state violence, and violence against civilians have become prominent forms of conflict. The targeting of children and adolescents for military recruitment has increased in recent years [13]. War and conflicts in resource-constrained low- and middle-income countries (LMIC) have become more protracted in nature [80]. Facing continuous exposure to economic hardships, limited options, and humanitarian and political complexities, four out of five refugees flee to neighboring countries, mostly LMIC [88]. For displaced children, climate-related extreme weather events and the competition over depleted natural resources further compound the precarity of their situations and

E. Stein
Department of Global Health and Social Medicine,
Harvard Medical School, Boston, MA, USA
e-mail: edith_stein@hms.harvard.edu

S. J. Song (✉)
Department of Psychiatry and Behavioral Sciences,
George Washington University, Washington, DC, USA
e-mail: suzan.song@post.harvard.edu

© Springer Nature Switzerland AG 2021
A. R. Dyer et al. (eds.), *Global Mental Health Ethics*,
https://doi.org/10.1007/978-3-030-66296-7_14

may expose them to conflict or secondary displacement. Rather than living in refugee camps or dispersed rural areas, almost two-thirds of all forcibly displaced people reside in urban environments more scattered and difficult to reach [88]. Meeting displaced children's needs for protection and access to adequate mental health care remains a formidable task. The vast majority of refugees are displaced for over 5 years and about one-fifth of all refugees for more than 20 years [88]. The impact of climate change, environmental degradation, and extreme weather conditions increasingly interrelate with armed conflicts by compounding the risk for disputes due to inequity, heightening the vulnerability of those already displaced [87]. The ostracism of particularly vulnerable groups, unaccompanied minors, children with disabilities, survivors of sexual violence, and those suffering mental disorders, for example, makes them prone to experience continuous, high levels of distress that may hamper their development. The reality of displaced children and their migration trajectories has become even more appalling. In the context of rising anti-immigrant sentiments, children have become central targets of dehumanizing and detrimental immigration policies that deliberately expose them to protracted uncertainty, forced separations, confinement, encampment, and expedited removal proceedings that undermine their basic human and children's rights. Border enforcement policies have harshened, with some adopting a core strategy of deterrence based on the infliction of trauma [10]. Adding interpersonal violence and torture as cumulative risk factors to their already strained mental health is damaging [29, 68]. Critical protection mechanisms are withheld from displaced children who are left in a limbo of "waithood" [92]. The uncertainty about the outcome of their asylum application and the ever-present risk of forced deportation to conditions of threat, insecurity, and persecution is of grave concern to the mental health and wellbeing of displaced children [29].

Nonmaleficence in Providing Mental Health Care for Forcibly Displaced Youth

The provision of competent care amidst conditions of precarity and instability to attend to displaced children's needs is of utmost relevance within an ethical discussion [31]. Determining and meeting their mental health needs based on individual resources and vulnerabilities, differing trajectories, and future aspirations is challenging. The ethical principle of *nonmaleficence*, or ensuring one does not intentionally or unintentionally harm, should be at the forefront of every practitioner's mind when interacting with forcibly displaced children— from diagnosis to intervention and beyond. Ethical challenges surrounding the provision of mental health services to displaced children are manifold, as previous research has outlined [3, 31, 96]. Power imbalances, or differentials, and scarce resources give rise to a myriad of unintended adverse consequences [30,

78]. Conflicting perspectives between an organization's mandate, the ethos of the clinician, and the local's prospects are frequent dilemmas in humanitarian emergencies [18]. A lack of consideration for the structural and political forces impacting humanitarian work or the cultural insensitivity of diagnostic criteria, screening tools, and interventions is another concern [86]. All too often, ethics are considered as a disjuncture from practical work. Instead, they should give direction to any action taken in humanitarian settings [2]. This is particularly important when working with children who have had adverse experiences during childhood that may have a dire impact on the subsequent development of the child [11]. Hence, advocating for ethical considerations within and across humanitarian organizations and their actors is critical not to aggravate pre-existing complexities [15].

The Intersection of Humanitarian Principles and Ethical Obligations

Often, humanitarian workers and clinicians working in complex humanitarian emergencies may find themselves experiencing a tension between their ethical obligations and their fulfillment of humanitarian principles. Mental health-care providers are at the forefront of witnessing and collecting evidence on human rights violations against displaced children. In many humanitarian emergencies, the repercussions of human rights violations on displaced children and their families are so substantial that advocacy and political activism are critical to the delivery of effective treatment programs [30]. This need is evident where the political disregard or the failure of global resettlement strategies leaves children and their families in protracted uncertainty and insecurity, often under inhumane, appalling conditions not suitable to children [35]. Security and safety concerns for children who are vulnerable to suffer exploitation, abuse, kidnapping, and military recruitment under such restrained conditions become major concerns [89].

Ethical dilemmas also arise frequently as part of resource allocation. The humanitarian principle of neutrality could be in tension with the ethical obligation to support the fair distribution of benefits when deciding which population to work with—providing care to refugees but not to local children of the host community, for example. Ideally, humanitarian assistance should include both displaced populations and host communities. However, limited resources may not always allow for it, posing an ethical dilemma. The precarity of LMIC, where most of the displaced children reside, increases that conundrum.

Humanity, neutrality, impartiality, and independence, as laid out in the 1991 United Nations General Assembly Resolution 46/182 and 58/114, constitute the underlying principles guiding all humanitarian actions. *Neutrality* is commonly

Case example: SJS (author) was conducting a mental health and psychosocial assessment for displaced Syrian adolescents in a refugee camp in Jordan. The camp was 1 year old, and many Jordanians were open to helping their neighbors manage the negative effects of the war. The next year, while conducting a follow-up study of displaced Syrian adolescents in the camp and non-camp settings of Jordan, the Jordanian community had a different response toward the displaced Syrians. With more than 3 years of experiencing the influx of displaced Syrians, many Jordanians felt competition over resources in education, food, and housing, which all increased the price and decreased accessibility. The study, therefore, included both displaced Syrian adolescents as well as Jordanian adolescents to attempt to not further stigma, discrimination, or perceived competition over resources [90].

referred to as the provision of humanitarian assistance on a needs-based approach in an impartial, independent matter. *Impartiality* reflects the humanitarian doctrine of providing care to anyone in need, regardless of their political or social background. *Independence* refers to the provision of *humanitarian* assistance independent of any political or strategic objectives [62]. To translate these principles into practice, pivotal humanitarian frameworks—the 1992 ICRC's Code of Conduct, the Sphere standards, and the Core Humanitarian Standard on Quality and Accountability—outline key provisions and minimum standards for humanitarian assistance to ensure quality and accountability.

Similarly, the dramatic rise of intrastate and ethnic conflicts constitutes another serious challenge. When clinicians who work for a humanitarian organization closely consult with a local population to best understand the child to provide effective clinical care; if the local population is considered to be on one side of the conflict, that association could be perceived to infringe neutrality. Aid and care can be interpreted as political. Increasingly, humanitarian actors are pushed to compromise humanitarian principles for political means [62] or may even be hindered or legally targeted for providing humanitarian assistance to displaced children in need [54]. Their mandate of protecting the life, health, and dignity of displaced children must never be compromised by any means. Protecting humanitarian principles is fundamentally pivotal to the effectiveness of humanitarian coordination, domestically and internationally.

Clinical and Public Health Ethics

The principles of biomedical ethics proposed by Beauchamp and Childress [5]—*autonomy, beneficence, nonmaleficence, and justice*—provide systematic, practical guidance on moral decision-making for clinicians worldwide. While the focus of clinical ethics lies in the moral responsibility of a clinician toward the patient, public health predicaments concern the individual's right versus the benefit for the community [91]. Public health ethics are based on a variety of philosophical underpinnings, foundational values, and guiding principles; ethical frameworks are numerous [46]. Similar to the moral governance required in humanitarian emergencies, the public health ethics discourse is underpinned by values such as promoting respect for people while protecting public health, social justice, equity, accountability, cost-effectiveness, and absolute versus acceptable standards [46]. However, there is no formal ethics framework that can help identify and support ethical decision-making for children in humanitarian settings systematically [46]. The complexity of the humanitarian context is enormous and involves multidirectional relationships and diverging values. Stakeholders may prioritize substantive values such as impartiality or religious beliefs or rather focus on procedural values mirroring a needs-based approach, accountability, and transparency [15]. Yet, clinical decisions must follow a professional biomedical ethical approach. The challenge humanitarian emergencies pose is that impactful decisions occasionally must be made very quickly and might have complex and far-reaching consequences. Although different in perspective, clinical ethics focuses on the individual versus public health ethics on the population. Both fields require efficient, stringently argued responses. Drawing upon both frameworks, Clarinval and Biller-Andorno [15] have incorporated key features of numerous ethical decision-making tools in "a ten-step approach to ethical decision-making in humanitarian aid" that could support clinical and complex decisions to be made in the humanitarian context (Box 8.1).

Box 8.1 A Ten-Step Approach to Ethical Decision-Making in Humanitarian Aid

1	Gathering evidence	Conduct a situational analysis of all humanitarian actors involved, and nominate a person in charge of the ethical decision-making
2	Specifying values, norms, or principles	Outline core values, norms, and principles at stake at the individual, organizational, legal, and social level
3	Critical examination	Carefully analyze points at stake, including the definition of ethical discord
4	Defining options	Detail possible options including their consequences and potential interferences
5	Weighing	Weigh on available options
6	Elaborating decisions	Consent on the most feasible course of action
7	Providing justification	Explain the rationale behind the decision ensuring transparency
8	Implementation	Specify indicators and outcome measures for monitoring and evaluation
9	Monitoring and evaluation	Assess the chosen decision's positive and negative impacts in general and on all actors involved
10	Recommendations	Provide recommendations for future avenues

Adapted from Clarinval and Biller-Andorno [15]

Reaching consent upon dissenting ethical values is demanding, mainly where there is no institutional culture for doing so [15]. Clinicians engaged in humanitarian work must strengthen their capacity to identify and address possible ethical dilemmas. In a concerted effort, clinicians need to collaborate in establishing a culture for discussing ethical disputes openly. Particularly in humanitarian assistance, where ethical values may be driven by strategies and interests and may collide, displaced children's interests must be put at the heart of the debate. Clinicians with expert proficiency are obliged to clinical ethics and have a moral responsibility to put children's interests first. Upholding the dictum *primum non nocere* ("first, do no harm") must be clinician's primary consideration to avoid unintended adverse consequences.

Contextually Inappropriate Interventions

Humanitarian ethics in the provision of child and adolescent mental health care has gained little scholarly attention so far [38]. To avoid violations of the "do no harm" imperative, understanding and addressing children's distinct individual needs within the context of a changing ecology of conflict and displacement is key.

Utilizing an *ecological model* [12] provides a useful framework in humanitarian response; it depicts the child's development and wellbeing in the center influenced fundamentally by familial, communal, and societal factors. Hence, effective mental health interventions must not only address the individual but include the family, community (peers and school), and structural aspects (child protection system, politics, cultural and societal norms) shaping a child's mental health [24]. Child psychiatrists know the value of taking an ecological approach that takes into account the abilities and availability of parents, peers, teachers, schools, and other influential people in the child's life since they are more reliant upon their environment, dependent on significant adults, physically and psychologically [6]. Interventions that aim at enhancing social support and cohesion, reducing family violence, and creating social and economic opportunities are critical [55, 56]. An ecological model attributes distress in displaced populations not only due to individual factors but also ongoing stressors in their social ecology, exerting to the distress caused by war-related exposure. Determining the resettlement factors that influence displaced children's adaptive behavior and positive mental health is vital in designing successful intervention strategies [56]. Parenting programs, school-based mental health interventions, and skills-based training are promising avenues for preventive interventions. They should address the most vulnerable children exposed to parental mental illness and those with pre-existing developmental or mental health impairments [28].

Structural violence through poverty, inequity, social exclusion, and discrimination are pertinent to displaced children's lived experiences. Framing structural disenfranchisement as psychiatric may consolidate displaced children's stigma and deprive them of their moral aptitude. The medicalization of life stressors may divert attention to mental health problems where, in fact, child protection needs, legal support, livelihood, and education are primary concerns.

Case example: M. is a 17-year-old boy from Honduras who crossed the US border seeking asylum after being exploited for labor by his family and persecuted by a local gang. He was held in immigration detention for 3 months and was transferred to inpatient psychiatric care due to aggressive behaviors toward detention staff. At the inpatient facility, the psychiatrist gave M. a diagnosis of bipolar disorder and started him on an antipsychotic. He had no episodes previously of major depressive episodes, and his "manic symptoms" were aggression and irritability due to detention conditions, insomnia due to flashbacks, and fear due to past persecution, the uncertainty of his future safety, and detention conditions. The inpatient team was aware he was an unaccompanied minor under immigration custody but had not asked about the effects of current detention conditions on his mental health nor his past experience being trafficked. As such, he was returned to immigration custody on antipsychotic medication and with a diagnosis of bipolar disorder—a misguided treatment. Had the context of his immigration detention been explored, his experiences of violation, physical and sexual assault, and adverse effects of isolation in confinement, could have been prevented and identified in treatment planning.

A humanitarian approach through a *contextually sensitive* lens examines the pathways of structural and political forces affecting displaced children's mental health and well-being. Translating a humanitarian and public health ethical approach to a clinical ethical approach should be the goal for mental health clinicians working with displaced children. Rather than viewing challenges of forced migration as psychiatric and, therefore, individual clinicians may use a contextual lens to uncover linkages between the social and the individual.

Sidelining of Existing Evidence on Mental Health Interventions

Conducting research under logistical, clinical, and safety barriers led many researchers to avoid this needed field. A combination of chaos, mass influx of refugees and humanitarian agencies, uncoordinated response, resource scarcity, and people in need may invite for the application of non-evidence-based interventions. Despite these, studies on the mental health of displaced children as well as the effectiveness of interventions continue to grow [7, 28, 37, 39, 40, 63, 84]. As most studies on displaced children have been conducted by researchers from high-income countries (HIC), there has been a recent interest in capacity building, collaboration, and promotion of researchers from the Global South in leading research in the field. Currently, local communities and organizations may have interventions that are effective but do not have the resources for rigorous studies. Such "practice-based evidence" should be explored and supported to inform current interventions better [85].

There is a consensus of shifting from an individual-, and psychopathology-oriented model towards a multi-leveled, resource-oriented approach incorporating care across the entire social ecology of children (family, peers, school, and the broader community) to tackle "daily stressors" adding up to displaced children's ongoing distress in displacement [55], including the strengthening of child protection services and school-based mental health interventions for displaced children [28, 38, 40, 56]. Empirical evidence overall is supportive to individual- as well as group-based counseling for children in need of specialized care [37, 40, 63, 84], with cognitive behavioral therapy (CBT) showing the most robust evidence [63]. Positive treatment effects are mostly restricted to certain subgroups of children (age- or gender-related) and a few treatment modalities such as trauma-focused CBT or narrative exposure therapy (NET). Occasionally, interventions show negative effects, mostly, where interventions contain numerous components and are broadly applied to children in armed conflict [40]. Hence, advancing the targeted adjustment and conceptualization of interventions is key.

Rigorous, systematic feasibility studies have primarily been evaluating trauma-focused interventions [85]. Comparably little evidence is available on the effectiveness of interventions that are more likely to be implemented in practice and target at facilitating community support mechanisms for the displaced child, including the provision of child-friendly spaces [85]. The generalizability of such results is limited due to common methodological constraints [37]. Moreover, the longer-term efficacy of interventions has rarely been assessed [7]. There is a scarcity of evidence for mental health and psychosocial support interventions in humanitarian emergencies applied to non-clinical settings in LMIC [4, 38]. The shortfall of mental health professionals requires capacity building through task-sharing with non-specialists and lay health workers through community-based mental health interventions [60, 65]. There is growing acknowledgment about the importance of tackling parenting quality, parental mental health, and the familial environment [57, 86], including intrafamilial violence in post-conflict settings [64]. Parental support and monitoring are critical for strengthening resilience in displaced children [86]. Hence, family-based interventions aiming to improve the child-caregiver attachment relationship and reduce intrafamilial violence through parenting interventions are key [57, 77], albeit the existing limited evidence on parenting interventions so far shows inconsistent intervention results [22, 49, 61, 67, 86]. School-based mental health interventions are the most widely implemented and evaluated [7] and provide a suitable avenue for preventive interventions [7, 28; outcomes are mixed and lean toward the improvement of social cohesion and peer support rather than specific disorder-related symptoms [28, 40]. School-based mental health interventions in LMIC show good-quality evidence, especially multicomponent community-based interventions focusing on peer support, life-skills, and vocational training combined with components improving health literacy or adding fitness and physical health [4]. Moreover, education in itself is an "intervention" foundational to displaced children's wellbeing reestablishing safe and supportive spaces for children amid the often chaotic conditions of displacement [32]. Despite the importance of implementing child protection measures in humanitarian settings that pose a significant risk for abuse, violence, and trafficking [79], a one size fits all approach toward the reflexive, large-scale implementation of community-based child protection groups runs the risk of being contextually insensitive and eroding the child protection system strengthening of the host country [95].

A Narrow Focus on Symptom Checklists

What constitutes evidence on the effectiveness of interventions in humanitarian emergencies is another challenging concern. Albeit existing Inter-Agency Standing Committee (IASC) standards on monitoring and evaluation encourage the participation of children in the process [34], mostly, interventions focus on decreasing psychopathology; very few evaluation studies take into account child-centered outcome measures that prioritize what is important to the child and are contextually and culturally sensitive [40, 63]. The exclusion of culture and context, as well as children as active participants in their lives, may risk failing what matters to them, impacting the acceptance and effectiveness of interventions. We should measure functional outcomes inherently natural to a displaced child's environment and life instead of statistical cut-offs or diagnostic criteria based on populations in HIC to evaluate clinically significant change. Statistical significance does not mean clinical significance, which is based on other factors, such as clinical benefits. Research has shown that displaced children's wellbeing may be discordant to their score in psychiatric symptom checklists. This could result in pathologizing children's wellbeing, but most importantly, it may exclude those children in need who are not capable of expressing their malaise in symptomatic terms [36].

Humanitarian organizations planning for clinical programming should be cautious following a symptom-based approach for needs assessments in displaced children [36], which may be bound to a single diagnostic construct and confined in presenting the full complexity of post-conflict distress [20]. When measuring psychopathology in children utilizing diagnostic constructs that do not recognize the developmentally specific symptom presentation in children, a symptomatic approach may present a distorted picture of displaced children's mental health that lacks accuracy. Still, most scholarship follows a clinical, biomedical approach and investigates the level of psychopathologies—foremostly post-traumatic stress disorder (PTSD), depression, and anxiety—in displaced children [37, 70, 94]. However, these terms insufficiently capture the elaborate symptom presentation in children, the developmental impairments, emotional and relational dysregulation, and attachment-related disturbances [16, 17, 58]. Many forcibly displaced children in emotional despair and suffering may not present with the typical diagnostic symptoms required for a diagnosis, which leads to the potential of excluding them from needed care. Not identifying children in need of specialized care has severe consequences to the subsequent development of a child and their family and broader community impacting social cohesion, socioeconomic factors, and the reinforcement of adversity through intergenerational transmission [8, 51]. Utilizing a diagnostic construct that insufficiently accounts for the impairment in functioning and social skills in complex traumatized children and adolescents that frequently leads to problems with family, peers, and the educational, legal, and health systems is problematic [93]. Although a developmentally appropriate understanding of mental health care provision to displaced children and adolescents in practice has become state of the art, we still lack valid diagnostic categories mirroring that transition. Establishing formal diagnostic criteria that capture the complex symptom presentation in displaced children's mental health will be fundamental to inform the development of urgently needed screening tools and interventions that address the distinct needs of displaced children [28]. However, to understand the full consequences of the changing reality of displacement in children, including their clinical needs, psychiatric symptom checklists may well have to be combined with non-symptom-focused, narrative approaches that allow for non-stigmatizing, culturally sensitive ways of expressing distress [36].

Cultural Illiteracy

The provision of culturally sensitive care is considered standard in humanitarian emergencies [33, 83]. *Cultural sensitivity* is commonly understood as care responsive to local modes of suffering, coping, and resilience. It is critical to understand the complexity and highly dynamic nature of culture at the intersection of individual, communal, and structural forces. Understanding how factors in the context of forced and distress migration such as violence, insecurity, displacement, fractured social networks, discontinuing education, and altering gender roles affect individual children, their families, and communities—and thus *culture*—is essential. Hence, operating in humanitarian emergencies requires specific skills and adequate training of mental health clinicians from HIC. Griffith et al.'s [30] training module on global mental health that aims at preparing mental health clinicians for work in humanitarian settings and LMIC outlines key aspects—if disregarded, it may well present frequent causes of unintended adverse consequences (refer to Box 8.2):

Box 8.2 Key Considerations in Conducting Global Mental Health

1. *Social suffering* [44] is a common cause of illness and might not translate into psychiatric symptom presentation in the biomedical sense but presents as non-specific somatic symptoms utilizing local idioms of distress and cultural symptom explanation [19, 48].
2. Acknowledging, addressing, and including the social ecology of local idioms of distress and traditional ways of healing are critical [19].

3. Egalitarian engagement with local communities is essential, particularly where identity may be understood collectivistic based upon identification with a family, clan, religion, or ethnicity, rather than being individualistically oriented [19, 45, 69]. Training in systemic family therapy is imperative [45]—especially for child psychiatrists.

4. Psychopharmacological treatment must be sensitive to biological alterity determined by differences in genetics, environmental factors, and psycho-neuro-immuno-endocrinological responses that impact not only psychiatric symptom expression but also pharmacokinetics and drug metabolism [98].

5. The shortfall of mental health capacity in LMIC requires task-sharing with non-specialists and lay health workers that are trained to provide community-based mental health interventions. The role of a clinical psychiatrist in resource-limited settings differs from the one in HIC and is much more of being a trainer, supervisor, and capacity builder [19, 43]. Due to the scarcity of mental health professionals, interventions may also be more community rather than individual oriented [23].

6. Advocacy for human rights, activism, and engagement on a policy level in order to address structural violence must be integral to a clinician's engagement in humanitarian emergencies.
Adapted from Griffith et al. [30]

The comprehensiveness of such training illustrates the complexity of what *culture* comprises. An attitude of modesty of the HIC clinician in a low-resource context might be appropriate.

Dismissing Children's Agency and Resilience

Cultural adaption should reflect upon the specific dynamics of the culture of youth-hood. Including children and adolescents in the process of cultural adaption will not only help to get a more nuanced understanding of the perspectives, needs, and challenges of children and adolescents over different ages, but a participatory approach equals to create empowerment and shared social meaning. A *child-centered approach* understands displaced children as competent actors with resources and social capital; they are not merely seen as victims of adversities and repressive structures but as resilient survivors.

Case example[1]: T. is a 10-year-old boy from a family of a religious minority in Ethiopia. Due to religious persecution, his family fled their home country to seek asylum in the United Kingdom. Shortly after arrival, he began to have defiant behavior toward adults, was often instigating physical fights with peers, and began to urinate at night in his bed. His school referred him to a mental health counselor who tried to engage with T. but was quickly discouraged by his disrespectful behavior. The counselor then chose to instead speak at length with T.'s teacher, mother, and peers. T. was determined to have oppositional defiance and was encouraged to have CBT, which, after 5 months, was not effective. His counselor happened to transition out of the school, and a new counselor was able to engage with T.'s defiant behavior, understanding the effects of persecution and cultural dislocation on T. developmentally. The new counselor asked T. what was bothering him the most and what he needed. T. was able to describe the fears he had sleeping alone in a room since he had not done so before, his deep longing for his grandmother who raised him in Ethiopia, and his feeling teased by others since he did not speak English well. The counselor then asked T. what he thought would help and implemented those changes (sleeping in the room next to his mother, having routine calls with his grandmother, and having an individual tutor for English). Within 2 months, his defiant behavior subsided, and he was more engaged in school and with family.

Clinicians may pathologize the survival struggle of displaced children, thereby enforcing their disempowerment. Research and clinical work typically focus on examining vulnerabilities and the level of psychopathologies of displaced children [70, 94]. Albeit of growing interest, less attention has been diverted to a *resilience- and resource-oriented approach* that acknowledges displaced children's survival struggle despite their susceptibility [25, 96]. *Resilience*, defined as the ability to do well in the face of adversities [50, 71, 72], is not characterized by an absence of adversity-related psychopathology [52, 73]. Resilience is a dynamic process shaped by time-dependent and contextual determinants [86] based on individual genetic traits and environmental factors operating via biological processes [53, 74, 97]. What constitutes meaningful, resilient coping behavior or a vulnerable identity must be continuously negotiated between the child, the community, and the (host) society. Applying a contextual perspective to resilience [42] is vital in understanding the present situation of displaced children and adolescents—it means situating their individual resilience and vulnerability in the context of structural and political forces, of deep-rooted marginalization, systemic oppression, and disenfranchisement while not invalidating their agency.

The changing conception of displaced children as active agents must be situated in the broader arena of an emerging rights-based perspective on displaced children

---

[1] Clinical case of SJS adapted to protect the patient's identity

[94]. Initially legally driven through the wide ratification of the 1989 United Nations Convention on the Rights of the Child, a *rights-based approach* has gradually impacted the humanitarian agenda. Ever since, displaced children have become subjects of concern to international law, deserving attention and state protection in the same way as domestic children do [9]. The challenge of a humanitarian approach that aims at alleviating social suffering and treats children as competent agents and best experts on their own wellbeing and mental health is to identify those children who fall by the wayside; who do not have the individual, familial, and communal resources; and who are left victims in need of specialized care [94].

The *Dual Loyalty* Conflict

The guidance of existing codes of ethics may be limited for care delivery in complicated situations. For example, clinicians provide mental health services to children who are detained in immigration detention centers that pose a serious threat to the health and integrity of the child, either due to political negligence or purposeful intention to target displaced children. Are clinicians facilitating the detainment or placement of children under conditions that are known to themselves cause mental health distress? Providing mental health care on behalf of a governmental agency that is perpetuating the adverse experiences of children can have moral and ethical challenges. Torn between being complicit to the government and wanting to alleviate the suffering of children in detention, this is a *dual loyalty* conflict sui generis. While the clinician's intention is to do what is in the best interest of the child, it is not always clear how to best accomplish that in such an intricated situation. It further may not be unambiguous what the best interest of the child is—should a toddler be detained with its parents or rather be separated from them to avoid the harmful environment for children in detention? Should clinicians administer care as usual or rather advocate for their detained children's release [27]? While some have argued it is the clinician's moral imperative to document and publish the harmful effects of immigration detention on children [82], advocating on behalf of detainees to be released or to improve, services may run the risk to jeopardize the contractual relationship with the governmental agency at all [26]. The daunting dilemma of conflicting loyalties, complicity, and how many tradeoffs are tolerable has been discussed in scholarship, e.g., in the context of Australia's harsh immigration policies to detain children and families for extended periods in offshore camps under conditions detrimental to children [21, 75, 76, 99].

Clinical independence and autonomy, as well as a clinician's moral ethos for a rights-based approach might conflict with the governmental agency's position impairing the provision of effective care [81]. How should clinicians pacify their professional responsibility to provide the highest excellence of care under suboptimal conditions where treatment recommendations are likely to be compromised [27]? Essex [26] provides an interesting analysis referring to Lepora and Goodin's [47] work on complicity and compromise. He examines the issue of complicity, exploring how clinicians may act as a buffer in abusive systems by contributing to maintaining order and security within thereof. One way to resolve the problem of dual loyalty might be to move beyond clinical care and engage in collective advocacy to speak out against an inhuman system [99]. Zion introduces Porter's concept of "politics of compassion" [66], which builds upon the ethics of care but moves beyond the level of interpersonal therapeutic relationships. A compassionate response is facilitated by engaging with the individual's suffering and demoralization of vulnerable people through active listening and acknowledging their needs [66, 100]. An ethical analysis utilizes moral engagement with suffering, lifting it to the political level, which "links the universal and the particular in that it assumes a shared humanity of interconnected, vulnerable people and requires emotions and practical, particular responses to different expressions of vulnerability" ([66]:99).

Conclusion

Clinicians and humanitarian workers should consider using public health and clinical ethical frameworks when engaging with displaced children globally and domestically. They should seek to agree upon ethical frameworks that transcend disciplinary and political boundaries and are set out to close scrutiny and monitoring. To avoid violations of the "do no harm" imperative, addressing the distinct needs of children in the context of the changing ecology of conflict and displacement is critical. Unintentional adverse consequences are particularly devastating for children due to their formative nature and should be avoided at any cost. The vulnerability and resilience of displaced children are shaped by a complex interaction of individual, environmental, structural, and political forces. Hence, mental health care for displaced children in humanitarian emergencies demands a systemic approach. Individual symptom presentation in children should be situated not only in the socio-ecological context of familial and communal violence but in the broader realm of social suffering through systemic oppression, disenfranchisement, and political neglect. If not taken into consideration, power imbalances and differences, paternalism, and resource scarcity easily give rise to unintended consequences. A collaborative approach can build upon local resources and knowledge and sustain cultural identity and children's agency. Operating in humanitarian emergencies requires a distinct set of skills; therefore, adequate training of clinical psychiatrists is key. A clinician in humanitarian emergencies requires reflexivity, an attitude of humility, and one of a "co-learner" rather than expertise [14, 78]. The controversial political dimension surrounding displaced children is mirrored in the ethically conflicting dissenting positionalities of political engagement versus the humanitarian neutrality actors are obliged to. Advocacy has become an inevitable part of humanitarian engagement where violations of basic children's and human rights shed light upon structural issues that need to be addressed through legislative, regulatory, and policy amendments to align with international human rights standards and ensure the best interest of the child.

References

1. Abel, K. M., Hope, H., Faulds, A., & Pierce, M. (2019). Promoting resilience in children and adolescents living with parental mental illness (CAPRI): Children are key to identifying solutions. *The British Journal of Psychiatry, 215*(3), 513–515. https://doi.org/10.1192/bjp.2019.118.
2. Ahmad, A., & Smith, J. (2018). *Humanitarian action and ethics*. London: Zed Books Ltd.
3. Allden, K., Jones, L., Weissbecker, I., Wessells, M., Bolton, P., Betancourt, T. S., Hijazi, Z., Galappatti, A., Yamout, R., Patel, P., & Sumathipala, A. (2009). Mental health and psychosocial support in crisis and conflict: Report of the Mental Health Working Group. *Prehospital and Disaster Medicine, 24*(Suppl 2), s217–s227. https://doi.org/10.1017/S1049023X00021622.
4. Barry, M. M., Clarke, A. M., Jenkins, R., & Patel, V. (2013). A systematic review of the effectiveness of mental health promotion interventions for young people in low and middle income countries. *BMC Public Health, 13*(1), 835. https://doi.org/10.1186/1471-2458-13-835.
5. Beauchamp, T. L. (1979). *Principles of biomedical ethics*. Oxford: Oxford University Press.
6. Belitz, J., & Bailey, R. A. (2009). Clinical ethics for the treatment of children and adolescents: A guide for general psychiatrists. *Psychiatric Clinics of North America, 32*(2), 243–257. https://doi.org/10.1016/j.psc.2009.02.001.
7. Betancourt, S., Meyers-Ohki, E., Charrow, P., & Tol, A. (2013). Interventions for children affected by war: An ecological perspective on psychosocial support and mental health care. *Harvard Review of Psychiatry, 21*(2), 70–91. https://doi.org/10.1097/HRP.0b013e318283bf8f.
8. Betancourt, T. S., Mcbain, R. K., Newnham, E. A., & Brennan, R. T. (2015). The intergenerational impact of war: Longitudinal relationships between caregiver and child mental health in postconflict Sierra Leone. *Journal of Child Psychology and Psychiatry, 56*(10), 1101–1107. https://doi.org/10.1111/jcpp.12389.
9. Bhabha, J. (2014). *Child migration & human rights in a global age*. Princeton and Oxford: Princeton University Press.
10. Bhabha, J, Basset MT. (2019). Trauma as a border control strategy. https://fxb.harvard.edu/2019/07/22/trauma-as-a-border-control-strategy/.
11. Bick J, Nelson CA. (2015). Early adverse experiences and the developing brain. *Neuropsychopharmacology, 41*(1), 177–196. https://doi.org/10.1038/npp.2015.252.
12. Bronfenbrenner, U. (1979). *The ecology of human development: Experiments by nature and design*. Cambridge, MA: Harvard University Press.
13. Child Soldiers International. (2019). Child soldier levels doubled since 2012 and girls' exploitation is rising. https://reliefweb.int/report/world/child-soldier-levels-doubled-2012-and-girls-exploitation-rising.
14. Chiumento, A., Rahman, A., Frith, L., Snider, L., & Tol, W. (2017). Ethical standards for mental health and psychosocial support research in emergencies: Review of literature and current debates. *Globalization and Health, 13*(1), 8. https://doi.org/10.1186/s12992-017-0231-y.
15. Clarinval, C., & Biller-Andorno, N. (2014). Challenging operations: An ethical framework to assist humanitarian aid workers in their decision-making processes. *PLoS Currents, 6*. https://doi.org/10.1371/currents.dis.96bec99f13800a8059bb5b5a82028bbf.
16. Cloitre, M., Stolbach, B. C., Herman, J. L., Kolk, B. V. D., Pynoos, R., Wang, J., & Petkova, E. (2009). A developmental approach to complex PTSD: Childhood and adult cumulative trauma as predictors of symptom complexity. *Journal of Traumatic Stress, 22*(5), 399–408. https://doi.org/10.1002/jts.20444.
17. D'Andrea, W., Ford, J., Stolbach, B., Spinazzola, J., & Van Der Kolk, B. A. (2012). Understanding interpersonal trauma in children: Why we need a developmentally appropriate trauma diagnosis. *The American Journal of Orthopsychiatry, 82*(2), 187–200. https://doi.org/10.1111/j.1939-0025.2012.01154.x.

18. Darcy, J., & Hofmann, C. (2003). *According to need? Needs assessment and decision-making in the humanitarian sector.* Humanitarian Policy Group, ODI. http://www.odi.org.uk/hpg/papers/hpgreport15.pdf.
19. de Jong, J. T. V. M. (2014). Challenges of creating synergy between global mental health and cultural psychiatry. *Transcultural Psychiatry, 51*(6), 806–828. https://doi.org/10.1177/1363461514557995.
20. de Jong, K., Mulhern, M., Ford, N., van Der Kam, S., & Kleber, R. (2000). The trauma of war in Sierra Leone. *Lancet, 10,* 2067–2068.
21. Dudley, M. J., Newman, L. K., & Dudley, M. J. (2015). Ethical challenges for doctors working in immigration detention. *The Medical Journal of Australia, 202*(1), 16–17.
22. Dybdahl, R. (2001). Children and mothers in war: An outcome study of a psychosocial intervention program. *Child Development, 72*(4), 1214–1230. https://doi.org/10.1111/1467-8624.00343.
23. Dyer, A. R., & Bhadra, S. (2012). Global disasters, war, conflict and complex emergencies: Caring for special populations. In *21st century global mental health.* Burlington, MA: Jones and Bartlett.
24. Elbedour, S., Ten Bensel, R., & Bastien, D. T. (1993). Ecological integrated model of children of war: Individual and social psychology. *Child Abuse & Neglect, 17*(6), 805–819. https://doi.org/10.1016/S0145-2134(08)80011-7.
25. Eruyar, S., Huemer, J., & Vostanis, P. (2018). Review: How should child mental health services respond to the refugee crisis? *Child and Adolescent Mental Health, 23*(4), 303–312. https://doi.org/10.1111/camh.12252.
26. Essex, R. (2016). Healthcare and complicity in Australian immigration detention. *Monash Bioethics Review, 34*(2), 136–147. https://doi.org/10.1007/s40592-016-0066-y.
27. Essex, R. (2019). Do codes of ethics and position statements help guide ethical decision making in Australian immigration detention centres? *BMC Medical Ethics, 20*(1), 52. https://doi.org/10.1186/s12910-019-0392-8.
28. Fazel, M., & Betancourt, T. S. (2018). Preventive mental health interventions for refugee children and adolescents in high-income settings. *Lancet Child Adolesc Health, 2*(2), 121–132. https://doi.org/10.1016/S2352-4642(17)30147-5.
29. Fazel, M., Reed, R. V., Panter-Brick, C., & Stein, A. (2012). Mental health of displaced and refugee children resettled in high-income countries: Risk and protective factors. *Lancet, 379*(9812), 266–282. https://doi.org/10.1016/S0140-6736(11)60051-2.
30. Griffith, J., Kohrt, B., Dyer, A., Polatin, P., Morse, M., Jabr, S., Abdeen, S., Gaby, L., Jindal, A., & Khin, E. (2016). Training psychiatrists for global mental health: Cultural psychiatry, collaborative inquiry, and ethics of alterity. *Academic Psychiatry, 40*(4), 701–706. https://doi.org/10.1007/s40596-016-0541-z.
31. Hunt, M., Pal, N., Schwartz, L., & O'Mathúna, D. (2018). Ethical challenges in the provision of mental health Services for Children and Families during Disasters. *Current Psychiatry Reports, 20*(8), 1–10. https://doi.org/10.1007/s11920-018-0917-8.
32. Inter-Agency Network for Education in Emergencies. (2018). Strategic framework 2018-2023. http://s3.amazonaws.com/inee-assets/resources/INEE_Strategic_Framework_2018-2023_ENG.pdf.
33. Inter-Agency Standing Committee. (2007). *IASC guidelines on mental health and psychosocial support in emergency settings.* Geneva: IASC.
34. Inter-Agency Standing Committee (IASC) Reference Group for Mental Health and Psychosocial Support in Emergency Settings. (2017). *A common monitoring and evaluation framework for field test version mental health and psychosocial support in emergency settings.* Geneva: IASC.
35. International Rescue Committee. (2018). *Unprotected, unsupported, uncertain.* Recommendations to improve the mental health of asylum seekers on Lesvos. https://www.rescue-uk.org/sites/default/files/document/1792/unprotectedunsupporteduncertain24092018finalen.pdf.

36. Jones, L., & Kafetsios, K. (2002). Assessing adolescent mental health in war-affected societies: The significance of symptoms. *Child Abuse & Neglect, 26*(10), 1059–1080. https://doi.org/10.1016/S0145-2134(02)00381-2.
37. Jordans, M. J. D., Tol, W. A., Komproe, I. H., & de Jong, J. T. V. M. (2009). Systematic review of evidence and treatment approaches: Psychosocial and mental health care for children in war. *Child and Adolescent Psychiatry and Mental Health, 14*(1), 2–14. https://doi.org/10.1111/j.1475-3588.2008.00515.x.
38. Jordans, M. J., van den Broek, M., Brown, F., Coetzee, A., Ellermeijer, R., Hartog, K., Steen, F., & Miller, K. E. (2018). Supporting children affected by war: Towards an evidence based care system. In *Mental health of refugee and conflict-affected populations.* Cham: Springer Nature Switzerland. pp. 261–281.
39. Jordans, M., Komproe, I. H., Tol, W. A., Kohrt, B. A., Luitel, N. P., Macy, R. D., & de Jong, J. T. V. M. (2010). Evaluation of a classroom-based psychosocial intervention in conflict-affected Nepal: A cluster randomized controlled trial. *Journal of Child Psychology and Psychiatry, 51*(7), 818–826. https://doi.org/10.1111/j.1469-7610.2010.02209.x.
40. Jordans, M. J. D., Pigott, H., & Tol, W. (2016). Interventions for children affected by armed conflict: A systematic review of mental health and psychosocial support in low- and middle-income countries. *Current Psychiatry Reports, 18*(1), 1–15. https://doi.org/10.1007/s11920-015-0648-z.
41. Kazdin, A. E. (2006). Arbitrary metrics: Implications for identifying evidence-based treatments. *The American Psychologist, 61*(1), 42–49. https://doi.org/10.1037/0003-066X.61.1.42.
42. Kirmayer, L., Dandeneau, S., Marshall, E., Phillips, M. K., & Williamson, K. J. (2012). *Toward an ecology of stories: Indigenous perspectives on resilience.* New York: Springer.
43. Kirmayer, L. J., & Pedersen, D. (2014). Toward a new architecture for global mental health. *Transcultural Psychiatry, 51*(6), 759–776. https://doi.org/10.1177/1363461514557202.
44. Kleinman, A., Das, V., & Lock, M. (1997). *Social suffering.* Berkeley: University of California Press.
45. Kohrt, B., & Griffith, J. L. (2015). Global mental health praxis: Perspectives from cultural psychiatry on research and interventions. In *Re-visioning psychiatry: Cultural phenomenology, critical neuroscience, and global mental health.* Cambridge: Cambridge University Press. pp. 575–612.
46. Lee, L. M. (2012). Public health ethics theory: Review and path to convergence. *The Journal of Law, Medicine & Ethics, 40*(1), 85–98. https://doi.org/10.1111/j.1748-720X.2012.00648.x.
47. Lepora, C., & Goodin, R. E. (2013). *On complicity and compromise.* Oxford: Oxford University Press.
48. Lewis-Fernández, R., Aggarwal, N. K., Hinton, L., Hinton, D., & Kirmayer, L. J. (2016). *DSM-5 handbook on the cultural formulation interview.* Washington, DC: American Psychiatric Publishing.
49. Loughry, M., Ager, A., Flouri, E., Khamis, V., Afana, A. H., & Qouta, S. (2006). The impact of structured activities among Palestinian children in a time of conflict. *Journal of Child Psychology and Psychiatry, 47*(12), 1211–1218. https://doi.org/10.1111/j.1469-7610.2006.01656.x.
50. Luthar, S. S., Cicchetti, D., & Becker, B. (2000). The construct of resilience: A critical evaluation and guidelines for future work. *Child Development, 71*(3), 543–562. https://doi.org/10.1111/1467-8624.00164.
51. Masten, A., & Narayan, A. (2012). Child development in the context of disaster, war, and terrorism: Pathways of risk and resilience. *Annual Review of Psychology, 63*(1), 227–257. https://doi.org/10.1146/annurev-psych-120710-100356.
52. Masten, A. S. (2011). Resilience in children threatened by extreme adversity: Frameworks for research, practice, and translational synergy. *Development and Psychopathology, 23*(2), 493–506. https://doi.org/10.1017/S0954579411000198.

53. Meaney, M. J. (2010). Epigenetics and the biological definition of gene x environment interactions. *Child Development, 81*(1), 41–79. https://doi.org/10.1111/j.1467-8624.2009. 01381.x.
54. Migration Policy Institute. (2018). Pushback to the resistance: Criminalization of humanitarian actors aiding migrants rises. https://www.migrationpolicy.org/article/ top-10-2018-issue-5-pushback-resistance-criminalization-humanitarian-actors-aiding.
55. Miller, K. E., & Rasmussen, A. (2010). War exposure, daily stressors, and mental health in conflict and post-conflict settings: Bridging the divide between trauma-focused and psychosocial frameworks. *Social Science & Medicine, 70*(1), 7–16. https://doi.org/10.1016/j. socscimed.2009.09.029.
56. Miller, K. E., & Rasmussen, A. (2017). The mental health of civilians displaced by armed conflict: An ecological model of refugee distress. *Epidemiology and Psychiatric Sciences, 26*(2), 129–138. https://doi.org/10.1017/S2045796016000172.
57. Miller, K. E., & Jordans, M. J. D. (2016). Determinants of children's mental health in war-torn settings: Translating research into action.(report). *Current Psychiatry Reports, 18*(6), 1–6. https://doi.org/10.1007/s11920-016-0692-3.
58. Montgomery, E., & Foldspang, A. (2006). Validity of PTSD in a sample of refugee children: Can a separate diagnostic entity be justified? *International Journal of Methods in Psychiatric Research, 15*(2), 64–74. https://doi.org/10.1002/mpr.186.
59. Morgan, G. A., Gliner, J. A., & Harmon, R. J. (2007). Understanding research methods and statistics: A primer for clinicians. In *Lewis's child and adolescent psychiatry. A comprehensive textbook*. Philadelphia, PA: Lippincott Williams & Wilkins. pp. 104–124.
60. Morris, J., Van Ommeren, M., Belfer, M., Saxena, S., & Saraceno, B. (2007). Children and the sphere standard on mental and social aspects of health. *Disasters, 31*(1), 71–90. https:// doi.org/10.1111/j.1467-7717.2007.00341.x.
61. O'Callaghan, P., Mcmullen, J., Shannon, C., Rafferty, H., & Black, A. (2013). A randomized controlled trial of trauma-focused cognitive behavioral therapy for sexually exploited, war-affected Congolese girls. *Journal of the American Academy of Child and Adolescent Psychiatry, 52*(4), 359–369. https://doi.org/10.1016/j.jaac.2013.01.013.
62. OCHA. (2012). What are humanitarian principles? https://www.unocha.org/sites/dms/ Documents/OOM-humanitarianprinciples_eng_June12.pdf.
63. O'Sullivan, C., Bosqui, T., & Shannon, C. (2016). Psychological interventions for children and young people affected by armed conflict or political violence: A systematic literature review. *Intervention, 14*(2), 142–164. https://doi.org/10.1097/WTF.0000000000000110.
64. Panter-Brick, C., Goodman, A., Tol, W., & Eggerman, M. (2011). Mental health and childhood adversities: A longitudinal study in Kabul, Afghanistan. *Journal of the American Academy of Child and Adolescent Psychiatry, 50*(4), 349–363. https://doi.org/10.1016/j. jaac.2010.12.001.
65. Patel, V., Flisher, A. J., Nikapota, A., & Malhotra, S. (2008). Promoting child and adolescent mental health in low and middle income countries. *Journal of Child Psychology and Psychiatry, 49*(3), 313–334. https://doi.org/10.1111/j.1469-7610.2007.01824.x.
66. Porter, E. (2006). Can politics practice compassion? *Hypatia, 21*(4), 97–123. https://doi. org/10.1111/j.1527-2001.2006.tb01130.x.
67. Puffer, E. S., Annan, J., Sim, A. L., Salhi, C., & Betancourt, T. S. (2017). The impact of a family skills training intervention among Burmese migrant families in Thailand: A randomized controlled trial. *PLoS One, 12*(3), e0172611. https://doi.org/10.1371/journal. pone.0172611.
68. Reed, R. V., Fazel, M., Jones, L., Panter-Brick, C., & Stein, A. (2012). Mental health of displaced and refugee children resettled in low-income and middle-income countries: Risk and protective factors. *Lancet, 379*(9812), 250–265. https://doi.org/10.1016/ S0140-6736(11)60050-0.
69. Roberts, L. (2013). *Community-based participatory research for improved mental healthcare: A manual for clinicians and researchers* (1st ed.). New York: Springer. Imprint: Springer.
70. Rutter, J. (2006). *Refugee children in the UK*. Maidenhead: Open University Press.

71. Rutter, M. (2006). Implications of resilience concepts for scientific understanding. *Annals of the New York Academy of Sciences, 1094*, 1–12.
72. Rutter, M. (2007). Resilience, competence, and coping. *Child Abuse & Neglect, 31*(3), 205–209. https://doi.org/10.1016/j.chiabu.2007.02.001.
73. Rutter, M. (2012). Resilience as a dynamic concept. *Development and Psychopathology, 24*(2), 335–344. https://doi.org/10.1017/S0954579412000028.
74. Rutter, M., Sonuga-Barke, E. J., Beckett, C., Castle, J., Kreppner, J., Kumsta, R., Schlotz, W., Stevens, S., Bell, C. A., & Gunnar, M. R. (2010). Deprivation-specific psychological patterns: Effects of institutional deprivation. *Monographs of the Society for Research in Child Development, 75*(1), 1–252.
75. Sanggaran, J.-P., Haire, B., & Zion, D. (2016). The health care consequences of Australian immigration policies.(essay). *PLoS Medicine, 13*(2), e1001960. https://doi.org/10.1371/journal.pmed.1001960.
76. Silove, D. (2002). The asylum debacle in Australia: A challenge for psychiatry. *Australian and New Zealand Journal of Psychiatry, 36*(3), 290–296. https://doi.org/10.1046/j.1440-1614.2002.01036.x.
77. Slone, M., & Mann, S. (2016). Effects of war, terrorism and armed conflict on young children: A systematic review. *Child Psychiatry and Human Development, 47*(6), 950–965. https://doi.org/10.1007/s10578-016-0626-7.
78. Song, S. (2011). An ethical approach to life-long learning: Implications for global psychiatry. *Academic Psychiatry, 35*(6), 391–396. https://doi.org/10.1176/appi.ap.35.6.391.
79. Sphere Child Protection Working Group. (2012). *Minimum standards for child protection in humanitarian action (CPMS)*. Geneva: The Sphere Project.
80. Spiegel, P. B., Checchi, F., Colombo, S., & Paik, E. (2010). Health-care needs of people affected by conflict: Future trends and changing frameworks. *Lancet, 375*(9711), 341–345. https://doi.org/10.1016/S0140-6736(09)61873-0.
81. Spiegel, P., Kass, N., & Rubenstein, L. (2019). Can physicians work in US immigration detention facilities while upholding their Hippocratic oath? *JAMA, 322*(15), 1445–1446. https://doi.org/10.1001/jama.2019.12567.
82. Steel, Z., Momartin, S., Bateman, C., Hafshejani, A., Silove, D. M., Everson, N., Roy, K., Dudley, M., Newman, L., Blick, B., & Mares, S. (2004). Psychiatric status of asylum seeker families held for a protracted period in a remote detention Centre in Australia. *Australian and New Zealand Journal of Public Health, 28*(6), 527–536. https://doi.org/10.1111/j.1467-842X.2004.tb00042.x.
83. The Sphere Project. (2011). *Humanitarian charter and minimum standards in humanitarian response*. Geneva: The Sphere Project.
84. Tol, W. A., Barbui, C., Galappatti, A., Silove, D., Betancourt, T. S., Souza, R., Golaz, A., & van Ommeren, M. (2011a). Mental health and psychosocial support in humanitarian settings: Linking practice and research. *Lancet, 378*(9802), 1581–1591. https://doi.org/10.1016/S0140-6736(11)61094-5.
85. Tol, W. A., Patel, V., Tomlinson, M., Baingana, F., Galappatti, A., Panter-Brick, C., Silove, D., Sondorp, E., Wessells, M., & Ommeren, M. v. (2011b). Research priorities for mental health and psychosocial support in humanitarian settings. *PLoS Medicine, 8*(9), e1001096. https://doi.org/10.1371/journal.pmed.1001096.
86. Tol, W. A., Song, S., & Jordans, M. J. D. (2013). Annual research review: Resilience and mental health in children and adolescents living in areas of armed conflict – a systematic review of findings in low- and middle-income countries. *Journal of Child Psychology and Psychiatry, 54*(4), 445–460. https://doi.org/10.1111/jcpp.12053.
87. UNHCR. (2015). UNHCR, the environment & climate change. https://www.unhcr.org/en-us/540854f49.
88. UNHCR. (2019). Global trends forced displacement in 2018. https://www.unhcr.org/5d08d7ee7.pdf.
89. UNHCR. (2020). UNHCR emergency handbook. Child protection. https://emergency.unhcr.org/entry/43381/child-protection.

90. UNICEF, & International Medical Corps. (2014). Mental health psychosocial and child protection for Syrian Adolescent Refugees in Jordan. https://data2.unhcr.org/en/documents/download/42632.
91. Upshur, R. (2002). Principles for the justification of public health intervention. *Canadian Journal of Public Health, 93*(2), 101–103. https://doi.org/10.1007/BF03404547.
92. Vacchiano, F. (2018). *Desiring mobility: Child migration, parental distress and constraints on the future in North Africa*. In: Research handbook on child migration. Cheltenham: Edward Elgar Publishing. pp. 82—97.
93. Van der Kolk B, Pynoos R, Cicchetti D, Cloitre M, D'Andrea W, Ford JD, Liebermann AF, and Putnam F. (2009). Proposal to include a developmental trauma disorder diagnosis for children and adolescents in DSM-V. http://www.traumacenter.org/announcements/DTD_papers_Oct_09.pdf.
94. Watters, C., & Derluyn, I. (2018). *Wellbeing: Refugee children's psychosocial wellbeing and mental health*. In: Research handbook on child migration. Cheltenham: Edward Elgar Publishing. pp. 369—380.
95. Wessells, M. (2009). *What are we learning about protecting children in the community? An inter-agency review of the evidence on community-based child protection mechanisms in humanitarian and development settings*. The Save the Children Fund. https://www.unicef.org/protection/files/What_We_Are_Learning_About_Protecting_Children_in_the_Community_Full_Report.pdf.
96. Wessells, M. G. (2009b). Do no harm: Toward contextually appropriate psychosocial support in international emergencies. *The American Psychologist, 64*(8), 842–854. https://doi.org/10.1037/0003-066X.64.8.842.
97. Wilkinson, P. O., & Goodyer, I. M. (2011). Childhood adversity and allostatic overload of the hypothalamic–pituitary–adrenal axis: A vulnerability model for depressive disorders. *Development and Psychopathology, 23*(4), 1017–1037. https://doi.org/10.1017/S0954579411000472.
98. Worthman, C. M., & Kohrt, B. (2005). Receding horizons of health: Biocultural approaches to public health paradoxes. *Social Science & Medicine, 61*(4), 861–878. https://doi.org/10.1016/j.socscimed.2004.08.052.
99. Zion, D. (2013). Extending the clinical contract: Advocacy as a part of ethical health care for asylum seekers. *The American Journal of Bioethics, 13*(7), 19–21. https://doi.org/10.1080/15265161.2013.794878.
100. Zion, D., Briskman, L., & Loff, B. (2012). Psychiatric ethics and a politics of compassion. *Journal of Bioethical Inquiry, 9*(1), 67–75. https://doi.org/10.1007/s11673-011-9346-7.

Part V

Global Mental Health and Human Rights

Human Rights and Global Mental Health: Reducing the Use of Coercive Measures

15

Kelso R. Cratsley, Marisha N. Wickremsinhe, and Tim K. Mackey

Introduction

The application of human rights frameworks is an increasingly important part of efforts to accelerate progress in global mental health. Most recently, influential appeals to the "right to health" have helped make the case for strengthening and expanding services in low-resource settings. Such an approach foregrounds an important rights claim; namely, the responsibility of multilateral agencies, national health ministries, and local health systems to ensure the provision of public goods that improve health and well-being. This has taken on a significant degree of urgency given the prevailing burden of mental disorder and the widespread treatment gap [83]. There is also growing awareness of the social determinants of health and mental health, many of which are the product of inequities and thus important targets of social justice and rights-based approaches to global health [132]. The United Nations (UN) Special Rapporteur on the Right to Health has recently endorsed these commitments, characterizing human rights as a "determinant" of mental health [113].

K. R. Cratsley (✉)
Department of Philosophy & Religion, American University, Washington, DC, USA
e-mail: cratsley@american.edu

M. N. Wickremsinhe
Ethox Centre and Wellcome Centre for Ethics and Humanities, University of Oxford, Oxford, UK
e-mail: marisha.wickremsinhe@ethox.ox.ac.uk

T. K. Mackey
Department of Anesthesiology and Division of Global Public Health, School of Medicine, University of California San Diego, San Diego, CA, USA
e-mail: tmackey@ucsd.edu

© Springer Nature Switzerland AG 2021
A. R. Dyer et al. (eds.), *Global Mental Health Ethics*,
https://doi.org/10.1007/978-3-030-66296-7_15

This chapter takes up a closely related challenge, equally important for global mental health, that of strengthening protections against human rights violations.[1] The problem takes many forms. The most egregious are the following: stigma and discrimination, which can impact everything from educational and employment opportunities to basic rights such as the right to travel, marry, and have children; neglect, abuse, and torture, including inhumane living conditions in many treatment centers and harmful practices under the guise of treatment; and the use of a range of coercive measures, including arbitrary detention, forced medication, seclusion, and restraint [26]. These are ongoing problems, across high-income and low- and middle-income countries (LMICs), and there are a number of international legal and policy instruments that address them. Most prominent is the UN's *Convention on the Rights of Persons with Disabilities* (CRPD) [108]. The World Health Organization (WHO) drew directly on the CRPD in its own *QualityRights Took Kit* [125], which provides guidelines for evaluating and improving mental health facilities, and in its groundbreaking *Mental Health Action Plan 2013–2020* [126], recently extended to 2030 [120].

These serve as blueprints for development, with explicit prioritization of human rights. They carry the potential to strengthen the link between human rights obligations and actionable legal protections, particularly the call to reform mental health legislation worldwide. This underscores the importance of what have been termed the "legal determinants" of global health [41]. Such initiatives also have the power to influence the funding and design of national health systems, with direct implications for local service capacity.[2] However, it is fair to say that progress on all of these fronts has been slow, as recognized by the WHO's own dedicated reporting mechanism, the *Mental Health Atlas* [128]. Not enough has been done to institute robust human rights monitoring and enforcement mechanisms. There is a pressing need for more substantial progress on human rights as an essential part of broader development efforts in global mental health.

The focus of this chapter is on a critical component of this broader challenge, which is the question of how best to regulate and reduce the use of coercive measures. The mitigation or outright elimination of coercion is increasingly seen as a moral imperative across the field of mental health [10, 44, 93, 101]. More generally, human rights violations have traditionally been an under-researched topic in global mental health, with the majority of reporting coming from NGOs, government agencies, and the media. Documentation and first-hand accounts are widely

---

[1] There has been some concern that an over-emphasis on rights violations has come at the expense of legal responses to the problem of limited access to services [8, 111]. For the UN High Commissioner for Human Rights [111], the "right to health" of mental health service users encompasses both negative freedoms – from coercive interference – and positive entitlements. Effective advocacy will require working towards securing all fundamental human rights [70].

[2] This is particularly important given the disproportionately low levels of funding for mental health within global health [54].

available in the grey literature,[3] but there remains a pressing need for more academic research. Fortunately, certain topics have begun to receive sustained attention, particularly stigma [34], and there is now a large literature on coercion. Much of this research has been the work of research groups in high-income countries that have tracked the prevalence of involuntary admission, forced medication, seclusion, and restraint (e.g. [56]). This research represents a potentially useful resource to draw upon when responding to the current challenges in policymaking and implementation, although it also raises important questions about how well such findings generalize to LMICs.

In what follows, the need to regulate and reduce the use of coercive measures is situated within a broader human rights perspective. First, relevant legal and policy instruments are described, with particular attention to the work of the UN and WHO ("Global Health Law and Policy"). Next, domestic legislation is discussed, with an emphasis on efforts to bring mental health laws in line with international human rights standards ("Domestic Legislation"). Some of the most recent data on coercion in psychiatry are then briefly considered, including strategies that can help reduce the use of coercive measures ("Coercive Measures"). Finally, drawing on all of these considerations, several general recommendations are made in order to help improve monitoring and enforcement, guide national-level mental health legislation, and strengthen health systems ("General Recommendations"). The reduction of coercion must be a key target of efforts at all of these levels in order to protect human rights and further advance the goals of global mental health.

Global Health Law and Policy

In broad terms, protecting and promoting the human rights of service users involves a commitment to the principles of *entitlement*, or access to services; *equality*, or freedom from discrimination; *liberty*, or freedom from unwarranted detention; and *dignity*, or humane living conditions ([40]; also see [27]). These basic rights are captured by several of the core articles of the CRPD [108]. Particularly important are the following, listed in corresponding order: Article 25 ("the right to the enjoyment of the highest attainable standard of health without discrimination on the basis of disability"); Article 5 ("all persons are equal before and under the law and are entitled without any discrimination to the equal protection and equal benefit of the law"); Article 14 ("the right to liberty and security of person…not deprived of…liberty unlawfully or arbitrarily"); Article 15 ("freedom from torture or cruel, inhuman or degrading treatment or punishment"); and Article 16 ("freedom from exploitation, violence and abuse"). The CRPD thus provides a legal framework that should be directly applied to rights claims in global mental health, and each of these principles is at stake in various coercive practices. However, the application of the CRPD's standards has been anything but straightforward.

---

[3] For example, see reports by Human Rights Watch [41, 42, 48] and the Mental Disability Advocacy Center [61].

Debate Over the CRPD

While the CRPD is widely regarded as an important step forward for disability rights, debate has ensued over its implementation. Part of the problem has been interpretation of the core articles, with much of the debate centering on the requirement of legal capacity and equal recognition before the law in Article 12 ("persons with disabilities have the right to recognition everywhere as persons before the law"), a key principle of the CRPD that was further defended by the UN Committee's General Comment on Article 12 [109]. This later document explicitly affirms the presumption that individuals necessarily retain their legal standing before the law, regardless of mental incapacity or incompetence. This effectively precludes the possibility of involuntary commitment or treatment on the grounds of mental incapacity while signaling a shift away from "substituted" decision-making (service users have treatment decisions made for them if necessary) to a requirement of "supported" decision-making (service users are assisted with the process of consenting to treatment) [4]. Responses to this directive have been varied and contentious.

The critics' main charge is that in barring considerations of mental capacity, the CRPD is at risk of violating the right to treatment and the "highest attainable standard of health" [1, 33]. This perspective takes the position that there are cases where involuntary treatment may be the only route to recovery, which includes regaining the capacity to consent to or decline treatment. For some, this suggests that a more "realistic" interpretation of the CRPD may be preferable, in which certain predetermined, exceptional circumstances allow for involuntary treatment and substitute decision-making [24]. In addition, there are concerns that requiring a standard of absolute capacity may undercut the use of advance directives, increase the risk of undue influence in the process of supported decision-making, and complicate the assignment of criminal responsibility [18, 33, 95].[4] More research on its impact is needed [100], but concerns about Article 12 have hindered its implementation in some countries [45]. While the CRPD has been ratified by 181 member states, a number have submitted reservations or interpretive declarations with regard to Article 12.[5]

Less debate has surrounded the other articles of the CRPD, although several are directly relevant to coercion in mental health. Articles 15 and 16 have probably received the least amount of attention in the literature. But there are arguments for considering forced medication, seclusion, and physical restraint to be direct violations of either article, depending upon whether such measures are viewed as forms of torture or violence. For example, given the harms that can result from seclusion

---

[4] For more recent contributions to the debate, see the commentaries on Szmukler [96].

[5] For example, Canada – "To the extent Article 12 may be interpreted as requiring the elimination of all substitute decision-making arrangements, Canada reserves the right to continue their use in appropriate circumstances and subject to appropriate and effective safeguard" – or the Netherlands, "The Kingdom of the Netherlands interprets Article 12 as restricting substitute decision-making arrangements to cases where such measures are necessary, as a last resort and subject to safeguards" [108]

and restraint, they might be characterized as violence and abuse and thus contraventions of Article 16 [68]. The application of the CRPD, then, has the potential to help regulate such practices. Article 14 is perhaps the most relevant to involuntary commitment. As the UN Special Rapporteur on the CRPD confirms in a recent report, Article 14 requires an "absolute ban" of any denial of liberty based upon impairment or disability [114]. This is part of a broader commitment to the repeal of discriminatory mental health legislation and elimination of coercive interventions.

WHO QualityRights and Mental Health Action Plan

Despite the ongoing debate over the CRPD, it has been highly influential, particularly in its direct incorporation into the guidelines of the WHO. In both the *Mental Health Action Plan* [126] and the ongoing *QualityRights* initiative [129], the WHO has called for policies, legislation, and services that are consistent with the CRPD. This commitment is most explicit in the WHO's *QualityRights Tool Kit* [125], which is intended as resource for assessing and strengthening mental health services based upon human rights principles. It takes as its core themes the aforementioned Articles 12, 14, 15, 16, and 25, along with Article 19 ("the right to live independently and be included in the community") and Article 28 ("the right to an adequate standard of living and social protection"). The broader QualityRights initiative has the following stated objectives: strengthen efforts to curb stigma and discrimination while promoting human rights and recovery; improve human rights conditions and quality of care in mental health services; develop community-based and recovery-oriented services; help support a civil society movement that can advocate for policy change; and reform national mental health policies and legislation [129].[6]

The WHO's *Mental Health Action Plan* reflects similar commitments. Its first stated objective is "to strengthen effective leadership and governance for mental health," with two specific targets related to human rights: for 80% of countries to have mental health policies or plans consistent with human rights standards and for 50% of countries to bring their mental health laws in line with human rights standards.[7] This framework thus sets important standards relevant to the protection of the rights of service users. But according to the WHO's *2017 Mental Health Atlas* [128], recent efforts by member states to meet these expectations have fallen short.

Of the countries responding to select portions of the survey, 79% ($n = 175$) have stand-alone mental health policies and plans, with 120 countries reporting that updates were made in the past 5 years and 68% ($n = 151$) reporting full compliance

---

[6] The QualityRights initiative recently published a new set of training materials [118].

[7] The Plan's other objectives are (2) a 20% increase in service coverage, including provision of integrated mental health and social care services in community-based settings; (3) the implementation of promotion and prevention programs, with targets of 80% of countries with at least two such programs, and a 10% reduction of the suicide rate; and (4) the strengthening of information systems and evidence/research, with a target of 80% of countries collecting and reporting on mental health indicators every two years [115]

with human rights indicators.[8] This represents progress, but there is still a great deal of work left to be done. Ultimately only roughly half of all member states are in full compliance with human rights standards (though of the 36 countries reporting a lack of stand-alone mental health policies/plans, 22 noted that they were incorporated into broader health or disability policies/plans). Another notable feature of these reports concerned financial and human resource commitments, with 55% ($n = 169$) of surveyed countries indicating that estimates of such resources were explicitly included in mental health policies and plans; of those, only 53% ($n = 93$) reported that such allocation had actually taken place.

UN Sustainable Development Goals

Further progress on these indicators will require prioritization of human rights as part of a broader push for development goals specific to mental health. The UN's *2030 Agenda for Sustainable Development* [110] – also known as the Sustainable Development Goals (SDGs) – now includes mental health within Goal 3 ("ensure healthy lives and promote well-being for all at all ages") in a target focused on reducing premature mortality from non-communicable diseases (3.4), with an indicator of suicide mortality rate (3.4.2). Another target addresses substance abuse (3.5), with indicators on service coverage (3.5.1) and per capita consumption of alcohol (3.5.2). Inclusion of these targets came after sustained advocacy from within the field of global mental health, including unsuccessful calls for an additional indicator on service coverage [105]. More recently, the Lancet Commission on Global Mental Health and Sustainable Development has called for a comprehensive set of indicators, tied to mental health determinants, systems and services (including policies consistent with human rights protections), and outcomes and risk protection [83].[9]

The fact remains that including mental health in development frameworks is meaningless without actual targets and indicators, including those pertaining to human rights. The SDGs have been criticized for failing to prioritize human rights more generally [122]. That said, human rights are mentioned multiple times throughout the SDGs, including a foundational appeal to the *Universal Declaration of Human Rights* and a consistent emphasis on the principles of equality and non-discrimination. Many of the goals themselves include reference to human rights; thus the case can be made that all of the SDGs have direct relevance for economic, social, and cultural rights as well as civil and political rights [115]. Nonetheless,

---

[8] Compliance of policies/plans is scored by self-report on five criteria: promotion of transition toward community-based mental health services; explicit attention to respect for human rights; promotion of independent living and inclusion in the community; promotion of a recovery approach; and participation of persons with mental disorders in decision-making processes [117].

[9] The Commission's proposal also emphasizes the cross-cutting nature of mental health, as progress in mental health will impact – and be impacted by – progress on any number of SDGs. At the very least, more comprehensive indicators would make for increased policy coherence with the WHO's frameworks [16]. For further discussion of mental health and the SDGs, see Davidson [20].

within Goal 3 there is no explicit mention of the right to health (although target 3.8 calls for universal health coverage), and no direct connection is drawn between human rights and mental health. Protections against abuse and exploitation are most clearly articulated in Goal 16 ("promote peaceful and inclusive societies for sustainable development, provide access to justice for all and build effective, accountable and inclusive institutions at all levels"), as are calls for stronger and more accountable institutions and non-discriminatory laws and policies. Once again, though, there is no reference to health or mental health.

Domestic Legislation

On the national level, there is a marked lack of consistency in the implementation of human rights standards in domestic legislation. Indeed, the degree of variation makes comparative analysis difficult, with a wide range of legal frameworks governing the use of coercive measures in mental health. Recent reviews note varied criteria for involuntary detention and treatment across jurisdictions in countries from a range of income groups [87, 94, 119 ,121]. The vast majority of mental health laws are comparable, however, simply by virtue of authorizing involuntary hospitalization (if under divergent criteria). There have been significant efforts at reform, but new legislation tends to fall short of the CRPD's strict requirements.[10]

Need for Reform

The need to reform mental health legislation in many countries was recognized well before the introduction of the CRPD. For example, in Commonwealth countries that were colonized by Britain, the relevant legislation available to "protect and promote" the rights of individual with mental disorders was often based on colonial-era "Lunacy Acts" [98], which tended to be particularly discriminatory, punitive, and custodial in nature [11]. Fortunately, some countries have successfully replaced these outdated laws, e.g., Bangladesh's recent legislative victory in enacting the Mental Health Act of 2018 to replace the Lunacy Act of 1912 [46]. But there are also countries that lack mental health legislation altogether.

According to the WHO's *Mental Health Atlas* [128], only 63% ($n = 175$) of responding member states have dedicated mental health laws in place. There has been recent progress, with 66 countries updating legislation in the past 5 years. But many countries still lack mental health legislation altogether, up to 83 of all member states, if including countries that did not respond to this portion of the *Atlas* (of the 64 countries that reported a lack of mental health legislation, 34 have broader health or disability laws that include mental health). In response to additional survey questions, 75% ($n = 118$) of countries described their legislation as fully compliant with

---

[10] There are regional human rights instruments that also influence domestic mental health legislation, such as the *European Convention on Human Rights* [14].

international human rights instruments, although this represents less than half of all member states.[11] Member states were also asked about the presence of an independent body responsible for evaluating the compliance and implementation of mental health legislation: 40% ($n = 159$) of countries lack such an authority, and only 28% ($n = 159$) have an authority that provides regular inspections of mental health facilities.

These findings from the WHO *Atlas* are significant because without robust, dedicated legislation, there is an increased risk of arbitrary detention, without legal procedure, judicial oversight, or formal avenues for appeal or complaint (and often without basic treatment). This risk is pronounced in LMICs, where there is a greater risk for coercive measures to be used merely as a form of abuse or punishment [26, 40]. But to be absolutely clear, the lack of robust human rights-based mental health legislation is not restricted to LMICs. There is a general need for legal frameworks that adequately address the human rights of service users. For those jurisdictions where mental health laws are in place, policymaking should focus on clarifying the rules that govern the use of coercive measures.

Unresolved Ethical Issues

As the debate over the CRPD illustrates, the use of coercive practices in psychiatric care is subject to important questions about not only whether coercion is justified (if at all), but how and under what circumstances. Such questions are not easily resolved; regardless, attention must continue to be paid to the ethical defensibility of criteria required by law to justify the use of coercive measures. In many jurisdictions, the criteria that are legally permitted – particularly for involuntary commitment and treatment – are highly contested, difficult to predict, and often unevenly applied.

Debates regarding the ethical acceptability of certain criteria used to justify involuntary admission are yet to be settled, taking issue with a range of considerations, especially with respect to discrimination and the possibility of abolition. Regarding discrimination, some argue that the very nature of mental health law is discriminatory, leading to the proposal of a generic "fusion law" that treats involuntary treatment decisions for mental or physical illness equally, based upon assessments of capacity and best interests [25]. As for the possibility of abolition, some argue for a strict reading of the CRPD, with any form of involuntary commitment or treatment prohibited [72].

Further, analysis of available empirical data raises serious questions about the ethics of criteria for compulsory admission as they currently stand in many

---

[11] Compliance of legislation is defined by the following criteria: promotion of transition toward community-based mental health services; promotion of rights of people with mental disorder to exercise their legal capacity; promotion of alternatives to coercive practices; procedures to protect rights and the ability to file complaints to an independent body; and regular inspections of human rights conditions in mental health facilities by an independent body [117].

jurisdictions. In short, there is evidence to suggest that risk assessment tools are no better at predicting risk of violence than a simple coin toss [30]. This is problematic due to the fact many jurisdictions rely upon risk as a determining factor for involuntary commitment, compounded by concerns that even when capacity assessments are legally required – in place of or supplementing ascriptions of risk – they can devolve into a form of risk assessment [77]. In addition, evidence suggests that the criteria for justifying the use of coercion is subject to existing social and cultural biases, given, for example, the disproportionate use of forced admission amongst Black, Asian, and minority ethnic communities in the UK [6].[12]

Notable Examples

Several countries have tried to better align their mental health legislation with prevailing human rights standards, although there are still implementation challenges. Predating the CRPD by several decades, the most notable example is probably Italy's Law no. 180 of 1978 [38], the "Basaglia Law," which established a clear set of criteria for compulsory admission, requiring a need for treatment rather than attributions of risk. The law drastically changed the provision of psychiatric care and may partially explain why Italy now has the lowest rate of involuntary hospitalization in Europe [87]. Challenges persist, however. For example, a recent study found that some compulsory admissions were pursued not due to the need for treatment of a psychiatric condition, but rather as a product of brief, alcohol- or drug-related behavior change [81]. This is consistent with larger concerns about the role of extra-legal factors in decisions to involuntary commit [65].

Northern Ireland's Mental Capacity Act of 2016 (MCA) [78] is a more recent example of legal reform, considered a form of "fusion" legislation [43]. While an important step toward preventing human rights violations and coercive practice, the MCA "retains a 'diagnostic' element" where capacity is assessed as lacking according, in part, to "an impairment of, or a disturbance in the functioning of, the mind or brain" [64, 78]. Because this diagnostic element is present the MCA has been critiqued as not fully compliant with the CRPD [64], while others argue that, according to certain readings of the CRPD, the law is adequately aligned with its principles [43]. Future studies on the law's impact on the use of coercion, using service-level data, will give a better sense of the ways in which a more human rights-oriented legal framework can reduce coercive practice.

India's Mental Health Care Act of 2017 (MHCA) [71] represents another important point of progress in developing legislation that more closely aligns with the CRPD [28, 29]. The use of advanced directives is a key feature of MHCA, intended

---

[12]Another set of important issues concerns the regulation of discharge from hospital and commitment appeals. In some jurisdictions the regulations for discharge are so restrictive that even voluntary admission is arguably not truly voluntary [30]; in others it's interesting to note that there appears to be a decrease in appeals of involuntary admissions, despite relatively stable rates of commitment [3].

to fulfill the CRPD's mandate that individuals living with mental disability are afforded constant legal capacity [91]. The MHCA also makes provisions for supported – as opposed to substitute – decision-making, in order to further respect service user choice [74]. However, the legislation has been criticized for lack of full compliance with the CRPD, particularly its use of a biomedical definition of disability, which contradicts the CRPD's definition [75].[13]

Coercive Measures

Coercive measures are pervasive in mental health and represent the most significant challenges to human rights protections. Coercion is a term used variously; for the purposes of mental health, it is best understood inclusively as the use of threats or physical force as a form of treatment pressure, typically associated with involuntary commitment, forced medication, seclusion, and restraint [103]. Such practices involve restrictions on the right to exercise one's legal capacity, thus rendering them objectionable by the terms of the CRPD, or, at the very least, subject to ethical consternation and requiring substantial justification. There had been few efforts to investigate coercion in psychiatry until relatively recently, when an upsurge of research started to detail the nature of coercive practices (for overviews, see [20, 56, 73]). Much of this research has originated in Europe, and so there are lingering questions about whether its findings generalize to LMICs. But until a broader empirical picture is available, these data represent a potentially valuable resource.

Prevalence and Correlates of Coercion

The prevalence of coercive practices varies widely depending upon the jurisdiction and health system in question. In Europe, Australia, and New Zealand, where the most data is available, there is significant variation across countries [87]. There is evidence that commitment rates have increased in certain jurisdictions since the end of deinstitutionalization, such as in England [12].[14] Once detained, up to 40% of service users are subject to seclusion, restraint, or forced medication during hospitalization, though here there is also considerable variation between jurisdictions [54, 66]. Individuals who are involuntarily hospitalized tend to have more severe symptoms, suffer from psychotic disorders, and have lower scores on global

---

[13] Scotland's mental health legislation is another notable attempt at reform [91]. The prohibition of forced medication in Germany during 2011 and 2012 is also worth noting; it was associated with increased use of other coercive measures in some hospitals [32], although not in one regional health service [121]. As it happens, research groups in Europe have been working on the development of shared clinical guidelines for the use of forced medication [55].

[14] The reasons for this increase are the subject of ongoing debate about the effects of deinstitutionalization, transinstitutionalization, and legislation focused on risk management in the service of public safety (e.g., [84]). There is interesting new data implicating economic factors [89].

functioning; those most frequently subjected to seclusion, restraint, and forced medication have been linked to the same characteristics, along with aggressive behavior [54].

Research on the clinical effects of coercion has resulted in equivocal findings. Involuntary commitment is associated with better clinical outcomes for some service users, and a proportion retrospectively describe their treatment as necessary and justified [55, 57, 84, 85]. But this certainly does not hold for the majority of service users, and some studies have found relatively few health and social benefits associated with involuntary hospitalization [86]. This is particularly true for those who are subjected to seclusion, which appears to be associated with significantly longer inpatient stays, as well as forced medication, which greatly decreases the likelihood of retrospective assent [66]. In addition, in extreme cases coercive measures can lead to post-traumatic stress, cardiac arrest, and death [14, 59].[15]

There is also a good deal of research on the subjective experiences of service users in relation to treatment pressure, often referred to as "perceived coercion" or "informal coercion" (reviewed in [47, 76]). Much of this data describes frequent experiences of humiliation, lack of autonomy, and powerlessness on the part of both voluntary and involuntary service users. For example, a significant minority of voluntary service users report experiencing disrespect, exclusion from participation in treatment decisions, a lack of fair and clear decision-making processes (or "procedural justice"), and threats, including the implicit threat that they will be detained *in*voluntarily if they do not comply [58, 79]. They tend to have less symptomatic improvement than those who are involuntarily committed and are more likely to consider their treatment ineffective [58].

Reduction Strategies

Just as the current literature reveals the prevalence of coercion, it also describes a complicated picture regarding potential reduction strategies. Systematic reviews have identified promising new approaches to care planning, therapeutic intervention, and inpatient procedures and practices [39], but more research is required [89]. The recent studies on prevalence rates and clinical correlates have given rise to several provisional recommendations. This starts with improving the treatment of acute symptomatology, given the clinical profile of most service users who experience coercion. Researchers have also called for improvements to the process of involuntary hospital admission [31]. This includes providing clear and accessible information to service users about the justification and duration of treatment. Initial encounters with mental health services appear to be crucial opportunities in this regard [79]. Increased family involvement and better communication between the hospital and community are also recommended. This is especially important given

---

[15] Involuntary treatment in the community also has equivocal outcome data, despite the fact that it is increasingly used internationally and remains a controversial form of intervention [65].

the disproportionate impact of coercion on ethnic minorities (not to mention other social determinants such as social class, employment, and urbanicity; [60]).

More recent research has focused on alternative interventions, both prior to initiation of the admission process and during the course of inpatient treatment [5]. The use of advance crisis plans has been found to be the most effective means of reducing rates of involuntary commitment, according to an influential meta-analysis [22]. Innovative forms of assertive community treatment have started to show promise as a means to reduce the need for involuntary hospitalization [96], and a recent randomized control trial found that a new psychoeducation program could help reduce involuntary readmissions to hospital while also reducing their duration [61].

There are fewer data available on coercion reduction strategies for use on inpatient wards [93]. More generally, de-escalation techniques suffer from a lack of empirical support [37]. And while there is some evidence that a combination of strategies can help decrease the use of seclusion [36], a recent review concluded that programs designed to reduce seclusion and restraint are relatively ineffective, though they can improve safety and quality of care [42]. Other research points in the direction of new and constructive solutions, much of it underscoring the need for increased training of mental health practitioners. For example, there is evidence that ward staff don't fully understand the subtleties of coercion [51] and that enhanced staff training can improve the experiences of the involuntarily hospitalized [131]. Consistent with this, the Safewards conflict reduction program has begun to gain empirical support as an effective approach to reducing the use of coercive measures on inpatient wards [9].[16]

Generalizing the Findings?

There remain serious questions concerning the extent to which any of these findings can be generalized from Western, high-income contexts. To date, there has been far less research on coercive practices in LMICs, although this is slowly changing. For example, one widely discussed recent study focused on the use of chains in a religious prayer camp, often the site of detention and "treatment" for mental health conditions in certain countries, in this case Ghana [80]. This study investigated whether the administration of first-line pharmaceutical treatment would help lessen the use of chained restraint by way of reduced symptomatology. Clinical improvement did not correlate with less restraint, however, leaving important questions unanswered. There are likely to be significant *social* and *cultural* variables at play in the use of various forms of coercion in any given context. This is an important part of the larger challenge to reduce coercive practices (and in global mental health more generally). But it need not undercut a fundamental commitment to protecting the rights of service users [82].[17]

---

[16] There is also interesting research on the effects of open wards [44] and various architectural strategies [45].

[17] For further discussion of mental health policy and legislation in Ghana, see Walker and Osei [110].

General Recommendations

In the service of improved governance for global mental health, with special attention to human rights and the reduction of coercive measures, several general recommendations are in order. From the broadest perspective, there should be continuing efforts to make mental health more central to international development. As discussed, mental health has a relatively marginal place within what is currently the most influential set of development guidelines – the UN's *Sustainable Development Agenda*. This should be remedied in future development initiatives, consistent with the proposal for comprehensive indicators put forward by the Lancet Commission [83]. More specifically, efforts to reduce the use of coercive measures will require progress on key objectives at various levels, including improved monitoring and enforcement, clearer guidance for domestic legislation, and health systems strengthening.

Monitoring and Enforcement

For a start, more needs to be done to improve monitoring and enforcement. The Committee on the Rights of Persons with Disabilities is tasked with assessing implementation of the CRPD (per Article 34) and has a mandate to investigate alleged violations of the Convention. The WHO, for its part, is fulfilling important reporting functions with its *Atlas* surveys. They provide a regular review of progress on the targets set out in the *Action Plan*. This is essential, particularly as it includes tracking human rights indicators. But more robust monitoring is required, and the possibility of enforcement of some type needs to be available. Violations of the rights of service users continue to be widely documented, and without proper mechanisms for oversight and action, this population can be subjected to even more discrimination, neglect, and abuse [26].

One option that has been considered is the creation of a global commission on mental health institutions, responsible for monitoring the prevailing conditions in psychiatric facilities worldwide [15]. If housed within the UN, such a commission could have the necessary strength to enact reforms with real implications for treatment centers in member states that fall below acceptable human rights standards. A similar proposal from the Lancet Commission calls for the establishment of an independent oversight body, supported by a multisectoral partnership between UN agencies, non-governmental organizations, academic institutions, civil society groups, private sector representatives, and service users and their families [83]. The partnership's responsibilities would involve monitoring progress on global mental health targets, including reducing human rights violations and the use of coercive measures, and could run in parallel with national-level oversight mechanisms.

What is abundantly clear is that the current state of many mental health facilities is unacceptable, and so a more robust monitoring and enforcement process is required. One other mechanism that has been discussed is application of the UN's

Optional Protocol to the Convention against Torture and other Cruel, Inhuman or Degrading Treatment or Punishment [107], which can provide oversight of psychiatric institutions [102]. An important part of any of these processes must be the involvement of service users. As the Committee on the Rights of Persons with Disabilities has emphasized [112], Article 33 of the CRPD requires the active participation of civil society groups and service users in the monitoring of the Convention.

Guidance for National Legislation

There is a strong case for better governance to support jurisdictions with longstanding mental health legislation, as well as those where legal frameworks are lacking or absent altogether. Further guidance is needed, which can ultimately play an important role in regulating and reducing the use of coercive measures. The ongoing debates over Article 12 of the CRPD will not be easily resolved, but the Committee on the Rights of Persons with Disabilities must stay actively engaged with all stakeholders, including member states and civil society groups representing service users. There are a number of different paths forward that have been discussed; here only a few are briefly mentioned.

There have been calls for member states to interpret the CRPD in ways that are more consistent with capacity-based legislation, in line with critics who have worried that a strict reading of General Comment #1 precludes the possibility of involuntary treatment and thus may violate the right of service users to health and recovery [24, 104]. A stronger response would be for the Committee to make an amendment to the CRPD itself, which is allowed by Article 47 of the Convention [2, 95]. Coming from the opposite direction in these debates, there is also of course the possibility of reaffirming the original commitments of the Convention as standing international law. As others have noted, truly engaging and respecting the perspectives – or "will and preferences" – of service users might just require the type of paradigm shift represented by the CRPD [7, 77].

Ultimately, it may be that a uniform corrective is unlikely to work. The varied responses to the CRPD from member states bear this out. Each country may have to address these standards in ways specific to their own resources, legal precedents, and social and cultural standards. Research is needed to evaluate how mental health legislation is implemented – and can be improved – in different jurisdictions, including closely monitoring the effectiveness of recent attempts to reform domestic mental health legislation, such as in Northern Ireland and India. How exactly these new laws work in practice can help inform the design of new legislation in other jurisdictions requiring reform. This does not weaken the general point that there is a need for reform internationally, to ensure that substantial rights protections are in fact operationalized and implemented. More legal support is necessary, in the form of stronger multilateral guidance. For example, the WHO's mental health policy guidance [123] has not been updated since 2005, and its guidance for mental health legislation [124] was withdrawn due to noncompliance with the CRPD (though see [130]).

Health Systems Strengthening

In terms of health systems strengthening, some lessons from the recent research on coercive measures can be applied directly. System-level configurations appear to help reduce coercion, including more effective clinical interventions. The current evidence favors collaborative approaches that engage service users, their families, and the community during the process of hospitalization, as well as improved conditions throughout the course of treatment. Resources should be allocated accordingly. Increased funding is no guarantee of improved conditions, as rights violations regularly occur in well-financed health systems. But health systems strengthened in the right way, directed by the best available evidence, have a better chance of improving rights-related conditions.[18]

Perhaps most importantly, there is a need to expand the range of alternatives to hospitalization. The absence of such options has been identified as a key factor in commitment decisions [65].[19] This places an onus on community treatment, including the development of innovative forms of crisis team services and assertive community treatment.[20] Making advance statements more readily available is also necessary, as is an increased emphasis on supported decision-making [134], including influential approaches such as the Open Dialogue model [117]. A commitment to rights-based care and the reduction of coercion should also extend to hospitalization itself; an increased focus on community-based alternatives should not come at the cost of reforming psychiatric institutions. Here there is a need for more research on the most effective, least restrictive interventions on the ward. There is also recent progress worth noting, such as improvements to mental health services in Sri Lanka and Vietnam [16]. These efforts involved enhancements to rights-based care in both newly developed community services and reformed psychiatric institutions, driven by a combination of national-level political commitment and WHO support.

More effective capacity building will be an important part of these developments. This is another area where there is a dearth of knowledge, but initiatives like the "Emerging mental health systems in LMICs" (Emerald) program – in Ethiopia, India, Nepal, Nigeria, South Africa, and Uganda – have the potential to inform future efforts [106]. A key piece of this initiative is engagement with service users and caregivers, which, as previously mentioned, is increasingly recognized as essential for rights-based care and the reduction of coercion. For example, many service users report that coercive measures such as physical restraint can be avoided through improved engagement with the service users themselves [88]. In addition, there is a need for better understanding of the varied roles that families and caregivers play in coercive processes [90]. Just as service users and caregivers are increasingly involved in the design of mental health policy and legislation,

---

[18] The WHO's mhGAP initiative is an important resource for health systems strengthening [116].

[19] Surveys also suggest that there is concern among mental health professionals that community services suffer from significant limitations [11].

[20] This should include the expansion of preventive programming, though this comes with its own ethical challenges [18].

they should also be active collaborators in the structuring and implementation of clinical services.

Conclusion

Mental health remains an area within global health where human rights are routinely violated. To date, the response to this problem from international governing bodies has been inadequate. Legal and policy-based correctives are required. These initiatives should include explicit inclusion of indicators linking mental health and human rights in current development goals, as well as improved mechanisms for the monitoring and enforcement of human rights law and policy. Further guidance on domestic mental health law is also necessary, as there are countries that lack dedicated legislation and others where debate continues over the appropriate balance to strike between protecting the rights of service users and the authorization of compulsory detention and treatment. And finally, as in much of global mental health, there is a need for strategically targeted financial and human resources to help improve local health systems. A coordinated, multi-level approach is required, then, in order to strengthen human rights protections and reduce the use of coercive measures in global mental health.

Acknowledgments We would like to thank Peter Bartlett and Matthé Scholten for comments on earlier versions of this chapter.

References

1. Appelbaum, P. (2016). Protecting the rights of persons with disabilities: An international convention and its problems. *Psychiatric Services, 67*(4), 366–368.
2. Appelbaum, P. (2019). Saving the UN Convention on the Rights of Persons with Disabilities – from itself. *World Psychiatry, 18*(1), 1–2.
3. Arnold, B. D., Moeller, J., Hochstrasser, L., Schneeberger, A. R., Borgwardt, S., Lang, U. E., & Huber, C. G. (2019). Compulsory admission to psychiatric wards – who is admitted, and who appeals against admission? *Frontiers in Psychiatry, 10*, 544.
4. Arstein-Kerslake, A., & Flynn, E. (2016). The General Comment on Article 12 of the Convention on the Rights of Persons with Disabilities: A roadmap for equality before the law. *International Journal of Human Rights, 20*(4), 471–490.
5. Barbui, C., Purgato, M., Abdulmalik, J., Caldas-de-Almeida, J., Eaton, J., Gureje, O., et al. (2020). Efficacy of interventions to reduce coercive treatment in mental health services: Umbrella review of randomised evidence. *The British Journal of Psychiatry*, 1–11. https://doi.org/10.1192/bjp.2020.144.
6. Barnett, P., Mackay, E., Matthews, H., Gate, R., Greenwood, H., Ariyo, K., et al. (2019). Ethnic variations in compulsory detention under the Mental Health Act: A systematic review and meta-analysis of international data. *Lancet Psychiatry, 6*(4), 305–317.
7. Bartlett, P. (2019). Will and preferences in the overall CRPD project. *World Psychiatry, 18*(1), 48–50.
8. Battams, S. (2016). Editorial: Public mental health policy, mental health promotion, and interventions which focus on the social determinants of mental health. *Frontiers in Public Health, 4*, 285.

9. Baumgartner, J., Jackel, D., Helber-Bohlen, H., Stiehm, N., Morgenstern, K., Voigt, A., et al. (2019). Preventing and reducing coercive measures – an evaluation of the implementation of the Safewards model in two locked wards in Germany. *Frontiers in Psychiatry, 10*, 340.
10. Bhugra, D., Tasman, A., Pathare, S., Priebe, S., Smith, S., Torous, J., Arbuckle, M. R., et al. (2017). The WPA-Lancet Psychiatry Commission on the future of psychiatry. *Lancet Psychiatry, 4*, 775–818.
11. Bhugra, D., Pathare, S., Joshi, R., & Ventriglio, A. (2018). Mental health policies in Commonwealth countries. *World Psychiatry, 17*(1), 113–114.
12. Care Quality Commission. (2020). Monitoring the Mental Health Act in 2018/2019.
13. Chow, W. S., Ajaz, A., & Priebe, S. (2019). What drives changes in institutional mental health care? A qualitative study of the perspectives of professional experts. *Social Psychiatry and Psychiatric Epidemiology, 54*, 737–744.
14. Chieze, M., Hurst, S., Kaiser, S. & Sentissi, O. (2019). Effects of seclusion and restraint in adult psychiatry: A systematic review. *Frontiers in Psychiatry*, 10, 491.
15. Cohen, A., Chatterjee, S., & Minas, H. (2016). Time for a global commission on mental health institutions. *World Psychiatry, 15*(2), 116–117.
16. Cohen, A., & Minas, H. (2017). Global mental health and psychiatric institutions in the 21st century. *Epidemiology and Psychiatric Sciences, 26*, 4–9.
17. Council of Europe. (1952). *The European convention on human rights*. Strasbourg: European Court of Human Rights.
18. Craigie, J. (2015). Against a singular understanding of legal capacity: Criminal responsibility and the Convention on the Rights of Persons with Disabilities. *International Journal of Law and Psychiatry, 40*, 6–14.
19. Cratsley, K., & Mackey, T. K. (2018). Global mental health and the United Nations' sustainable development goals. *Families, Systems & Health, 36*(2), 225–229.
20. Cratsley, K. (2019). The ethics of coercion and other forms of influence. In R. Bluhm & S. Tekin (Eds.), *Bloomsbury companion to philosophy of psychiatry*. London: Bloomsbury.
21. Cratsley, K., & Radden, J. (Eds.). (2019). *Mental health as public health: Interdisciplinary perspectives on the ethics of prevention*. San Diego: Elsevier.
22. de Jong, M. H., Kamperman, A. M., Oorschot, M., Priebe, S., Bramer, W., et al. (2016). Intervention to reduce compulsory psychiatric admissions: A systematic review and meta-analysis. *JAMA Psychiatry, 73*(7), 657–664.
23. Davidson, L. (Ed.). (2019). *The Routledge handbook of international development, mental health and wellbeing*. London/New York: Routledge.
24. Dawson, J. (2015). A realistic approach to assessing mental health laws' compliance with the UNCRPD. *International Journal of Law and Psychiatry, 40*, 70–79.
25. Dawson, J., & Szmukler, G. (2006). Fusion of mental health and incapacity legislation. *The British Journal of Psychiatry, 188*, 504–509.
26. Drew, N., Funk, M., Tang, S., Lamichhane, J., Chavez, E., Katonoka, S., et al. (2011). Human rights violations of people with mental and psychosocial disabilities: An unresolved global crisis. *Lancet, 378*, 1664–1675.
27. Dudley, M., Silove, D., & Gale, F. (Eds.). (2012). *Mental health and human rights: Vision, praxis, and courage*. Oxford: Oxford University Press.
28. Duffy, R. M., & Kelly, B. D. (2019). India's Mental Healthcare Act, 2017: Content, context, controversy. *International Journal of Law and Psychiatry, 62*, 169–178.
29. Duffy, R.M. & Kelly, B.D. (2020). *India's Mental Healthcare Act, 2017: Building laws, protecting rights*. Singapore: Springer.
30. Fazel, S., Singh, J. P., Doll, H., & Grann, M. (2012). Use of risk assessment instruments to predict violence and antisocial behaviour in 73 samples involving 24,827 people: Systematic review and meta-analysis. *BMJ, 345*, e4692.
31. Fiorillo, A., De Rosa, C., Del Vecchio, V., Jurjanz, L., Schnall, K., Onchev, G., et al. (2011). How to improve clinical practice on involuntary hospital admissions of psychiatric patients: Suggestions from the EUNOMIA study. *European Psychiatry, 26*, 201–207.

32. Flammer, E. & Steinert, T. (2016). Association between restriction of involuntary medication and frequency of coercive measures and violent incidents. *Psychiatric Services*, 67, 12, 1315–20.
33. Freeman, M. C., Kolappa, K., Caldas de Almeida, J. M., Kleinman, A., Makhashvili, N., Phakathi, S., Saraceno, B., & Thornicroft, G. (2015). Reversing hard won victories in the name of human rights: A critique of the General Comment on Article 12 of the UN Convention on the Rights of Persons with Disabilities. *Lancet Psychiatry, 2*, 844–850.
34. Gaebel, W., Russler, W., & Sartorius, N. (Eds.). (2017). *The stigma of mental illness – end of the story?* Cham: Springer.
35. Garakani, A., Shalenberg, E., Burstin, S. C., Brendel, R. W., & Appel, J. M. (2014). Voluntary psychiatric hospitalization and patient-driven requests for discharge: A statutory review and analysis of implications for the capacity to consent to voluntary hospitalization. *Harvard Review of Psychiatry, 22*, 241–249.
36. Gaskin, C. J., Elsom, S. J., & Happell, B. (2007). Interventions for reducing the use of seclusion in psychiatric facilities. *The British Journal of Psychiatry, 191*, 298–230.
37. Gaynes, B. N., Brown, C. L., Lux, L. J., Brownley, K. A., Van Dorn, R. A., Edlund, M. J., et al. (2017). Preventing and de-escalating aggressive behavior among adult psychiatric patients: A systematic review of the evidence. *Psychiatric Services, 68*(8), 819–831.
38. Gazzetta Ufficiale della Repubblica Italiana. (1978). LEGGE. n. 180. Accertamenti e trattamenti sanitari volontari e obbligatori.
39. Giacco, D., Conneely, M., Masoud, T., Burn, E., & Priebe, S. (2018). Interventions for involuntary psychiatric treatments: A systematic review. *European Psychiatry, 54*, 41–50.
40. Gostin, L. O. (2008). 'Old' and 'new' institutions for persons with mental illness: Treatment, punishment or preventive confinement? *Public Health, 122*, 906–913.
41. Gostin, L. O., Monahan, J. T., Kaldor, J., DeBartolo, M., Friedman, E. A., Gottschalk, K., Kim, S. C., et al. (2019). The legal determinants of health: Harnessing the power of law for global health and sustainable development. *Lancet, 393*, 1857–1910.
42. Goulet, M. H., Larue, C., & Dumais, A. (2017). Evaluation of seclusion and restraint programs in mental health: A systematic review. *Aggression and Violent Behavior, 34*, 139–146.
43. Harper, C., Davidson, G., & McClelland, R. (2017). No longer 'anomalous, confusing and unjust': The Mental Capacity Act (Northern Ireland) 2016. *International Journal of Mental Health and Capacity Law, 2016*(22), 57–70.
44. Herman, H. (2019). Psychiatry, human rights and social development: Progress on the WPA Action Plan 2017-2020. *World Psychiatry, 18*(3), 368–369.
45. Hoffman, S. J., Sritharan, L., & Tejpar, A. (2016). Is the UN Convention on the Rights of Persons with Disabilities impacting mental health laws and policies in high-income countries? A case study of implementation in Canada. *BMC International Health and Human Rights, 16*, 28.
46. Hossain, M. M., Hasan, M. T., Sultana, A., & Faizah, F. (2019). New Mental Health Act in Bangladesh: Unfinished agendas. *Lancet Psychiatry, 6*(1), e1.
47. Hotzy, F. & Jaeger, M. (2016). Clinical relevance of informal coercion in psychiatric treatment – A systematic review. *Frontiers in Psychiatry* 7: 197.
48. Human Rights Watch. (2012). 'Like a Death Sentence': Abuses against persons with mental disabilities in Ghana.
49. Human Rights Watch. (2016). Living in hell. Abuses against people with psychosocial disabilities in Indonesia.
50. Human Rights Watch (2020). Living in chains: Shackling of people with psychosocial disabilities worldwide.
51. Jaeger, M., Ketteler, D., Rabenschlag, F., & Theodoridou, A. (2014). Informal coercion in acute inpatient setting – knowledge and attitudes held by mental health professionals. *Psychiatry Research, 220*, 1007–1011.
52. Jungfer, H.-A., Schneeberger, A. R., Borgwardt, S., Walter, M., Vogel, M., Gairing, S. K., et al. (2014). Reduction of seclusion on a hospital-wide level: Successful implementation of a less restrictive policy. *Journal of Psychiatric Research, 54*, 94–99.

53. Jovanovic, N., Campbell, J., & Priebe, S. (2019). How to design psychiatric facilities to foster positive social interaction – A systematic review. *European Psychiatry, 60*, 49–62.
54. Kalisova, L., Raboch, J., Nawka, A., Sampogna, G., Cihal, L., Kallert, T. W., & Fiorillo, A. (2014). Do patient and ward-related characteristics influence the use of coercive measures? Results from the EUNOMIA international study. *Social Psychiatry and Psychiatric Epidemiology, 49*, 1619–1629.
55. Kallert, T. W., Katsakou, C., Adamowski, T., Dembinskas, A., Fiorillo, A., Kjellin, L., et al. (2011). Coerced hospital admission and symptom change – A prospective observational multi-centre study. *PLoS One, 6*(11), e28191.
56. Kallert, T. W., Mezzich, J. E., & Monahan, J. (2011). *Coercive treatment in psychiatry: Clinical, legal and ethical aspects*. West Sussex: Wiley.
57. Katsakou, C., & Priebe, S. (2006). Outcomes of involuntary hospital admission – A review. *Acta Psychiatrica Scandinavica, 114*, 232–241.
58. Katsakou, C., Marougka, S., Garabette, J., Rost, F., Yeeles, K., & Priebe, S. (2011). Why do some voluntary patients feel coerced into hospitalization? A mixed methods study. *Psychiatry Research, 187*, 275–282.
59. Kersting, X. A. K., Hirsch, S., & Steinert, T. (2019). Physical harm and death in the context of coercive measures in psychiatric patients: A systematic review. *Frontiers in Psychiatry, 10*, 400.
60. Keown, P., Weich, S., Bhui, K. S., & Scott, J. (2011). Association between provision of mental illness beds and rate of involuntary admissions in the NHS in England 1988-2008: Ecological study. *BMJ, 343*, d3736.
61. Lay, B., Kawohl, W., & Rossler, W. (2018). Outcomes of a psycho-education and monitoring programme to prevent compulsory admission in psychiatric inpatient care: A randomized controlled trial. *Psychological Medicine, 48*(5), 849–860.
62. Liese, B. H., Gribble, R. S. F., & Wickremsinhe, M. N. (2019). International funding for mental health: A review of the last decade. *International Health, 11*, 361–369.
63. Luciano, M., De Rosa, C., Sampogna, G., Del Vecchio, V., Giallondardo, V., & Fabrazzo, M...& Fiorillo, A. (2018). How to improve clinical practice on forced medication in psychiatric practice: Suggestions from the EUNOMIA European multicentre study. *European Psychiatry, 54*, 35–40.
64. Lynch, G., Taggart, C., & Campbell, P. (2017). Mental Capacity Act (Northern Ireland) 2016. *BJPsych Bulletin, 41*(6), 353–357.
65. Mahler, L., Mielau, J., Heinz, A., & Wullschleger, A. (2019). Same, same but different: How the interplay of legal procedures and structural factors can influence the use of coercion. *Frontiers in Psychiatry, 10*, 249.
66. McLaughlin, P., Giacco, D., & Priebe, S. (2016). Use of coercive measures during involuntary psychiatric admission and treatment outcomes: Data from a prospective study across 10 European countries. *PLoS One, 11*(12), e0168720.
67. McSherry, B. (2014). Mental health laws: Where to from here? *Monash University Law Review, 40*, 175–197.
68. McSherry, B. (2017). Regulating seclusion and restraint in health care settings: The promise of the Convention on the Rights of Persons with Disabilities. *International Journal of Law and Psychiatry, 53*, 39–44.
69. Mental Disability Advocacy Center. (2014). Cage beds and coercion in Czech psychiatric institutions.
70. Mezzina, R., Rosen, A., Amering, M., & Javed, A. (2019). The practice of freedom: Human rights and the global mental health agenda. In A. Javed & K. N. Fountoulakis (Eds.), *Advances in psychiatry*. Cham: Springer.
71. Ministry of Law and Justice. (2017). The Mental Healthcare Act, 2017. The Gazette of India (Extraordinary), Part II Section I, 7th April 2017.
72. Minkowitz, T. (2011). Prohibition of compulsory mental health treatment and detention under the CRPD. https://doi.org/10.2139/ssrn.1876132.

73. Molodynski, A., Rugkasa, J., & Burns, T. (Eds.). (2016). *Coercion in community mental health care: International perspectives*. Oxford: Oxford University Press.
74. Namboodiri, V., George, S., & Singh, S. P. (2019). The Mental Healthcare Act 2017 of India: A challenge and an opportunity. *Asian Journal of Psychiatry, 44*, 25–28.
75. National CRPD Coalition–India. (2019). CRPD Alternate Report for India.
76. Newton-Howes, G., & Mullen, R. (2011). Coercion in psychiatric care: Systematic review of correlates and themes. *Psychiatric Services, 62*(5), 465–470.
77. Newton-Howes, G., & Gordon, S. (2020). Who controls the future: The Convention on the Rights of Persons with Disabilities from a service user focused perspective. *The Australian and New Zealand Journal of Psychiatry, 54*(2), 134–137.
78. Northern Ireland Assembly. Mental Capacity Act (Northern Ireland) 2016.
79. O'Donoghue, B., Roche, E., Shannon, S., Lyne, J., Madigan, K., & Feeney, L. (2014). Perceived coercion in voluntary hospital admission. *Psychiatry Research, 215*(1), 120–126.
80. Ofori-Atta, A., Attafuah, J., Jack, H., Baning, F., Rosenheck, R., & the Joining Forces Research Consortium. (2018). Joining psychiatric care and faith healing in a prayer camp in Ghana: Randomised trial. *The British Journal of Psychiatry, 212*, 34–41.
81. Oliva, F., Ostacoli, L., Versino, E., Portigliatti Pomeri, A., Furlan, P. M., Carletto, S., & Picci, R. L. (2019). Compulsory psychiatric admissions in an Italian urban setting: Are they actually compliant to the need for treatment criteria or arranged for dangerous not clinical condition? *Frontiers in Psychiatry, 9*, 740.
82. Patel, V., & Bhui, K. (2018). Unchaining people with mental disorders: Medication is not the solution. *The British Journal of Psychiatry, 212*, 6–8.
83. Patel, V., Saxena, S., Lund, C., Thornicroft, G., Baingana, F., Bolton, P., et al. (2018). The Lancet Commission on global mental health and sustainable development. *Lancet, 392*, 1553–1598.
84. Priebe, S., Katsakou, C., Amos, T., Leese, M., Morriss, R., Rose, D., & Yeeles, K. (2009). Patients' views and readmissions 1 year after involuntary hospitalization. *The British Journal of Psychiatry, 194*, 49–54.
85. Priebe, S., Katsakou, C., Glockner, M., Dembinskas, A., Fiorillo, A., Karastergiou, A., & Kallert, T. (2010). Patients' views of involuntary hospital admission after 1 and 3 months: Prospective study in 11 European countries. *The British Journal of Psychiatry, 196*, 179–185.
86. Priebe, S., Katsakou, C., Yeeles, K., Amos, T., Morriss, R., Wang, D., & Wykes, T. (2011). Predictors of clinical and social outcomes following involuntary hospital admission: A prospective observational study. *European Archives of Psychiatry and Clinical Neuroscience, 261*, 377–386.
87. Rains, L. S., Zenina, T., Dias, M. C., Jones, R., Jeffreys, S., Branthonne-Foster, S., et al. (2019). Variations in patterns of involuntary hospitalization and in legal frameworks: An international comparative study. *Lancet Psychiatry, 6*, 403–417.
88. Rose, D., Perry, E., Rae, S., & Good, N. (2017). Service user perspectives on coercion and restraint in mental health. *BJPsych Int, 14*(3), 59–61.
89. Rossler, W. (2019). Factors facilitating or preventing compulsory admission in psychiatry. *World Psychiatry, 18*(3), 355–356.
90. Rugkasa, J., & Canvin, K. (2017). Mental health, coercion and family caregiving: Issues from the international literature. *BJPsych International, 14*(3), 56–58.
91. Sachan, D. (2013). Mental health bill set to revolutionise care in India. *The Lancet, 382*(9889), 296.
92. Sashidharan, S. P., & Saraceno, B. (2017). Is psychiatry becoming more coercive? *BMJ, 357*, j2904.
93. Sashidharan, S. P., Mezzina, R., & Puras, D. (2019). Reducing coercion in mental healthcare. *Epidemiology and Psychiatric Sciences, 28*(6), 605–612.
94. Saya, A., Brugnoli, C., Piazzi, G., Liberato, D., Di Ciaccia, G., Niolu, C., & Siracusano, A. (2019). Criteria, procedures, and future prospects of involuntary treatment in psychiatry around the world: A narrative review. *Frontiers in Psychiatry, 10*, 271.

95. Scholten, M., & Gather, J. (2018). Adverse consequences of article 12 of the UN Convention on the Rights of Persons with Disabilities for persons with mental disabilities and an alternative way forward. *Journal of Medical Ethics, 44*, 226–233.
96. Schottle, D., Ruppelt, F., Schimmelmann, B. G., Karow, A., Bussopulos, A., Gallinat, J., et al. (2019). Reduction of involuntary admissions in patients with severe psychotic disorders treated in the ACCESS integrated care model including therapeutic assertive community treatment. *Frontiers in Psychiatry, 10*, 736.
97. Smith, S., Gate, R., Ariyo, K., Saunders, R., Taylor, C., Bhui, K., et al. (2020). Reasons behind the rising rate of involuntary admissions under the Mental Health Act (1983): Service use and cost impact. *International Journal of Law and Psychiatry, 68*, 101506.
98. Somasundaram, O. (1987). The Indian Lunacy Act, 1912: The historic background. *Indian Journal of Psychiatry, 29*(1), 3–14.
99. Stavert, J. (2018). Paradigm shift or paradigm paralysis? National mental health and capacity law and implementing the CRPD in Scotland. *Laws, 7*, 26.
100. Steinert, C., Steinert, T., Flammer, E., & Jaeger, S. (2016). Impact of the UN Convention on the Rights of Persons with Disabilities (UN-CRPD) on mental health care research – A systematic review. *BMC Psychiatry, 16*, 166.
101. Sugiura, K., Mahomed, F., Saxena, S., & Patel, V. (2020). An end to coercion: Rights and decision-making in mental health care. *Bulletin of the World Health Organization, 98*, 52–58.
102. Sveaass, N., & Madirgal-Borloz, V. (2017). The preventive approach: OPCAT and the prevention of violence and abuse of persons with mental disabilities by monitoring places of detention. *International Journal of Law and Psychiatry, 53*, 15–26.
103. Szmukler, G. (2015). Compulsion and 'coercion' in mental health care. *World Psychiatry, 14*(3), 259–261.
104. Szmukler, G. (2019). 'Capacity', 'best interests', 'will and preferences' and the UN Convention on the Rights of Persons with Disabilities. *World Psychiatry, 18*(1), 34–41.
105. Thornicroft, G., & Patel, V. (2014). Including mental health among the new sustainable development goals. *BMJ, 349*, g5189.
106. Thornicroft, G., & Semrau, M. (2018). Mental health capacity building in low and middle income countries: The Emerald Programme. *Epidemiol Psychiatr Services, 27*, 1–2.
107. United Nations. (2002). Optional protocol to the convention against torture and other cruel, inhuman or degrading treatment or punishment. A/RES/57/199.
108. United Nations. (2006). Convention on the rights of persons with disabilities.
109. United Nations. (2014). Committee on the rights of persons with disabilities. General comment no. 1: Article 12: Equal recognition before the law. CRPD/C/GC/1.
110. United Nations. (2015). Transforming our world: The 2030 Agenda for Sustainable Development. A/RES/70/1.
111. United Nations. (2017). Report of the High Commissioner for Human Rights. Mental health and human rights. A/HRC/34/32.
112. United Nations. (2018). Committee on the rights of persons with disabilities. General comment no. 7: On the participation of persons with disabilities, including children with disabilities, through their representative organizations, in the implementation and monitoring of the Convention. CRPD/C/GC/7.
113. United Nations. (2019). Report of the Special Rapporteur on the right of everyone to the enjoyment of the highest attainable standard of physical and mental health. A/HRC/41/34.
114. United Nations. (2019). Report of the Special Rapporteur on the rights of persons with disabilities. A/HRC/40/54.
115. United Nation. (2020). Office of the High Commissioner for Human Rights. Human rights and the 2030 Agenda for Sustainable Development. https://www.ohchr.org/Documents/Issues/MDGs/Post2015/HRAndPost2015.pdf
116. United Nations Treaty Collection. (2020). Status of treaties: Convention on the rights of persons with disabilities. https://treaties.un.org/pages/ViewDetails.aspx?src=TREATY&mtdsg_no=IV-15&chapter=4&clang=_en#EndDec

117. von Peter, S., Aderhold, V., Cubellis, L., Bergstrom, T., Stastny, P., Seikkula, J., & Puras, D. (2019). Open dialogue as a human rights-aligned approach. *Frontiers in Psychiatry, 10*, 387.

118. Walker, G. H., & Osei, A. (2014). Mental health law in Ghana. *BJPsych International, 14*(2), 38–39.

119. Wasserman, D., Apter, G., Baeken, C., Bailey, S., Balazs, J., Bec, C., et al. (2020). Compulsory admissions of patients with mental disorders: State of the art on ethical and legislative aspects in 40 European countries. *European Psychiatry, 63*(1), E82. https://doi.org/10.1192/j.eurpsy.2020.79.

120. WHO (2019). Fourth report of Committe A. A72/76.

121. Wickremsinhe, M. N. (2018). Emergency involuntary treatment law for people with mental disorders: A comparative analysis of legislation in LMICs. *International Journal of Law and Psychiatry, 56*, 1–9.

122. Winkler, I. T., & Williams, C. (2017). The sustainable development goals and human rights: A critical early review [special issue]. *International Journal of Human Rights, 21*(8), 1023–1028.

123. World Health Organization. (2005). Mental Health Policy, plans and programmes (updated version 2).

124. World Health Organization (2005). WHO resource book on mental health, human rights and legislation: Stop exclusion, dare to care.

125. World Health Organization. (2012). QualityRights tool kit: Assessing and improving quality and human rights in Mental Health and Social Care Facilities.

126. World Health Organization. (2013). Mental Health Action Plan 2013–2020.

127. World Health Organization. (2016). mhGAP intervention guide for mental, neurological and substance use disorders in non-specialized health setting.

128. World Health Organization. (2018). 2017 Mental Health ATLAS.

129. World Health Organization. (2019). QualityRights initiative – improving quality, promoting human rights.

130. World Health Organization & Calouste Galbenkian Foundation (2017). Policy options on mental health: A WHO-Gulbenkian Mental Health Platform collaboration.

131. Wykes, T., Csipke, E., Williams, P., Koeser, L., Nash, S., Rose, D., & McCrone, P. (2017). Improving patient experiences of mental health inpatient care: A randomized controlled trial. *Psychological Medicine, 48*, 488–497.

132. Yamin, A. E., & Constantin, A. (2018). The evolution of applying human rights frameworks to health. In B. M. Meier & L. O. Gostin (Eds.), *Human rights in global health: Rights-based governance for a globalizing world*. New York: Oxford University Press.

133. Zinkler, M. (2016). Germany without coercive treatment in psychiatry – A 15 month real world experience. *Laws, 5*, 15.

134. Zinkler, M. (2019). Supported decision-making in the prevention of compulsory interventions in mental health care. *Frontiers in Psychiatry, 10*, 137.

Interrogations, Torture, and Mental Health: Conceptualizing Exceptionalism

16

George David Annas

Introduction: Making Moral Decisions

Global crises cause many moral dilemmas. The devastation of war, famine, or pandemic illness causes mass migrations of desperate and often helpless people who are forced to make heart-breaking decisions. Yet even the most welcoming of neighbors will have limited resources with which to help. How do nations and individuals make decisions in these situations? When a country is faced with terror attacks and is on high-alert, what are the trade-offs their leaders make to preserve safety and sovereignty?

Two of the fundamental ways in which society, just like mental health professionals, approach moral decision making include Deontology, determining what is the moral duty, and Consequentialism, deciding based on the greatest good that will come to the most people. There are two classic thought experiments that demonstrate these two approaches, often referred to collectively as the "trolley problems" [13]. Multiple iterations exist, but the two scenarios below represent their basic structure and help demonstrate how the correct course of action is not always easy.

1. *A runaway trolley is hurtling down the tracks toward five people who are unable to escape. You can flip a switch to divert the trolley onto a side track and save the lives of the five, but one person on the side track will be killed. Should you flip the switch?*
2. *A runaway trolley is hurtling down the tracks toward five people who are unable to escape. You are standing on a footbridge over the tracks next to a large man. You can push the man onto the tracks to stop the trolley and save the lives of the five people, but the man will be killed. Should you push him?* [13].

G. D. Annas (✉)
Forensic Psychiatry Consulting, LLC, Syracuse, NY, USA

© Springer Nature Switzerland AG 2021
A. R. Dyer et al. (eds.), *Global Mental Health Ethics*,
https://doi.org/10.1007/978-3-030-66296-7_16

When faced with scenario 1, most individuals choose to flip the switch and divert the train, on the grounds that five lives will be spared at the expense of one. This response—around 80–90%—demonstrates a fairly simple means by which people make moral decisions: taking the action that saves more lives [9, 13].

Yet, when faced with the same consequences with one meaningful addition, significantly fewer individuals choose to push a man onto the tracks [9, 13]. Among the many analyses of this scenario, one unifying feature appears to be that most individuals do not hold to a strict philosophy of Consequentialism. Rather, there are times when actively killing someone is inherently wrong, even if it benefits more people.

In thought experiments, the available choices are simple. But real-world dilemmas involve higher levels of complexity and uncertainty. The civil war in Syria has contributed to countless refugees in desperate need, yet some look upon every refugee as a potential terrorist. Caught in the middle is a mental health professional performing an objective analysis of Posttraumatic Stress Disorder and risk of harm in the home country. What happens when the evaluator determines that the symptoms are feigned, yet still believes the person needs asylum? Global crises may force treatment professionals into roles they are unaccustomed. Moral decision making may consequently be difficult to achieve.

While one can justify using mental health experts to evaluate the presence of feigning, the question arises whether or not professionals should—or even can—aid in interrogating terror suspects. Taken to its extreme, would it ever be morally permissible for professionals to be involved in the torture of a suspect, or would it ever be just for any person—professional or not—to torture another?

After the events of 9/11/2001, there was a renewed debate in the West on the justification for torture. For some, torture could be justified if it prevented a similar terrorist attack. Often, during these debates, proponents of torture would use the "Ticking Time Bomb Scenario" (TTBS) to support their positions [21]. Developed from a postulate by Consequentialist philosopher Jeremy Bentham [18], the basic TTBS describes the following dilemma:

> Imagine that a terrorist has placed a bomb in some public place such that, if detonated, many lives will be lost. Further imagine that law enforcement has just apprehended a terrorist and has absolute certainty that the terrorist is responsible for the bomb, the terrorist knows the details that could lead to its defusing, absent the terrorist's confession there is no other way to defuse the bomb, if the information is provided, defusing is certain, absent torture, the terrorist will not divulge the relevant details, and, with torture, he will [accurately] divulge those details. What should law enforcement do? [1].

In this scenario, the justification for torturing the terrorist is that of saving many lives at the expense of one individual, shifting the risk-benefit calculation along Consequentialist lines. On its face, this choice seems preferable to the absolute Deontological prohibition against torture on moral grounds alone.

Treatment professionals and their organizations already assert that any involvement in torture is beyond any spectrum that one could ever reach. The ethical guidelines for the American Psychiatric Association, for example, explicitly state that a psychiatrist should never engage or be involved with torture (2013, section 7, #5). Objectively examining this statement, one might reasonably ask why such a guideline even needs articulation. Psychiatrists do not need a rule prohibiting rape or murder, so why is a public statement required for torture? The answer sheds light on a sad reality: Global crises and terrorism can cause even those in the health professions to lose sight of the basic standards of moral discourse.

For the purposes of this analysis, I will use the example of the forensic psychiatrist and the proper ways in which such a professional may ethically navigate new roles or circumstances. Although my focus will be on the challenges of the psychiatrist in these environments, much of the framework will also apply to mental health practitioners outside the field of medicine who work in nontreatment settings. Although Forensic Exceptionalism arose for court consultations in the USA, I will argue that the foundation in approaching moral dilemmas is universal and applies to global mental health as well.

Nontraditional Treatment Roles

Psychiatrists practice in a number of settings and roles. Some of these involve treatment in settings that may modify or limit the usual doctor–patient relationship. These include treating inmates in maximum security settings, working in a forensic unit dedicated to restoring the competency of a defendant who has been found incompetent to stand trial, or working for an agency screening refugees for asylum on medical grounds.

In treatment settings, medical ethicists have developed a number of models for approaching moral decision making. These include Casuistry (focusing on individual facts over theory), Virtue Ethics (determining what a "virtuous" person would decide), and Impartial Rules (using a set of moral rules to justify decision-making). However, in treatment settings the most widely used model in the West was developed by Thomas Beauchamp and James Childress [11], commonly referred to as "Principlism."[1] In this model, one determines the best course by weighing four main principles: Autonomy (respecting patients and their right of self-determination), Beneficence (acting to improve patients' well-being), Nonmaleficence (acting in a manner that avoids or minimizes harm), and Justice (applying equal treatment and overall fairness).

In the settings above, for example, treating someone to restore competency to stand trial, one may ethically operate using Principlism, provided certain disclosures are made to the patient [32]. In such an example, it is important to act in the person's best medical interests and provide appropriate medical care (beneficence), but also to disclose and periodically remind the person that the purpose of the hospitalization is to move forward in the legal process (autonomy). Because some may

---

[1] Additionally, the authors point out that proponents of some of the other models of medical ethics are not in conflict with theirs, but—in truth—advocate for the same general approach [10].

not be in a position to understand, such disclosures and educational efforts should be made regularly to remind the individual of the focus and purpose of treatment.

Ethical dilemmas in this setting may include restoring a person to competency on a charge that carries the death penalty. It may be difficult to justify restoring competency when the outcome could be the person's execution—a conflict with beneficence and nonmaleficence. On the other hand, the rights to trial and to face one's accusers are among some of the most fundamental to a defendant, so furthering those rights would respect the person's autonomy. In addition, restoration of competency could also lead to acquittal, a beneficent outcome. While controversy remains in these settings, most professional organizations recognize that it is ethical to work in capital cases, provided certain conditions are met (e.g., appropriate disclosures are given; medical decision making for restoration is also in the best medical interest of the individual.) [7]. Thus, Principlism may still be a workable model for some nontraditional treatment settings, as long as the balance is adjusted.

Treatment Professionals Working in Nontreatment Roles

Mental health professionals also work in settings in which they do not necessarily provide treatment or advocacy for the people they evaluate. One common example is working as an expert witness. In such a scenario, a psychiatrist may be asked to provide an opinion on a question or questions posed by an agency or court. For example, the expert may be asked whether or not a person was suffering from severe mental health symptoms at the time of a crime (i.e., an insanity evaluation). Alternatively, a psychiatrist might be asked to determine the presence of a mental illness consistent with oppression or torture in their homeland (i.e., an asylum evaluation). In such situations, one may be faced with a difference between what is just and what is objective. Commonly, there are PTSD symptoms, but insufficient data about their cause.

Ethics of Working as a Forensic Expert Witness

When working as an expert witness, one comes into conflict when attempting to apply the ethical model of Principlism. Professor Paul Appelbaum wrote a landmark article for forensic psychiatry, coming to the conclusion that a doctor cannot be held to all of these specific principles when working as an expert witness [7].

Regardless of their specific credentials, there are mental health professionals from different disciplines who may consult while applying a minimum set of core ethical principles. The code of ethics put forth by the American Academy of Psychiatry and the Law (AAPL) provides such direction for forensic psychiatrists [2], while serving as a framework that should apply to all those who do similar work. Before commenting on these guidelines, I will first briefly discuss how a doctor cannot employ the commonly used model of ethical treatment to a person being examined forensically.[2]

While doctors have a duty to act in their patients' best medical interests, a doctor who is an expert witness may not have this duty (outside of the rare instances where the evaluee requires emergency care during the encounter). This is primarily due to the principal purpose of the expert: to form an objective opinion in response to the question posed by a third party. For example, imagine a scenario wherein the expert witness is duty bound to act in the best interests of a person claiming a mental health disability, yet saw no evidence for a mental illness. The expert might opine that the person would benefit from the financial incentive, but would thereby disengage from the duty owed to the court (and result in fraudulent behavior). Therefore, the duty to act in the best interest of the evaluee would be in conflict with providing the court an objective opinion [7]. Such a conflict would not be resolved by balancing or adjusting the same principles, unlike in the prior examples.

However, simply because a clinician in the expert role has less of a duty of beneficence to the person evaluated, this does not mean that the doctor is released from standards of moral or professional behavior. In fact, performing work as an expert witness is a privilege in which one must take special precautions, binding the expert to a new set of principles. As noted in the Commentary for its "Guidelines for the Ethical Practice of Forensic Psychiatry," the American Academy of Psychiatry and the Law (AAPL), states: "…the practice of forensic psychiatry entails inherent potentials for complications, conflicts, misunderstandings and abuses." Due to this potential, the forensic psychiatrist needs to work in a way that honors the principles of "respect for persons, honesty, justice, and social responsibility." Additionally, there are four basic behaviors that a forensic psychiatrist should exhibit: Consent (obtaining consent for the evaluation when possible), Confidentiality (disclosing the limits to and staying within the confidential bounds of the case), Striving for Objectivity (putting all efforts into giving an unbiased opinion, while recognizing that no one is perfectly objective), and Qualifications (only proffering an opinion on matters in which one is qualified) (2005). Thus, an expert is reminded that largely absolving oneself of beneficence carries significant risks.

While debate may still exist over the obligation to nonmaleficence, this may be more of a gray area than beneficence. For example, if an expert were to examine a defendant for an insanity evaluation on behalf of the defense and determine there was no valid case for insanity, can such an expert be said to act in a manner that harms the defendant? One might argue that the actions would harm the defendant's *case* because it would contradict his defense. But is this harm maleficence or truth?

Consider, on the other hand, if the expert opines that there *is* a valid insanity defense, without believing it wholeheartedly. Would this action be less maleficent when this could encourage the defendant to move forward with a case that would be meritless and likely unsuccessful? By the same token, an honest and direct opinion could help the defendant realize there is no valid insanity defense, and thus

---

[2] For further reading, please see the citation noted at the end of the previous section: Appelbaum PS: A theory of ethics for forensic psychiatry. *J Am Acad Psychiatry Law* 25:233–47, 1997.

encourage a plea bargain for a lesser sentence. Therefore, striving for objectivity is paramount for the expert witness; it is arguably the best method to minimize harm in this scenario.

Law Enforcement Interviews with Criminal Suspects

A former AAPL president addressed the ethical problems inherent to extracting incriminating evidence or confessions, especially when they involve intentional efforts to deceive the suspect [27]. For example, it would not be uncommon for a law enforcement officer to tell a suspect falsely that he had been implicated by another witness— an attempt to elicit a confession with the full knowledge that no such implication had been made [24].

These techniques are so misleading that many European nations have banned their use [31]. The debate persists, however, over whether such practices are inherently immoral. Because of their wide use, as well as the hesitation of US courts to limit them, it is universally understood that such practices carry an empirical risk of false confession, mis-statements, and susceptibility to later manipulation by investigators.

Because AAPL states that forensic examiners must practice in a manner that respects the person being evaluated, and in a manner which strives for honesty and social responsibility, a psychiatrist who aids law enforcement in the practice of deception would violate fundamental principles [2, 27]. Thus, it is important to explore the possible situations one might face, prior to participating in a nontraditional role. In this way, one can anticipate areas of potential conflict with traditional principles which may either require setting limits on what the expert is asked to do, or applying a more rigorous set of principles. More important is to avoid some settings all together.

There are exceptions to the ethical prohibition of employing deception in a forensic evaluation. One of these is in the assessment of malingering.[3] In this instance, the deception is used to uncover the potential deception of the person being evaluated, not for the purposes of extracting a confession or collecting evidence to use against them. Ruling out the feigning of symptoms is important in obtaining an accurate diagnosis and is therefore allowed to further this aim.

Additionally, AAPL insists that professionals operate within their area of expertise. Regardless of how skilled a clinician may be in performing interviews, nothing in medical school, residency, or fellowship involves training in interrogating a criminal suspect. Forensic Psychiatry includes specialized training in detecting malingering, assessing risk of danger to others, writing reports for the courts, and testifying on legal matters. Yet, none of this qualifies a forensic professional for interrogating a suspect to extract a confession, even if it were ethical in the first place.

---

[3] Malingering is defined as the intentional production or exaggeration of psychiatric symptoms for the purpose of an external incentive (e.g., avoiding prosecution, avoiding military service, obtaining monetary damages).

Due to the fact that psychiatrists are trained to be empathic and to develop a therapeutic alliance with patients, this clinical approach can express itself in the forensic encounter. This is referred to as "therapeutic slippage" as the forensic examiner falls into a state of rapport building with the evaluee as is done in a doctor–patient encounter. The person being evaluated may consequently feel more relaxed and caught off-guard during these moments. While it is not unethical to maintain some level of rapport with those being evaluated (and a thorough assessment may even demand it), the examiner needs to be mindful about the potential to slip into a therapeutic stance. With this challenging concept in mind, one may see how the risk to an evaluee would be multiplied should a psychiatrist question a criminal suspect for purposes outside an objective forensic assessment. Consider another example: a suspect with additional vulnerabilities such as a language barrier or lack of education. The potential for exploiting such vulnerabilities is compounded by the active involvement of psychiatry. Therefore, as both a practical matter and moral matter, a psychiatrist is precluded from ethically assisting law enforcement in the interrogation of a criminal suspect. Such prohibition should also apply to others in the mental health field.

Such an ethical constraint need not necessarily preclude a psychiatrist from working in law enforcement interrogation after relinquishing one's medical license. Nor would it preclude a law enforcement officer from obtaining further education for the purposes of improving knowledge of the psychology of criminal behavior. However, in neither instance would such an individual ever introduce herself as "doctor," "psychologist" (or any other title commonly attributed to those in treatment roles). Additionally, a forensic evaluator may assist law enforcement in conducting research into criminal behavior, providing risk assessments, or in other roles that are not in conflict with honesty, respect, and striving to uphold professional principles.

New Global Realities and the Creation of New Professional Roles

In addition to housing and security needs, the global refugee crisis has increased the need for mental health workers. Many of those who flee war zones, conflict, or corruption have experienced intense trauma. One of the great challenges in this context is to develop trust, so an assessment can be completed. Barriers to trust include fear of strangers, skepticism about confidentiality, lack of resources for children, and a paucity of culturally sensitive and proficient interpreters. Such barriers compound the difficulties in explaining one's organizational or institutional role. Even in the USA, it can be difficult for native speakers to hear the phrase "I'm a doctor" and fully grasp that the doctor is not there to help, regardless of the statements that follow [8]. In scenarios where there is a significant language and cultural barrier, such disclosures require extraordinary care. Issues may yet arise when examinees disclose information that undermines their refugee status; their understanding of the limits of confidentiality may remain imperfect. The evaluation may even lead to a denial of their asylum claim despite their need for treatment.

These difficulties may nonetheless be overcome. It remains respectful and pro-tective to identify exactly who the evaluator is working for and what the primary duties and obligations are. One may need to set limits to the evaluations and opin-ions formed, for example, until proper interpretation, culturally sensitive, and robust communication can be assured. One may also need to be clear with the governing agency of the ethical obligations of the profession, regardless of whether or not the position involves treatment. This requires—at a minimum—that the ethical princi-ples of respect for persons and honesty be honored by disclosing the purpose of the evaluation and limits of confidentiality.

While dual roles are not new, it is notable that the USA' "global war on terror" has resulted in instances where national security has interfered with the proper treat-ment of terrorist suspects at the US Base in Guantanamo Bay, Cuba (GTMO). For example, the doctors who provide the care for GTMO detainees often see signs of Posttraumatic Stress Disorder in their patients, yet may be precluded from taking a full trauma history because it could uncover allegations of torture during US cus-tody [23] One cannot diagnose or properly treat trauma-related disorders without taking such a history. Thus, as one human rights worker notes, "PTSD does not exist in GTMO" [17].

There are consequently situations where there is no ethical role for a mental health professional. This is where some use Forensic Exceptionalism to justify behavior that falls outside of traditional moral principles. In the next sections, I will address how any connection to torture is universally immoral, regardless of the risk scenario created to justify its use.

Mis-Applied Ethics and the Torture "Question"

Between 2001 and 2006, the US Central Intelligence Agency (CIA) implemented a program to interrogate individuals suspected of being terrorists. The CIA refers to the methods used during these encounters as "Enhanced Interrogation Techniques" or "EITs." Yet, despite the many ways the intelligence services describe them, there are few—if any—who can find ways to distinguish these methods from torture.[4] The program was designed and implemented by two independently contracted psychol-ogists, Drs. James Mitchell and J. Bruce Jessen. The main sources for what we know about this include the partially redacted summary of the Senate Select Committee on Intelligence (SSCI) Report [34] and Dr., Mitchell's own words in his book *Enhanced Interrogation* (2016).

When one examines some of the arguments justifying mental health profession-als' participation in torture, it becomes clear how dangerous it can be to act without regard for a traditional moral or humanistic framework. One of the chief architects of the program attempted to justify his actions in the following ways [30]:

---

[4] In fact, the index to one of the main architects of the program, James Mitchell's book, under the entry for "Enhanced Interrogation Techniques" is "See also *torture* ..." (pg 305, italics in original).

1. It is acceptable to work outside treatment roles (pg. 128);
2. Forensic psychologists have experience in interviewing criminal suspects and therefore are qualified in performing interrogations (pgs. 14, 46–48, 52);
3. There was no way other than torture to obtain vital information (pg. 28);
4. It was legal (pgs. 231–232, 257, 287);
5. The acts were justified because they saved "thousands of lives" (pg. 49).

After a brief synopsis of some of the methods that were used on terror suspects during the program, I will explore the validity of these arguments.

"Enhanced Interrogation Techniques"

In an email from the main architect of the program[5] to an anonymous CIA official, the author describes 12 methods to force Guantanamo detainee Abu Zubaydah to give up information are proposed: (1) the attention grasp, (2) walling, (3) facial hold, (4) facial slap, (5) cramped confinement, (6) wall standing, (7) stress positions, (8) sleep deprivation, (9) waterboarding, (10) use of diapers, (11) use of insects, and (12) mock burial ([34], pg. 44).

Although some of these techniques are self-explanatory, a few descriptions from the redacted email clarify some of them further:

> [Due to Mr. Zubayda's fear of insects] … threaten to place stinging insects into the cramped confinement box with him, but instead place harmless insects. The purpose of this would be to play off his fears and increase his sense of dread and motivate him to avoid the box in the future by cooperating …

> …. Mock Burial: The individual is placed in a cramped confinement box that resembles a coffin ... The individual is moved to a prepared site where he hears digging. The site has a prepared hole, dug in such a way that the box can be lowered into the ground and shovels of dirt thrown in on top of it without blocking the air holes or actually burying the individual. This procedure would be used as part of a threat and rescue scenario where the "burial" is interrupted and the subject is rescued by a concerned party. The rescuers then use the subject's fear of being returned to the people trying to bury him as a means of pressuring the subject for information [35].

It Works, it's the Only Way to Get the Info, and it's Legal

When convincing the CIA that EIT methods would succeed in extracting accurate information from reluctant suspects, the designers provided no evidence to support their claims. The program was based on a theory loosely connected to Martin Seligman's well-known Learned Helplessness model for depression ([34], pg. 35). Intending to cause a depressed state of mind, they proposed using techniques

---

[5] Redacted in document.

developed in the military's SERE Training (Survival, Evasion, Resistance, Escape).[6] The hope was that detainees would eventually feel dependent on their captors and cooperate. Such an idea had not been tested nor studied, and even lacked a logical basis as a theoretical model for information-gathering.[7] In fact, the CIA determined that it would be a violation of "Federal Policy for the Protection of Human Subjects" to study empirically or test the hypothesis ([34], pg. 18). Nonetheless, they concluded that it was appropriate to use EITs. This suggests that their prisoners did not qualify as "human."

While a complete rebuttal of the efficacy of torture is beyond the scope of this chapter, I will underscore two critical points. First, the CIA itself had determined many years earlier that torture did not elicit useful information. This is highlighted by citations in the SSCI Report, itself ([34], pg. 32). Additionally, when pressed for evidence, the CIA claimed that torture led to the arrests of others who were planning attacks. Yet the SSCI report is clear that none of these claims were accurate. For example, (note "[--]" = a redacted source):

> ... According to OIG records, "[o]n the question of whether actual plots had been thwarted, [--] opined that since the operatives involved in many of the above plots had been arrested, [CTC had], in effect, thwarted the operation[s]." [--] provided a list to the OIG of terrorists captured and the plots with which they were associated. None of the individuals listed by [--] were captured as a result of reporting from CIA detainees ([34], pg. 159).

The arguments that "it works" and "it's the only way to get the information" (the former, of course, required for the latter) were initially brought up by government lawyers who were exploring a novel form of pre-emptive self-defense or "necessity" as a legal defense. In fact, it was a defense against prosecution for war crimes in the event the government decided to deviate from the Geneva Conventions ([20], pg. 68; [15], pg. 28). There was no evidence at the time (nor afterwards) that torture actually worked; therefore, any defense of "necessity" would logically be invalid. However, even if there were evidence of its efficacy, it would still have likely been illegal.

Yet, throughout his book, Mitchell argues that his methods were legal, or claims ignorance by saying he was "never told it was not" ([30], pg. 231–232, 257, 287)— as if that fact alone could justify his actions. This indicates that that he did not realize (or care) that an action can be unethical even if it is legal, not to mention that it was not legal to begin with.

The latter point is made clear in the Memorandum to Alberto Gonzales from Assistant Attorney General Jay S. Bybee of 1/22/2002 (the Bybee Memo) [15]. In this document, Bybee attempts both to argue that deviating from the Geneva

---

[6] A program that trains military personnel to resist interrogation in case of capture, sometimes including a carefully administered simulated torture method of simulated drowning or "waterboarding."

[7] For example, those with extreme depression often report experiencing memory and other cognitive deficits. Therefore to cause one to enter such a mental state runs counter to the goal of obtaining useful informaticausing depression may cause the victim to forget key details.

Conventions would be justified, as well as to claim that EITs were not torture to begin with. Specifically, the memo argues that "severe mental pain or suffering" as defined in the US Code's definition of torture did not arise from EITs.

> ...the prolonged mental harm caused by or resulting from ... the intentional infliction or threatened infliction of severe physical pain or suffering ... the administration or application, or threatened ... procedures calculated to disrupt profoundly the senses or the personality ... the threat of imminent death; or ... the threat that another person will imminently be subjected to death, severe physical pain or suffering... (18 U.S.C. § 2340).

For Bybee, acts that inflict prolonged mental harm must include "...only extreme acts." In fact he writes:

> ... Severe mental pain requires suffering not just at the moment of infliction but it also requires lasting psychological harm, such as seen in ... [PTSD] .... Because the acts inflicting torture are extreme, there is sufficient range of acts that though they might constitute cruel, inhuman, or degrading treatment or punishment fail to rise to the level of torture ([15], pg. 46).

Numerous legal scholars have criticized these arguments [19, 26], but one criticism stands out for mental health professionals. The legality of EITs was partially based on psychologists like Mitchell and Jessen assuring the DOJ that their methods would not cause significant psychological injury (DOJ Office of Professional Responsibility Report, 2009, pg. 56). Furthermore, Mitchell defends his actions with circular reasoning: He asserts that the DOJ told him his torture methods were legal, with the full knowledge that the DOJ decided they were legal based on his opinion minimizing EIT's long-term effects. Namely, "... and a report from CIA psychologists asserting that the use of harsh interrogation techniques in SERE training had resulted in no adverse long-term effects" ([20], Pg. 56). Although not stated explicitly in the DOJ's Office of Professional Responsibility Report, "CIA Psychologists" clearly refers to Mitchell and Jessen (Memorandum of 7/2 [28]; [29], pg. 325).[8]

Furthermore, Mitchell's assertion that the SERE techniques provided no significant trauma in service members overlooks the voluntary (and finite) nature of SERE training which is not an experience consistent with that of a detainee. The SSCI report references a redacted source from the CIA on this score, clearly delineating the difference between a volunteer who can stop the process at any time and a detainee, "...who will be made to believe this is the future course of the remainder of his life" ([34], pg. 232, reference 2563 (redacted)).

Additionally, the 2008 Senate Armed Services Committee Report (SASC Report) contains numerous reports that SERE techniques like waterboarding were even risky for the trainees who undertook them ([37], pgs. 5–6).

---

[8] In his deposition of 1/16/2017, Mitchell confirms that a reference to "IC SERE Psychologists" from a redacted cable was a reference to him and Jessen (pg. 325). The redacted memo describes the same language referred to in the OPR report regarding the supposed "safety" of waterboarding.

It's OK to Work Outside Treatment Roles

While forensic practitioners in fields related to psychiatry may follow a different written set of ethical guidelines, virtually all include language in their ethical codes related to the fundamental importance of honoring respect for persons ([2, 3, 5, 33]; American Psychological Association 2016). This is true for any mental health practitioner engaging in work either inside or outside the treatment realm. This is because to allow exceptions where the practitioner could disrespect persons would diminish the traditional healing practice as a whole. Even if it is acceptable for a clinician to operate without stringent nonmaleficence/avoidance of harm (such as when avoiding indirect harm conflicts with the primary duty to report an honest opinion), no one can argue convincingly that it is ethical to engage in the *intentional* harm of another person. Using Forensic Exceptionalism to justify psychologists implementing the EIT program disregards any reasonable moral approach to such a "dilemma" that the global war on terror might create. In fact, despite the initial hesitancy of the American Psychological Association to bar psychologists from assisting government officers in performing national security interrogations [16], their ethical principles already had included "Respect for People's Rights and Dignity" prior to this ban (1995).[9] Therefore, even without the governing association banning work in the field of interrogation, any involvement in torture, under any guise or definition, would be such an obvious conflict with this principle that participation in EITs would already have been prohibited. This highlights the importance of all individuals retaining inherent value that cannot be diminished, and indicates a universal line that no one should cross.

"Expertise" in Interrogating Suspects

Dr. Mitchell justifies his qualifications to design and lead the EIT program by indicating that he had extensive experience in interviewing criminal suspects ([30], pg. 48). Using the AAPL guidelines as a framework, this argument fails the prohibition against working outside one's expertise, as well as being honest about one's limitations. One's experience with a certain population does not automatically confer the same skill to work with a different population; it is a problem for many analyses where a test or model is not validated for a related group. Thus, Mitchell created the image of expertise where none truly existed. The SSCI report makes clear that neither Mitchell nor Jessen had any substantive expertise in the interrogation of criminal suspects ([34], pg. 15).

A psychologist purporting that torture "works" demonstrates another moral failing that of asserting information he cannot know to be true—especially when it cannot be verified by nonexperts. When an expert behaves this way in court, it is called *ipse dixit*: "It's true because I say it's true." This is ethically unsound because many laypersons—such as the members of a jury—might be quick to accept the

---

[9] General Principles D (1992) [4].

opinion of a seemingly authoritative expert, even when it is meritless. Similarly with EITs, many declassified documents demonstrate that intelligence agents and attorneys often took these psychologists at their word, whenever they needed "assurance" that the EIT program was effective and safe.

It's Not *Really* Torture

The mental gymnastics between DOJ attorneys, CIA contract psychologists, and others show that the definition of torture in the law ended up being meaningless. In his book, Mitchell downplays what occurred to the suspects in CIA custody: "In my mind nothing in *my* ethical code requires that I put the *temporary discomfort* of a handful of terrorists ahead of saving the lives of thousands of innocent Americans ...." (pg. 128, (emphasis added)).

Referring to the EIT program as "temporary discomfort" suggests that the tactics were benign and that the suspects were not – in fact – tortured. Descriptions from the SSCI report provide sufficient rebuttal to these equivocations:

> ... waterboarding [induced] convulsions and vomiting. Abu Zubaydah, for example, became "completely unresponsive, with bubbles rising through his open, full mouth." Internal CIA records describe the waterboarding of [KSM] as evolving into a "series of near drownings."

> Sleep deprivation involved keeping detainees awake for up to 180 hours... At least five detainees experienced disturbing hallucinations during prolonged sleep deprivation and, in at least two of those cases, the CIA nonetheless continued the sleep deprivation.

> At least five CIA detainees were subjected to "rectal rehydration" or rectal feeding without documented medical necessity. The CIA placed detainees in ice water "baths." .... (pg. 5)

Additionally, the comment "...nothing in *my* ethical code," suggests Mitchell is simply making up his own rules. Ethical decisions, acts, and behavior can never be based solely on one's personal code. In fact, in order to behave ethically, an individual must sometimes act in a manner that does not personally feel right. Virtually, every doctor who enters the medical field experiences this conflict. When a competent patient with a chronic illness decides to defer life-sustaining treatment, for example, a doctor may feel it is wrong to allow the patient to die, but is mindful of the patient's autonomy. Professionals behave ethically by integrating community and professional moralities into their behavior, not by ignoring them in favor of their own moral code.

But What About the Ticking Time Bomb?

Returning to the "Ticking Time Bomb Scenario" (TTBS) which has been used to justify torture, a few observations are in order. First, it should be noted that in order to justify torturing a suspect (i.e., using Consequentialism to justify the action on the basis that it "saves lives"), there are multiple assumptions which must be accepted with certainty. If *any* are incorrect, the rationale fails. The suspect:

1. The suspect... is a terrorist
2. The suspect... knows about a terror plot
3. The suspect… has knowledge that will help stop the plot
4. The suspect... will give information under torture, and only under torture
5. The suspect... will give information *in time* to stop the terror plot (i.e., you have time to use the information to stop the attack/bombing, etc.)

And

6. His detainment has gone *unnoticed* by his terrorist group.
7. You can find an expert torturer in time.

I will briefly examine these assumptions:

#1. In a real-life scenario, one can never be 100% sure before the interrogation begins that the captive is truly a terrorist, any more than a suspect is certain to be guilty before questioning.

#2. If #1 is true, there remains the question of whether or not he actually knows about a future attack on civilians. He may simply be associated with a terrorist group without knowledge of the plot.

#3. If #1 and #2 are true, there remains the question of whether or not he has vital information about the attack. He may only be a peripheral actor in the plot itself

#4. If #1-#3 are true, will the suspect yield the information if he is tortured, and in no other way? In reality, there is little evidence that torture works at all to elicit truthful information, and substantial evidence that it does not.[10]

#5. If #1-#4 are true, does one have enough time to torture the suspect for information and use it to prevent the attack?

#6. If #1-#5 are true, one is still be left with the question of whether or not the arrest had gone unnoticed by other conspirators. Consider that if one has detained and begun interrogating a suspect, it would be difficult to assume that he was acting alone. Therefore, it is relevant to consider the other actors in the plot and how they might react to one of their group being arrested. A reasonable assumption would be that if they noticed his absence, and were not able to get in touch with him, that they would conclude he had been arrested, and was in the process of interrogation. Therefore, they would certainly alter the plans.

#7. Even for those who believe torture *can* work to elicit good information from a suspect, few of would argue that torturing a person is an "easy" or "simple" job. In order for the TTBS to be valid one would need to ensure that someone with "expertise" in torturing others would be available. If not, it adds to the unknowable timeline. In truth, psychological trauma is something that perpetrators as well as victims of torture suffer from [16]. As far back as 1956, the psychiatrist Frantz Fanon, who did a significant amount of work in

---

[10] See prior sections (referencing SSCI Report, pg. 18, 159).

treating torture victims, also documented treating patients who suffered psychological trauma from perpetrating torture, themselves [22].

Even if all of the above conditions were met, no one could be certain that they were any step of the way closer to eliciting valid information. The TTBS is written in such a manner that it dangles a valid Consequentialist argument for torture. Yet few proponents consider the damage caused, beyond the victims themselves. State-sponsored torture has far-reaching effects, the extent of which may not be known for years. The possibilities include the fueling of terrorist recruitment, the risk of torture to one's own POWs, and delegitimization of a nation's moral authority [38]. Thus, the true Consequentialist argument is not as one-sided as it first appears.

Taking into account all of these considerations, it may be clear that the TTBS is at best an unrealistic scenario and, at worst, an impossible one. But, perhaps it's not required to be realistic, as thought experiments themselves are not meant to be. Rather, they are used to elicit ways in which people make judgments in the face of moral dilemmas. However, as such, thought experiments are not meant to provide a basis for implementing specific policy or law.

Consider the most famous two thought experiments, noted at the beginning of this chapter. Never in their long history has this led anyone to advocate for implementing the installation of periodic train track levers that the public can operate at will on the chance that someone might have to choose between saving one life or five. Neither has anyone advocated for laws that encourage overweight individuals to spend more time on bridges with the thought that one could save a life that way, someday, by pushing him over the side, as a train is approaching. In truth, the TTBS is no more realistic than either of the trolley scenarios, and therefore, it would be absurd to justify a specific program based on it.

Is There a More Realistic "Ticking Time Bomb Scenario"?

An advocate for the use of torture in some cases might still argue that *some* scenario *could* arise where torturing a suspect saves innocent lives. Yet, even if there were such a scenario, would it still be wrong? And—if so—why?

On October first, 2002, German citizen Magnus Gäfgen was picked up and interrogated by Frankfurt police on suspicion of kidnapping an 11-year-old boy. He was arrested after sending a ransom note and picking up the money. The facts of the interrogation are in dispute, except for one aspect: During the interrogation, Gäfgen was told that unless he divulged the boy's whereabouts, he would be subjected to "considerable pain" at the hands of a "specially trained" torturer who was en route. Ten minutes after the threat, Gäfgen confessed he had suffocated the boy 4 days earlier.

While the threat of torture in this instance did not save a life, it raised the spectre of a "realistic" TTBS that might result in the justification of torture [12]. In 2004, the Frankfurt Regional Court issued judgments against the officers involved, noting that the defense of "necessity" was unjustified because the method of threatening torture "violated human dignity." The court noted "the protection of human dignity was absolute, allowing no exceptions or any balancing of interests." When reviewing the case in 2010, The Grand Chamber of the European Court of Human Rights upheld the decision, concluding that Article 3 of the United Nations Convention against Torture was violated during Gäfgen's interrogation [25].

Article 3 of the UN Convention against Torture is revealing: "No one shall be subjected to torture or to inhuman or degrading treatment or punishment" [36]. The Chamber noted that all of the lower courts examining the case had agreed that Article 3 had been violated, adding:

> … such methods of investigation could not be justified as an act of necessity because "necessity" was not a defence to a violation of the *absolute protection of human dignity* under Article 1 of the Basic Law, which also lay at the heart of Article 3 ... (2010, emphasis added).

The officers involved did not receive significant punishment, nor did the majority court find that Gäfgen's confession under threat interfered with his ability to receive a fair trial. However, the court upheld the absolute ban on torture under the dignity of the person, regardless of whether or not there was the potential to save lives.

There is some debate over the scope of dignity in philosophy and medicine, with some arguing that autonomy or the respect for persons is adequate. Yet Yale's Alec Buchanan notes that respecting one's autonomy may not be enough to recognize the inherent value of the individuals whom professionals evaluate. Noting that dignity appears closer to the moral meaning of "worth," Buchanan and others keep this concept paramount to remind experts that each individual has a value that is "incapable of being abolished and that creates obligations in others" [14]. Thus, when searching for the fundamental reason why torture is wrong (beyond a visceral rejection of the practice), perhaps professionals should consider human dignity as absolute.

Conclusions

When the involvement of psychologists in the torture program was uncovered, it led to widespread condemnation by mental health professionals and laypersons alike. In fact, while the American Psychological Association was initially hesitant to denounce the practice of psychologists being involved in national security interrogations [6], even it finally realized such a ban was needed (2016). Yet, regardless of the ethical principles or guidelines of any organization, there may be some who ignore them in the pursuit of their own agendas. Mitchell and Jessen did not engage in torture because they "mis-read" the ethical guidelines of their profession, demonstrating that it takes more than a strong statement to prevent bad actors from doing harm. But, strong statements by professional organizations are at least a start.

In addition to the challenges of navigating some fields, and avoiding others, the torture program provides an opportunity to examine the weaknesses of all moral decision makers under the threat of terror: the exercise of poor judgment and inadequate reasoning. Even some in the clinical professions seemed comfortable with torture, provided they were not personally involved [27]. However, even a remote respect for human dignity dictates that it is not. The American Academy of Psychiatry and the Law is explicit regarding torture: "As is true for any physician, psychiatrists practicing in a forensic role should not participate in torture" (2005). However, perhaps, "any physician" should be replaced with "any human being," demonstrating that the act of torture demeans the human dignity of the victim as well as the actor.

References

1. Allhoff, F. (2005). A defense of torture: Separation of cases, ticking time-bombs and moral justification. *International Journal of Applied Philosophy, 19*(2), 243–264.
2. American Academy of Psychiatry and the Law. (2005). Ethics guidelines for the practice of forensic psychiatry. [Adopted May 2005]. Available at: http://aapl.org/pdf/ethicsgdlns.pdf. Accessed 15 June 2019.
3. American Psychiatric Association. (2013). *Principles of medical ethics with annotations especially applicable to psychiatry.* Washington, DC: American Psychiatric Association. Available at: https://www.psychiatry.org/FileLibrary/Psychiatrists/Practice/Ethics/principles-medical-ethics.pdf. Accessed 15 June 2019.
4. American Psychological Association. (1992). Ethical principles of psychologists and code of conduct. [12/1/1992]. Available at: https://www.apa.org/ethics/code/code-1992. Accessed: 4/7/2020.
5. American Psychological Association. (2017). Ethical principles of psychologists and code of conduct. [Adopted August 21, 2002], Effective June 1, 2003 (With the 2010 Amendments to Introduction and Applicability and Standards 1.02 and 1.03, Effective June 1, 2010) With the 2016 Amendment to Standard 3.04 Adopted August 3, 2016. Effective January 1, 2017 American Psychological Association. 2012. Specialty Guidelines for Forensic Psychology © 2012 American Psychological Association. 68(1):7–19.
6. American Psychological Association. (2005). *Report of the American Psychological Association Presidential Task Force on Psychological Ethics and National Security.*
7. Appelbaum, P. S. (1997). A theory of ethics for forensic psychiatry. *The Journal of the American Academy of Psychiatry and the Law, 25,* 233–247.
8. Appelbaum, P. S., Roth, L. H., & Lidz, C. (1982). The therapeutic misconception: Informed consent in psychiatric research. *International Journal of Law and Psychiatry, 5*(3–4), 319–329.
9. Bauman, C. W., McGraw, A. P., Bartels, D., & Warren, C. (2014). Revisiting external validity: Concerns about trolley problems and other sacrificial dilemmas in moral psychology. *Social and Personality Psychology Compass, 8*(9), 536–554.
10. Beauchamp, T. L. (1995). Principlism and its alleged competitors. *Kennedy Institute of Ethics Journal, 5*(3), 181–198.
11. Beauchamp, T. L., & Childress, J. F. (1979). *Principles of biomedical ethics* (1st ed.). New York: Oxford University Press.
12. Bernstein R. (2003). Kidnapping has Germans debating police torture. *The New York Times.* https://www.nytimes.com/2003/04/10/world/kidnapping-has-germans-debating-police-torture.html. Accessed: 4/20/2020.
13. Bostyn, D. H., Sevenhant, S., & Roets, A. (2018). Of mice, men, and trolleys: Hypothetical judgment versus real-life behavior in trolley-style moral dilemmas. *Psychological Science, 29*(7), 1084–1093.

14. Buchanan, A. (2015). Respect for dignity and forensic psychiatry. *International Journal of Law and Psychiatry, 41*, 12–17.
15. Bybee, J. S. (2002). Memorandum for Alberto R. Gonzales, Counsel to the President Re: Standards of Conduct for Interrogation 18 U.S.C. § 2340-2340A..
16. Costanzo, M., & Gerrity, E. (2009). Psychologists and the use of torture in interrogations. *Social Issues and Policy Review, 3*(1), 179–210.
17. Crosby, S. (2019). *Lies, Denial, and Fantasy in Guantanamo Bay*. As Part of: Annas GD, Annas GJ, Freitas C, Annas MF, Crosby SS. Presentation/panel: Top secrets, lies, and conspiracy theories: Navigating a sea of uncertainty in a delusional world. Presentation: Presented at the XXXVI International Congress on Law and Mental Health in Rome, Italy. July 25, 2019.
18. Davies, J. (2012). *The fire-raisers: Bentham and torture. 19: Interdisciplinary Studies in the Long Nineteenth Century, (15)*. Available at: https://doi.org/10.16995/ntn.643. Accessed: 8/27/2019.
19. Dean, J. W. (2005). *The Torture Memo by Judge Jay S. Bybee that Haunted Alberto Gonzales's Confirmation Hearings*. Findlaw.com. Available at: https://supreme.findlaw.com/legal-commentary/the-torture-memo-by-judge-jay-s-bybee-that-haunted-alberto-gonzalss-confirmation-hearings.html. Accessed 9/8/2019. Accessed: 12/9/2019.
20. Department of Justice. (2009). Office of professional responsibility report, investigation into the Office of Legal Counsel's Memoranda Concerning Issues Relating to the Central Intelligence Agency's Use of "Enhanced Interrogation Techniques" on Suspected Terrorists.
21. Erickson, E. (2014). Moral preening and the luxury of the hypothetical. RedState.com/Salem Media. Available at: https://www.redstate.com/erick/2014/12/16/moral-preening-and-the-luxury-of-the-hypothetical/. Accessed 4/21/2020.
22. Fanon, F. (1963). *The wretched of the earth* (trans: Farrington, C.). New York: Grove Weidenfeld A division of Grove Press, Inc. pp. 263–269.
23. Fink, S. (2016). Where even nightmares are classified. *The New York Times*. Available at: https://www.nytimes.com/2016/11/13/world/guantanamo-bay-doctors-abuse.html Accessed: 4/7/2020.
24. Forrest, K. D., Wadkins, T. A., & Miller, R. L. (2002). The role of pre-existing stress on false confessions: An empirical study. *Journal of Credibility Assessment and Witness Psychology, 3*, 23–45.
25. Gäfgen v. Germany. (2010). (Application no. 22978/05). Judgment of the European Court of Human Rights, Grand Chamber. Strasbourg. Rectified on 3 June 2010 under Rule 81 of the Rules of Court.
26. Ghosh, B. (2009). Partisan passions dominate interrogation hearings. *Time USA*. Available at: https://content.time.com/time/nation/article/0,8599,1898125,00.html. Accessed 9/8/2019.
27. Janofsky, J. S. (2006). Lies and coercion: Why psychiatrists should not participate in police and intelligence interrogations. *The Journal of the American Academy of Psychiatry and the Law, 34*(4), 472–478.
28. Memorandum of July 2, [Year, redacted], Subject: "Comments on proposed enhanced interrogation" [Sender and Receiver, redacted]. Available at: http://humanrights.ucdavis.edu/projects/the-guantanamo-testimonials-project/testimonies/prisoner-testimonies/prisoner-testimonies/comments-on-proposed-enhanced-interrogation-july-2002. Accessed: 2/28/2020.
29. Mitchell, J. Deposition Testimony, dated 1/16/2017. Case docket #2:15-CV-286-JLQ, Suleiman Abdullah Salim et al., vs. James Elmer Mitchell and John "Bruce" Jessen, U.S. District Court for the Eastern District of Washington. Location: Law Offices of Blank Rome, 130 N. 18th Street, Philadelphia, PA 19103.
30. Mitchell, J. E., & Harlow, B. (2016). *Enhanced interrogation: Inside the minds and motives of the Islamic terrorists trying to destroy America*. New York: Crown Publishing Group/Penguin Random House LLC.
31. Moore, T., & Fitszimmons, L. C. (2011). Justice imperiled: False confessions and the Reid technique. *Criminal Law Quarterly, 57*, 509–542.
32. Mossman, D., Noffsinger, S. G., Ash, P., Frierson, R. L., Gerbasi, J., Hackett, M., Lewis, C. F., Pinals, D. A., Scott, C. L., Sieg, K. G., Wall, B. W., & Zonana, H. V. (2007). Practice guideline

for the forensic psychiatric evaluation of competence to stand trial. *Journal of the American Academy of Psychiatry and the Law Online, 35*(Supplement 4), S3–S72.

33. National Association of Social Workers (NASW) Code of Ethics. Approved by the 1996 NASW Delegate Assembly and revised by the 2017 NASW Delegate Assembly. Available at: https://www.socialworkers.org/about/ethics/code-of-ethics/code-of-ethics-english. Accessed: 2/28/2020.
34. Senate Select Committee on Intelligence. (2014). The Senate Intelligence Committee Report on Torture: Committee Study of the Central Intelligence Agency's Detention and Interrogation Program [Paperback Edition]. Melville House Publishing, Brooklyn.
35. Email from [redacted]: to: [Redacted]. Description of Physical Pressures; dated: July 8, 2002, at 04:15:15 PM. Available at: https://www.cia.gov/library/readingroom/docs/0006552083.pdf. Accessed 2/28/2020.
36. United Nations. Convention against torture and other cruel, inhuman or degrading treatment or punishment, adopted by the United Nations General Assembly on 10 December 1984.
37. United States Senate Committee on Armed Services (SASC). (2009). *Inquiry into the Treatment of Detainees in U.S. Custody*, A Report, November 20, 2008. U.S. Government Printing Office.
38. Xenakis, S. (2014). The role and responsibilities of psychiatry in 21st century warfare. *The Journal of the American Academy of Psychiatry and the Law, 42*(4), 504–508.

Mental Health Under Occupation: The Dilemmas of "Normalcy" in Palestine

17

Samah Jabr and Elizabeth Berger

The Context of Palestine

The authors are psychiatrists—one based in East Jerusalem and one based in New York—who have worked together over many years developing clinical programs and writing articles on mental health in Palestine (for an overview of current mental health services in Palestine, see [9]). In this chapter as previously, we take a broad view of mental health—including not only considerations of diagnosed illness and syndromes which a given patient may present but also well-being more generally, especially as well-being reflects the individual's place in a communal fabric and in a particular moment in history. Following the psychiatrist Frantz Fanon, we believe that no human experience can be divorced from the social reality in which it is rooted [4]. Like Fanon, we believe that the ethical notion of justice is central to an understanding of human needs. Our current chapter thus focuses on mental health in Palestine viewed from an ethical perspective. This inquiry raises questions such as these: "Without justice, what can be normal in mental health? Without justice, what is reality itself?"

The apartheid social reality faced by the nearly five million Palestinians living in the West Bank, Gaza, and East Jerusalem does not lead to human flourishing [3]. The fundamental problems are political, stemming from the stateless and vulnerable status of the population living under military occupation with a consequent secondary inadequacy in all spheres of life: economic, social, judicial, educational, environmental, and cultural. Palestine has experienced generations of injury through the

S. Jabr
Department of Psychiatry and Behavioral Sciences at the George Washington University School of Medicine and Health Sciences, Washington, DC, USA

Palestinian Ministry of Health, Ramallah, Palestine

E. Berger (✉)
Department of Psychiatry and Behavioral Sciences at the George Washington University School of Medicine and Health Sciences, Washington, DC, USA

© Springer Nature Switzerland AG 2021
A. R. Dyer et al. (eds.), *Global Mental Health Ethics*,
https://doi.org/10.1007/978-3-030-66296-7_17

destruction of its physical infrastructure, military and community violence by Israelis against individuals, strangulation of its once-robust agricultural economy, enforced injury to its social structure, and denial of the rights to safety, education, legal protection, and human development.

These problems are longstanding. The establishment in 1948 of the state of Israel had been followed by widespread expulsion of the Palestinian population—known as the *Nakba* or catastrophe—and subsequent sequestration of fleeing communities in refugee camps and under conditions of chronic insecurity and disenfranchisement within historic Palestine, other countries in the Middle East, and elsewhere globally. Periodic onslaught of outright warfare against displaced Palestinian civilians living in the West Bank, Jerusalem, and Gaza has punctuated the ensuing 70 years, involving the routine shelling of schools and hospitals and the use of phosphorus bombs despite international prohibition. For these communities, ongoing human rights abuses form the backdrop of everyday experience: curfews and restrictions on human movement, checkpoints, home demolitions, extrajudicial assassinations, targeting of community leaders and human rights advocates, mass incarceration, detention without charges, and the pervasive use of torture—including the torture of children (for primary source documents, see the list of references in [9 and 12]).

The chronicity, scale, and intensity of these abuses have stimulated public outcry among the world at large and prompted various condemnations from the United Nations, from groups dedicated to human rights such as Amnesty International, and from notable individuals such as Desmond Tutu and Jimmy Carter. The Palestinian protest generated two large popular uprisings, the First Intifada of 1987–1993 and the Second Intifada of 2000–2005. Even within the state of Israel, there have been political action groups speaking out against these human rights abuses, among them B'Tselem, the Public Committee against Torture in Israel, the Israeli Committee Against Home Demolitions, Breaking the Silence, and Rabbis for Human Rights.

By and large, however, the voice of the Palestinian people in the midst of these violations has been silenced. Those who support them within Muslim and Arab communities globally have often suffered from their own troubles, and the world's attention is often captured by new dramas at the expense of longstanding ones. But the role of propaganda in shaping public opinion about Palestine is also crucial. The political goals of the state of Israel—a state which wants the land but does not want the people—have been supported by a propaganda narrative which renders the Palestinian perspective null and void. This propaganda narrative is an additional injustice that harms the well-being of Palestinians.

The narrative supporting the state of Israel draws upon the actual historical suffering of the Jewish people, especially the history of the European Holocaust of the twentieth century, as justification for the establishment of a safe haven for Jewish persons everywhere. From this historical perspective, and indeed we share this broad perspective, the Jewish people have been grievously victimized and are thus entitled to redress. But to deliver such a safe haven—as twentieth-century history unfolded—required a set of political decisions which redefined the geography of the Middle East in such a manner that the Jewish people were entitled to a portion of that geography in a special way. They were entitled to a safe haven that was safer for them than for others. This redefinition, the agenda of political Zionism, imposed a new set of wrongs through land seizures, massacres, and a large-scale program of ethnic cleansing; these wrongs were and remain concrete consequences of particular political choices. The consequences for the pre-existing indigenous non-Jewish population were then suppressed and only in recent times admitted by Israeli historians.

It is noteworthy that the ongoing suppression of the historical record (and the denial of the suppression) makes use of a specially constructed image of Palestinians as ethically defective. The goodness and rightness of the Israeli—while an important element of the official Israeli narrative—are perhaps not as fundamental to the success of the narrative as the badness of the Palestinian. The Israeli, after all, may be "only too human" or "all too human." It is the incompletely human or variously sub-human Palestinian whose aggression, untrustworthiness, hatred, irrationality, and intransigence characterize an enduring cast member within the narrative drama and drives the contours of its plot. What can one expect from such a Palestinian? How can one even deal with him at all? The state of Israel is thus in the eyes of the world permitted to be practical, pragmatic, realistic, and even ruthless in the face of an enemy who is virtually unredeemable as ethically inadequate.

The ethically defective Palestinian is an almost-indelible feature of Israeli official pronouncements and of official commentary from the USA, the time-honored supporter of Israel's policies. This debased image did not arise de novo from Israeli propaganda, but harkens back to stock features of non-Western populations viewed through the lens of Western colonial and imperial ambitions. The Westerner is logical, rational, forthright, practical, fair-minded, and future-oriented. The non-Westerner is credulous, greedy, irrational, dishonest, lazy, backward (perhaps especially with regard to human rights), and focused on a mythical past. Within a large literature of relevant historical, colonial, and cultural studies, Edward Said's *Orientalism* traces the evolution of this durable ethnic stereotype with a particular focus on the European view of Arab and Muslim populations [16]. More recent scholarly works, such as Stephen Sheehi's *Islamophobia,* describe and locate this debased image of Arabs and Muslims within the global political hegemony of the current moment [17]. We would assess the application of this stereotype of the Palestinian psyche, invoked very frequently by journalists, politicians, and members of the public, as a form of abuse. It is a stalwart aspect of the Israeli Right.

The Israeli Left, however, presents a different narrative, which we have described as the dilemma of liberal Zionism [8]. The narrative of the Israeli Left seeks to frame the status quo as a regrettable but insurmountable aspect of ordinary normal reality. Here, the claims of the Israeli and the Palestinian are given almost equal weight, as if they were two brothers passively trapped by fate in a tragically vexing paradox. There is sadness all around and even sympathy for both participants in this endless struggle. A portion of the academic literature written by Israelis in mental health fields appears to share this view. Although sometimes naively well-intentioned, the narrative of eternal conflict implicitly accepts the status quo as a given and aims for mutual understanding around the margins of that status quo. This normalizing narrative does not put justice and the restoration of human rights at its central point, an approach which would raise the question whether the status quo can be considered "normal" and—if not—what must be done about it.

Although seductive, the liberal narrative of Israel/Palestine is both misleading and unjust. The ethical situation, as we see it, is asymmetrical and cannot be asserted as a sorrowful conflict between two sets of equally valid competing claims. The ethical situation is one of the military occupation, in which nearly five million stateless persons live under conditions of imposed hardship, unremitting abuse, violation, and humiliation at the hands of one of the most powerful military forces on earth. While the language of the Israeli Right is a frontal attack on the characterological integrity of Palestinians, the attack by the Israeli Left is a delicate hypocrisy. The liberal view protests that it yearns to perceive Palestinians as fully human, and asserts that they are indeed human in some domains—but not others. The forbidden domain is the political arena, in which Palestinian claims to political rights as indivisible from human rights are undermined as unrealistic. Reality is defined by the status quo, however lamentable that status quo may sometimes appear.

We see mental health in Palestine therefore as compromised through contextual factors which form a complex matrix. Many of the detrimental military, social, and economic determinants that impinge upon well-being and mental health for Palestinians are clear enough, but interplay among these external factors is far-reaching and subtle; moreover, these external factors have impact upon internalized issues of identity, self-esteem, intimacy, and collective meaning. The following vignettes illustrate some of these themes.

Clinical Vignettes

The vignettes and the comments following the vignettes are based on patients whom the authors have treated or on cases we have supervised; certain details have been altered to protect confidentiality.

It should be noted that zones of war and conflict are typically characterized by high rates of prevalence for mental disorders [2]. Statistics in Palestine that have been gathered by the Department of Health, however, indicate that there are essentially no waiting lists for governmental mental health services, although these clinics provide the largest amount of psychiatric care with a small professional staff. Stigma about mental illness may play a minor role in this phenomenon, but we believe that it is the perception of the population that accounts for the lack of waiting lists: Psychological pain is not denied—yet by and large, it is not perceived as something that can be resolved through clinical care. Emotional suffering is perceived as the result of the occupation.

Case One

A depressed elderly woman was brought to see a psychiatrist by her adult children after her family doctor determined that her physical complaints of fatigue and malaise were not caused by a medical illness and suggested that they arose from psychological issues. When the psychiatrist inquired how many children the patient had had, she firmly replied, "Five." At the same moment, however, her children answered that their mother had had "Six." Exploration of this contradiction revealed that the patient currently refused to acknowledge one of her children, an adult daughter. The patient had recently disowned this daughter after the young women and her husband had sold their home in Jerusalem to an Israeli couple, an act which is viewed in Palestine as a particularly despicable form of collaboration. The daughter and her husband had then escaped to Canada. The disavowal of the daughter had been followed by depression.

Comment

This patient's depression reflects her grief and anger over the concrete loss of the daughter and also her grief and anger over the loss of the image of the daughter as an idealizable person who is steadfast in her loyalty to her Palestinian family, city, and people. Collective resistance to Israeli seduction is a prominent aspect of idealized Palestinian self-regard and part of the cultural value of *sumud* or steadfastness in the face of the occupation. The patient experienced her daughter as "selling out" in every sense, not only a loss but a shameful loss. Her denial of the daughter was not, of course, a psychotic defense against a painful reality but nevertheless a regressive defense insofar as there was a retreat to stubbornly held black-and-white conclusions: "I never had such a daughter!"

The inner battle between wishing for individual safety for one's children and wishing for one's children's steadfastness in the face of the occupation is commonplace in Palestine. It is part of the abnormal normal. This issue might be viewed as a projection onto one's children of the internalized conflict between identification with the unethical aggressor and identification with the heroically resisting victim. The ever-present tension between maintaining stable self-regard as a Palestinian, in the face of a reality that undermines that self-regard as hopeless and unrealistic, is both inescapable and exhausting.

Case Two

A man who worked for the Palestinian security system in the West Bank (a branch of the Palestinian government charged with police functions) complained of marital problems. Although his employment often required him to support official Israeli policies, his personal views were in conflict with these policies. He often quoted Marx and Hobbes, recognizing that he played the intermediate role of an armed security force that protected the corrupt rich from the desperate poor. In this context, he commented bitterly about the "dirty games" he saw all around him but was not fully aware of his own involvement in these "dirty games." It turned out that this man had a secret second marriage and that indeed his father had also maintained a similar situation.

Comment

Here, we see another version of internal conflict in the face of a debased reality. This man's intellect provided him with insight into the corruption of the "system" around him—an indictment of the governance of the West Bank in its collusion with the Israelis. He was not altogether alert to his own confusion with regard to social corruption and his partial identification with it, as he had not been fully alert to his identification with his father's dishonesty. The patient, while identifying intellectually with a critique of exploitation, was involved in his own exploitative relationship. He acted-out both victim and victimizer as a defense against experiencing directly the painful memories of his father's betrayal and his painful current helplessness within an unethical social terrain.

Case Three

A family brought their adult daughter, a withdrawn and paranoid woman who had exhibited "crazy" ideas since her husband had been killed. The husband had lived in a city remote from the woman during their marriage, and due to movement restrictions within Palestine, the couple had met in person on only a few occasions. Most of their relationship had taken place online. She described her deceased husband in idealized terms and claimed that her emotional problems were the result of her grief.

The family reported a very different story. According to the patient's parents, her husband had been a collaborator with the Israelis and was in fact directly responsible for assassinating a person of importance who had been a significant community leader within Palestine, as part of his work on behalf of the Israelis. The husband had then been executed as a collaborator. The family had attempted to convince her of the facts by showing her well-publicized online videos and television news items which described the details of the deceased husband's actual actions. The patient, in turn, maintained that the family's presentation of videos and reports on television were elaborate fabrications and falsehoods.

The psychiatrist attempted to clarify the reality with the patient, but could not shake the patient's delusional beliefs. Apart from her assessment of her late husband, the patient presented no other psychological abnormalities. She was otherwise sane. Eventually, the psychiatrist came to the conclusion that the woman's psychotic denial of reality could not be altered; the psychiatrist negotiated a solution with the family in which the family agreed not to challenge the patient's ideas about her deceased husband. The psychiatrist observed that this case evoked a great deal of countertransference anxiety because of the multiple layers of deceit.

Comment

This case illustrates some of the grotesque psychological consequences generated by the Israeli exploitation of Palestinian collaborators. The system of collaboration is longstanding, entrenched, and pervasive throughout Palestine. Collaborators are often recruited through the use of torture and/or credible threats of capture, torture, and murder of their family members; collaborators then secretly carry out the agendas of their handlers while appearing to lead ordinary lives within the community. The system of collaboration thus hangs like a toxic cloud over Palestine, interfering with ordinary trust among the population and infiltrating human relationships both casual and intimate with suspicion and fear.

The work of the collaborator is often involved with extrajudicial assassination and other forms of political violence; not infrequently, the unmasked collaborator himself comes to a violent end. The intense danger implicit in the collaboration system—and the necessity of secrecy and hypocrisy throughout—sets the stage for extreme psychological reactions. We have seen mothers and wives especially to be vulnerable to psychotic responses to the death of family members who have been sucked into these arrangements.

Case Four

A woman employed within the office of a very high-ranking official in Palestine reported depressed mood and obsessive thoughts related to what she initially described as problems with her superior at work. She appeared to be a hardworking and conscientious person; her immediate boss was a close relative of the high-ranking official, an untrained individual who appeared to have no interest in meeting the demands of his position. The patient's devoted work was ignored, and responsibilities which rightly belonged to others were habitually heaped upon her. The more effort she put forth, the more numerous the extraneous jobs that were assigned. The therapist, a psychologist whose own situation in her place of employment shared many of the features of the patient's workplace, had considerable difficulty resisting the impulse to share her own story with the patient.

Comment

The situation of the patient and also the situation of her psychologist illustrate ethical problems arising from the widespread lack of legitimate authority in Palestine under the circumstances of occupation. There is understandable mistrust among the population for the governmental structure and the political parties which participate in it; no party has earned respect for championing the public good. This in itself is a source of cynicism and despair for the public overall. Government office work is frequently painful to conscientious and hardworking individuals employed there due to disorganization, nepotism, inadequacy, waste, and outright corruption at the workplace at every level. People who take a strong ethical stand, in our experience, are often particularly victimized, ostracized, and demeaned. The problem of illicit personal attacks within official agencies and institutions in Palestine looms large, as the legitimate flow of authority, responsibility, and justice is denied.

In addition to the domain of officialdom, Palestine suffers from pervasive problems due to the omnipresent economic system within which many human services are brokered through third-party relationships involving local and international non-governmental organizations (NGOs) and international donors. The role of the NGO in Palestinian life is huge. Indeed, the presence of foreign bureaucrats and consultants has shifted much of the Palestinian economy from its once-traditional agricultural base—now long-decimated by the occupation's land seizures, road closures, destruction of villages, diversion of water, and violence perpetrated by the Israeli forces and the Israelis living in the ever-expanding illegal settlements—to a service sector dependent upon large hotels and conference spaces filled by visiting foreigners.

Impaired dynamics between the NGO donor and the recipient are common-place. Consultants are often Westerners who come to Palestine for brief visits. For example, within a mental health training program for family medicine, the local psychiatrists were trained by Westerners who have little understanding of Palestinian culture or its typical idioms of distress. International donors, although often well-intentioned, have diverse agendas which are frequently at odds with local perceptions of need. Policy planning and service delivery within the realm of healthcare or education are often engineered from patchwork arrangements underwritten by short-term financing administered through governmental, private, religiously based, entrepreneurial, local, and/or international agencies and entities—all of which may be nullified at the will of the Israelis. There are also at times allegations of corruption within these agencies; even allegations aimed at large and well-respected agencies such as United Nations Relief and Works Agency [5].

In this fragmented picture, multiple factors driven by the occupation cause the infrastructure of Palestinian institutions to founder in dysfunction and neglect.

Case Five

An adolescent boy was brought to a social worker by his family for withdrawal from school and from social participation following his release from a three-week detention by the Israeli forces. The family described that the boy had been taken from his home during a nighttime incursion during which his father had been especially humiliated in front of the family and that thereafter the youngster had been held without charges while interrogated. He had been blindfolded and beaten, leaving permanent marks on his neck and back. The boy refused to speak a single word with the social worker during the initial interview and thereafter would not even enter her office. However, the family indicated with great shame and anguish that they suspected sexual violation of some kind had taken place during the period of detention based on the narrative that the adolescent had shared with them immediately after his release. The family soon dropped out of treatment, citing that travel to the social worker's office was extremely difficult. The social worker experienced great anxiety in relation to this case with insomnia and intrusive obsessional thoughts and observed that she did not think she had the capacity to deal with cases of torture in the future.

Comment

This case underscores the key role of detention by the Israeli forces. The use of detention is so pervasive that since 1967, approximately one-third of all Palestinian men have experienced detention. The Palestinian Central Bureau of Statistics observes that as a result, almost every Palestinian family has suffered the detention of at least one member and that many families have had several members detained (Palestinian Central Bureau of Statistics [14]. Mistreatment, human rights violations, and outright torture are frequently documented. Children are often detained, and there are reports of torture of children including sexual abuse [6].

The acute and chronic mental health effects of detention and/or torture are manifold, both for the survivor and for their families. Those left behind suffer chronic grief in relation to the missing family members as well as baffling issues reintegrating family members who may return home—having endured significant harm—after a period of many years. The sum of these implications poses a major public health problem; detention and torture are enduring fixtures within daily life in Palestine, part of its normalcy. These violations distort the values and significance of social experience: What is the meaning of one's personal suffering in such a terrain? When torture is an everyday experience, the survivor wonders, "Can I even complain about my 'normal' experience with torture when another person was tortured far more severely?"

This case also illustrates the problem of secondary trauma experienced by others, including accidental bystanders, witnesses, human rights workers, and mental health clinicians. Such workers in particular take on considerable psychological risk to themselves within contexts of overwork that often offer little in the way of support. In addition, clinicians may wrestle with countertransference issues arising from their own burden of suffering that interferes with the capacity to ask, listen, and see the patient's trauma in its entirety [7].

Discussion

What is normal in Palestine is the fact that nothing is normal. The reality of Palestine is one of the ongoing injustice through the occupation—abuse which is inseparable from every other aspect of psychological life. In particular, the occupation sees to it that social structures that in normal circumstances provide security and moral meaning are purposefully undermined. We emphasize here four interrelated aspects of normal living which sustain moral meaning in ordinary circumstances and describe how the occupation assaults these foundations of an ethical reality.

The first is the notion of home. The idea of home in Palestine is under perpetual attack at every level. The homeland itself is without boundaries, dissolved, annexed, and claimed by others. Language, history, culture, and artifacts have been debased, appropriated, and destroyed from priceless antiquities to ordinary home furnishings and rugs. The concrete process of home demolition by Israeli forces is indeed progressing at an accelerating rate as this chapter is being written [20].

The second is the notion of the family. Displacement of neighborhoods and restriction of human movement impedes the contact and communication between extended families, the traditional basis of Palestinian life. The home and family within it are perpetually vulnerable not only to displacement but terrifying nighttime incursions in which one or more family members are beaten, bound, and taken away. The capacity of fathers and mothers to protect their children from harm is undermined, and the helpless humiliation of parents damages their image in the eyes of their sons and daughters. In this way, the honorable role of parenthood is harmed and debased, as is the relation between men and women. What is the meaning of marital vows when a man has been in detention for a decade, now released to his family to come face to face with strangers? A child last seen as a toddler is now a teenager; a wife is at a loss how to react to the older man now returned to her.

The third is the notion of genuine authority. With all aspects of governance in Palestine under the control of the state of Israel, the people of Palestine lack recourse for social regulation at every level. Although the population supports equal rights for women in the workplace and within family life, for example, the feeble Palestinian executive, legislative, and judicial systems are unable to answer to the will of the people through supporting these rights and often is not even able to convene [19]. The occupation thus stymies the process of justice and social renewal in Palestine at the root of its most basic functioning. In informal ways as well, Palestine lacks the presence of culture heroes, spokespersons, and community leaders—a group which has always been especially targeted for intimidation, imprisonment, and assassination. Many legitimate heroes are falsely smeared by the Israelis as violent terrorists. In their place, one frequently finds puppets of the occupation and collaborators. The corruption of everyday institutions causes all visible sources of authority to be viewed with suspicion. The workplace is subject to jealousies and resentments, because the prevalence of special favors and nepotism undermine group cooperation and foster cynicism and despair.

The fourth is the notion of a future. With an ever-shrinking landscape of physical and—as it were—mental space, the hope for a future in Palestine is continually diminishing. The fear that one's best efforts are liable to be wasted and that one's children are likely to face increasingly deteriorated circumstances is pervasive in Palestine, a normal reaction to bitter realities. The population of Gaza offers poignant contrasts in this regard; while Gaza is perhaps the most literate of all of the cities of the world, its youth faces one of the highest rates of unemployment in the world (for primary source documents, see the list of references in [12]). The gap between aspiration and disappointment is staggering. It is a testament to the patience and dignity of the young people of Gaza that the acquisition of knowledge through its five colleges and universities remains a deep commitment.

At the most fundamental level, the processes of the occupation have robbed Palestinians of their system of values and sense of agency, such that ambivalence and psychological fragmentation have become a way of life. In an unethical landscape, it is impossible to find secure moral footing.

Recommendations

The challenges to the field of mental health posed by Palestine are thus profound and daunting. We offer recommendations to clinicians and policy makers within the global mental health community, as pathways to constructive involvement on behalf of the people of Palestine. These are, in ascending order of importance, meeting the need for assistance with clinical and research program implementation in Palestine, meeting the need for international solidarity, and meeting the need for justice.

Clinical and Research Program Implementation

There are numerous programs and agencies utilizing the support of international professionals, workers, and donors to address mental health in Palestine. Difficulties with coordination of programs in line with established local needs and with other programs have at times diminished the effectiveness of these efforts, although their motivations have been admirable. We welcome and encourage further support by internationals of the processes of mental health program planning and development in Palestine through the leadership of Palestinian professionals and in a manner that is consistent with the Palestinian National Health Strategy. Programs which benefit women, children, and underserved populations are especially valued, as are programs demonstrating evidence-based outcomes, cost-effectiveness, vertical and horizontal integration of services, stakeholder participation, and transparency; programs should embody as core values the principles of public health and human rights.

The toolkit of mental health too is in need of reinvention in order to address the deformations of experience endured by Palestinian individuals and communities. It is clear that there is still considerable usefulness in our established system of diagnostic categories and evidenced-based therapies that treat symptoms of these conditions—systems of medical practice developed in the West. It is equally clear that the established definitions of many syndromes such as Post Traumatic Stress Disorder, Depressive Disorders, and Anxiety Disorders are inadequate to describe the phenomena presented by captive populations facing ongoing violence in both physical and emotional domains. We are encouraged by the emergence of research initiatives within Palestine have contributed to our understanding of these phenomena through an examination of lived experience. There is a need for more research and the development of new conceptual schemes that capture more adequately the Palestinian experience as well as the experience of similarly beleaguered and oppressed populations elsewhere.

Further, we propose that the fields of healthcare and mental health overall work harder to integrate the wisdom and best practices of the other social sciences—the lessons of history, anthropology, sociology, and economics—to develop a more complete understanding of the collective aspects of psychological development. What we know about the individual psychology of children, adolescents, and adults far outstrips what we know about the relationship between individuals and larger groups. Our incomplete insight into human needs in relation to the social collective remains a notable gap in our intellectual foundation. The psychology of power relations and especially asymmetrical power relationships is another such gap, and particularly relevant to injustice and abuse, whether such injustice is apparently isolated or population-based.

Related to our hope for the future growth of greater theoretical understanding of the development of the individual in relation to the group is our impression that mental health treatments involving groups have much to offer, beyond the obvious considerations of their lower cost and greater efficiency. Many distressed individuals in Palestine suffer incomplete syndromes, failing to "meet criteria" of mental disorders, and indeed view themselves not as patients but as survivors of injustice—ex-prisoners and survivors of torture are perhaps particularly representative of these persons. Involvement in groups, led by a local person who has experienced similar circumstances, may be more beneficial than traditional mental health treatment by professionals. Along these lines, we believe that the psychological benefits of group activities and group social action as an antidote to pervasive social injustice deserve more exploration in both research and practical settings (for further discussion of clinical and research programs currently active in Palestine, see [9, 10], and [12]).

Solidarity

Involvement in solidarity campaigns supporting Palestine is our second recommendation. There are already a number of such movements in various countries and international umbrella organizations that have provided invaluable support. In addition to these, the field of mental health itself has recently become the focus of a global initiative uniting national solidarity movements such as the well-established UK-Palestine Mental Health Network and the USA-Palestine Mental Health Network [18, 21]. There is a newly formed Palestine Mental Health Network in Belgium and similar networks under construction in other countries [11].

Recently, a Palestinian network has been established unifying the multidisciplinary community of mental health clinicians in the West Bank, Gaza, and East Jerusalem as well as those living elsewhere throughout the Palestinian diaspora—the Palestine-Global Mental Health Network [15]. This network aims to articulate a human rights agenda with a global focus as well as particular emphasis on Palestine.

These international networks have coordinated various projects with the guidance of Palestinian clinicians, developing websites with links to news items, academic articles, films, online media, and other resources relevant to Palestine. Some of these network organizations have held conferences and film tours in their home countries and sponsored tours for international mental health workers that bring them to Palestine to meet their professional counterparts involved in both clinical and solidarity activities. These organizations have also launched "Don't Go" campaigns asking professional organizations in mental health to reconsider the choice of Israel as the location of future conferences and to hold them elsewhere instead [1].

Through these networks, fueled by the volunteerism of their clinician members, there has been growth of awareness globally on multiple aspects of the situation in Palestine. Various petitions launched by the networks have gathered huge numbers of signatures internationally from mental health clinicians and professionals. The target audience for the networks has remained for the most part mental health workers such as psychologists, psychiatrists, social workers, and occupational therapists; however, clinicians on the front line of primary care such as family doctors, nurses, and physician assistants also participate, as do many in related fields such as public health and medical research. Alliances have been formed with other activist organizations focused on Palestine as well as related social issues such as racism, colonialism, sexism, minority rights, and liberation psychology generally.

The establishment of these networks has permitted the international voice of protest to counter the forces that have often divided mental health workers supporting Palestine. By sharing information and advocacy initiatives across borders, the global movement has become stronger in its resolve and larger in its scope internationally. We hope that the newly established Palestine-Global Mental Health Network can play a central role in setting the broad agenda for action as well as encouraging interaction between Palestinian colleagues and their counterparts elsewhere. This global activist community offers all of its participants pathways to counter helplessness, hopelessness, and isolation. It is a way to lift the spirits of Palestinian colleagues who work under the burdens of chronic hardship, as well as to engage mental health workers in privileged circumstances who are alienated by the injustice of their circumstances. It provides to all of its global participants a sense of fellowship as well as information and the opportunity to actively shape and to inhabit an ethical community. Most important, solidarity among the mental health community contributes to the development of broader solidarity initiatives internationally that support Palestine and human rights.

Justice

Our third recommendation, and the most important, is the restoration of justice—which must include the end of the occupation, the recognition of equal civil rights to Palestinians, and respect for the rights of displaced Palestinians to return to their homes and properties. This agenda cannot be achieved without a major force of international pressure and commitment that has so far been lacking.

The injustice of Palestine should concern all of us, not only for the sake of the human beings directly harmed by the occupation, but for the sake of human rights everywhere. Palestine offers a vision of malevolent control of one population by another, the Haves crushing the Have-Nots into the dust. It has been observed indeed that Palestine—and particularly the unlivable Gaza—has provided a learning laboratory for the exploration and perfection of just such means of control through diverse means including water restriction, pervasive prison conditions, and extrajudicial assassination [13]. The lessons that Israelis have mastered through their experience of domination and control are commodities currently being exported elsewhere. Israeli expertise in paramilitary control of populations has provided consultation, for example, to the control of poor (typically African-American) communities in the USA by local police; the huge wall built by the Israelis lends inspiration to the USA' efforts to control the flow of people (often refugees from violence) at the walled border of Mexico. Sadly, among these lessons is the impunity with which the world has permitted the Israelis to act.

Meanwhile, we observe that the problem of global warming threatens the world with the prospect of hundreds of millions of new refugees generated by rising seas and rising temperatures, victims of the processes of industrialized "progress" that have benefitted the few to the detriment of the many over the past century. These new refugees will be residents, for the most part, of the global South—persons of color and inhabitants of poor nations. Their exodus is likely to pose an unprecedented challenge to rich nations: Can the human race find new ways to share cooperatively the resources of the earth, so that there is well-being for all? Or will rich nations continue to deny the poor an ethically fair share of water, land, and well-being? What will the world look like, when the despoliation of Palestine forebodes the fate of the majority of the planet?

Justice on a global scale is already gravely past due. To take an ethical stand with the Have-Not people of the earth is imperative, before conditions intensify to a point of unimaginable global crisis. The people of Palestine have long been the prototype of the Have-Not people, and their suffering so far has fallen on deaf ears. But to right this wrong could provide a model of problem-solving in a constructive direction and demonstrate that human beings have the capacity to create a livable planet after all. With justice, there is hope for our future and for a normal life for all of our children. Without a robust defense of justice, the line between reality and nightmare may be very thin indeed.

References

1. Berger, E., & Jabr, S. (2020). Silencing Palestine: Limitations on free speech within mental health organizations. *International Journal of Applied Psychoanalytic Studies, 17*(2), 193–207.
2. Charlson, F., van Ommeren, M., Flaxman, A., Cornett, J., Whiteford, H., & Saxena, S. (2019). New WHO prevalence estimates of mental disorders in conflict settings. *Lancet, 394*(10194), 240–248. Retrieved 1 Sept 2019 from https://www.thelancet.com/journals/lancet/article/PIIS0140-6736(19)30934-1/fulltext.
3. Falk, R., & Tilley, V. (2017). *Israeli practices towards the Palestinian people and the question of apartheid.* Report commissioned by the United Nations Economic and Social Commission on Western Asia. Retrieved 1 Sept 2019 from https://onlinelibrary.wiley.com/doi/full/10.1111/mepo.12265.
4. Fanon, F. (2008). *Black skin, white masks* (trans: Philcox R.). New York: Grove.
5. Holmes, O. (2019). Officials at UN agency for Palestinians accused of ethical abuses. *The Guardian.* Retrieved 1 Sept 2019 from https://www.theguardian.com/world/2019/jul/29/officials-at-un-agency-for-palestinians-accused-of-ethical-abuses.
6. International Middle East Media Center. (2014). Sexual abuse against Palestinian child detainees reported. Retrieved 1 Sept 2019 from https://imemc.org/article/69791/.

7. Jabr, S. (2019). Palestinian barriers to healing traumatic wounds. *Middle East Monitor*. Retrieved 1 Sept 2019 from https://www.middleeastmonitor.com/20190820-palestinia n-barriers-to-healing-traumatic-wounds/.

8. Jabr, S., & Berger, E. (2015). An occupied state of mind: Clinical transference and coun-tertransference across the Israeli/Palestinian divide. *Psychoanalysis, Culture, and Society, 21*(1):21–40. Retrieved 1 Sept 2019 from https://link.springer.com/epdf/10.1057/ pcs.2015.46?shared_access_token=I5Ajl9gGKxCVvypFGM0X8FxOt48VBPO10Uv7D6sAg HtJ_kteR2YM4chn-MPGydynF5bM9sls5VjlozkeX873wLoxNb7kc3ArUYO4G9OUCnOow bSKDZJaNCK3nMXamWHRZT6gl0MJs1FcSkezYqyXPA5SVIuHvXFjtjzU4NznTX0%3D.

9. Jabr, S., & Berger, E. (2016). The survival and well-being of the Palestinian people under occupation. In H. Tiliouine & R. J. Estes (Eds.), *The state of social progress of Islamic societies: Social, political, economic, and ideological challenges*. Dordrech: Springer, Book Series in Quality of Life Research.

10. Jabr, S., & Berger, E. (2017). The trauma of humiliation in the Occupied Palestinian Territory. *Arab Journal of Psychiatry, 28*(2):154–59. Retrieved 1 Sept 2019 from http://arabjournalpsy-chiatry.com/wp-content/uploads/2017/11/%D8%A7%D9%84%D8%B9%D8%AF%D8%AF-%D8%A7%D9%84%D9%86%D9%87%D8%A7%D8%A6%D9%8A-%D9%84%D9%84 %D9%85%D8%AC%D9%84%D8%A9.pdf.

11. Jabr, S., & Berger, E. (2019). Palestine mental health network launches in Belgium. Washington Report on Middle East Affairs. Retrieved 1 Sept 2019 from https://www.wrmea.org/2019-june-july/palestine-mental-health-network-launches-in-belgium.html.

12. Jabr, S., & Berger, E. (forthcoming). The children of Palestine: Struggle and survival under occupation. In G. Rees, D. Benatuil, M. Lau, & H. Tiliouine (Eds.), *Handbook of children's security, vulnerability, and quality of life: Global perspectives*. Dordrecht NL: Springer, Book Series in Quality of Life Research.

13. Li, D. (2006). The Gaza strip as laboratory: Notes in the wake of disengagement. *Journal of Palestine Studies, 35*(2):38–55. Retrieved 1 Sept 2019 from https://www.palestine-studies.org/ jps/fulltext/41640.

14. Palestinian Central Bureau of Statistics. (2014). *Current status of Palestinian detainees in Israeli prisons*. Ramallah, Palestine: Press release; Retrieved 1 Sept 2019 from http://www. pcbs.gov.ps/Portals/_pcbs/PressRelease/Detainees_in_Israeli.pdf.

15. Palestine-Global Mental Health Network. (n.d.) website. Retrieved 1 Sept 2019 https://www. pgmhn.org/.

16. Said, E. (1978). *Orientalism*. New York: Vintage Books.

17. Sheehi, S. (2011). *Islamophobia: the ideological campaign against Muslims*. Atlanta: Clarity.

18. UK-Palestine Mental Health Network. (n.d.) website. Retrieved 1 Sept 2019 from https:// ukpalmhn.com/.

19. United Nations Development Programme. (2010). *Palestinian human development report,2009/2010: Investing in human security for a future state*. Retrieved 1 Sept 2019 from http://hdr.undp.org/sites/default/files/nhdr_palestine_en_2009-10.pdf.

20. United Nations Office for the Coordination of Humanitarian Affairs. (2019, June 20). *Wadi Yasul: A community at risk of mass displacement*. Retrieved 1 Sept 2019 from https://www. ochaopt.org/location/east-jerusalem.

21. USA-Palestine Mental Health Network. (n.d.) website. Retrieved 1 Sept 2019 from https:// usapalmhn.org/.

LGBTQ Global Mental Health: Ethical Challenges and Clinical Considerations

18

Rajkaran Sachdej

Abbreviations

AIDS	Acquired immunodeficiency syndrome
DSM	Diagnostic and Statistical Manual
FtM	Female to male
GRID	Gay-related immune deficiency
HIV	Human immunodeficiency virus
LGBTQ	Lesbian, gay, bisexual, transgender, and queer
LMIC	Low- and middle-income countries
MSM	Men who have sex with men
MtF	Male to female
PTSD	Post-traumatic stress disorder
STI	Sexually transmitted infection
WSW	Women who have sex with women

It is well-known in the field of psychiatry that lesbian, gay, bisexual, transgender, and queer (LGBTQ) populations are at elevated risk for a variety of mental health concerns. Yet, there are many LGBTQ persons around the world who knowingly or unknowingly are suffering from mental illness. Though interest in focused LGBTQ health is relatively new, there is very limited information already available for LGBTQ global mental health. As a niche population, LGBTQ persons around the world, who also have mental health concerns, are a unique, vulnerable population subset whose health needs have been overlooked.

R. Sachdej (✉)
Department of Psychiatry and Behavioral Sciences, George Washington University, Washington, DC, USA
e-mail: sachdej@gwu.edu

© Springer Nature Switzerland AG 2021
A. R. Dyer et al. (eds.), *Global Mental Health Ethics*,
https://doi.org/10.1007/978-3-030-66296-7_18

This chapter, written in response to the lack of focused research on LGBTQ global mental health, has multiple aims. In the first portion, the information presented is intended to shed light on a poorly researched and poorly understood topic. This will be accomplished by presenting what is already known from the little available research. This will hopefully help familiarize the reader with this population. The second portion of the chapter looks at ongoing challenges in this field of research and clinical practice setting. This includes notable ethical dilemmas typically encountered when discussing and/or caring for this population. This is presented with the intention of identifying gaps in knowledge as well as initiating conversation around LGBTQ global mental health so as to have the reader look at this group of individuals more critically and closely. The chapter will also discuss appropriate clinical considerations that may be applied by practitioners. Though not meant to be an evidence-based or comprehensive guide for clinical practice, these considerations are presented to challenge the reader to approach this population in a way to provide more comprehensive and compassionate care.

A crucial starting point is to first recognize many are not familiar with the terms regularly used in LGBTQ populations. Knowing the appropriate terms helps care providers better understand their patients, reduces ambiguity, can de-mystify certain concepts, and can clarify many misconceptions providers might have. More importantly, providers familiar with everyday terms reflect the provider's willingness to understand, and care for, this unique group.

Sexual Orientation An individual's sexual attraction, intimate relations, and/or emotional connection with individuals of a different or same gender.

- Lesbian—A woman who has a physical, romantic, or emotional attraction to other women.
- Gay—A man who has physical, romantic, or emotional attraction to other men.
- Bisexual—An individual who has physical, romantic, or emotional attractions to both men and women.
- Men who have sex with men (MSM)—Men who may or may not identify as gay or bisexual but have sexual encounters with other men.
- Women who have sex with women (WSW)—Women who may or may not identify as lesbian or bisexual but have sexual encounters with other women.
- Queer—An umbrella term for a variety of sexual orientations and gender identities but excluding heterosexuality.
- Questioning—Those individuals who are unsure of their sexual orientation and/or gender identity but may also engage in physical or emotional relationships with others of the same or different gender.

Gender Identity Refers to each person's profound individual experience of gender, which may or may not match with the person's sex assigned at birth.

- Transgender—Those whose gender identity and/or gender expression is different from their sex assigned at birth.
  - MtF—A male-to-female transgender individual.
  - FtM—A female-to-male transgender individual.
- Transition—The process in which a transgender person aligns their physical appearance with their gender identity.

Arif Khan (AK) is a 31-year-old Afghan male born in 1984. He is from the outskirts of Kandahar. AK's native language is Pashto and is able to speak some English. At the age of 12, AK was sexually assaulted multiple times by one of his father's friends, an "uncle". Upon the Taliban insurgency in his town, AK witnessed the hanging of his father, "uncle", and others in 2000 at the age of 16. His mother was beaten by the Taliban for unknown reasons. AK was a refugee displaced by war who was transferred to an Afghan refugee camp near Peshawar, Pakistan in 2003 at the age of 19 along with his mother and younger sister. They are now in the United States where AK works in construction and hopes to improve his English and complete his education. Although AK would identify himself as heterosexual, AK experiences shame and guilt around finding other men attractive. AK is referred to psychiatry clinic for post-traumatic stress disorder (PTSD), depression, and psychotherapy.

Part One: Background and Research

History is filled with various ways in which LGBTQ persons were viewed and dealt with in the past. In ancient Greece, homosexuality, or at least men having sex with other men, was viewed as commonplace in society. Chemical castration was used in the past as a punishment for homosexuality. Sadly, death sentences were also seen as a means to deal with LGBTQ persons. Even the field of medicine has alienated LGBTQ persons by confounding sexual practice with illness. At the beginning of its understanding in 1982, what is now known as AIDS was initially proposed to be called gay-related immune deficiency, or GRID [6]. Having been previously described as a "paraphilia" and "sexual orientation disturbance" in the earlier editions of The Diagnostic and Statistics Manual of Mental Disorders (DSM), non-heterosexual practices have only recently been narrowed to disorders, like Gender Dysphoria, in which persistent distress or impairment is necessary for diagnosis. How sexual orientation was regarded evolved over decades. The first DSM in 1952 classified homosexuality as a sociopathic personality disturbance before it was recategorized as a sexual deviation or sexual orientation disturbance in the DSM-II in 1968. Stonewall Riots in 1969 sparked controversial academic discussions eventually leading to addition and subsequent removal of ego-dystonic homosexuality in the DSM-III and DSM-III-R, respectively. The DSM-V now includes gender dysphoria considered outside of mental disorders (*The History of Psychiatry & Homosexuality; Working with LGBTQ Patients* [27]). Regardless of the era or locations, LGBTQ persons have had difficulty seamlessly integrating into the fabric of society or being seen as equal with their contemporaries.

The state of affairs for LGBTQ persons today is still antiquated in many ways. Research highlights various instances of clear discrimination. At least 72 members of the United Nations criminalize same-sex practices and/or homosexuality ([28]; see Fig. 18.1). Uganda is a country that has gone as far as introducing an anti-Homosexuality bill in 2014 in which an individual may be jailed for life for "aggravated homosexuality." The bill even criminalizes those who fail to report homosexual activity [30]. Globally, prominent negative stigma towards LGBTQ persons and practices is widespread, leading to dire health and psychosocial consequences. This ranges from religious excommunication [20], negative portrayals in media [30], and segregated medical services [24]. The poor distinction between illness and sexual orientation persists today in certain countries such as Dominica, Turkmenistan, and Indonesia where there is evidence to suggest same-sex practices can be "cured" with psychiatric intervention [3]. However, attitudes towards LGBTQ persons are not all binary or bleak. In some countries, certain factions of LGBTQ persons are more readily accepted by society based on religious or cultural factors. In Thailand, *kathoey*, or transgender women, are more readily accepted and visible than *tom*, transgender men [9]. Though often socially ostracized, transgender women known as *hijra* in South Asia hold religious significance in Hinduism. Same-sex practices are also being welcomed by some countries like Taiwan which recently legalized same-sex marriages [28]. Moreover, Pride marches around the world are attracting more and more positive attention towards LGBTQ matters.

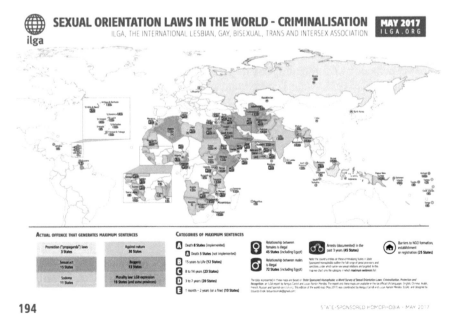

Fig. 18.1 Mapping out criminalization of LGBTQ practices (Source: Carroll and Mendos [3], page 194)

The available research looking specifically at mental health for LGBTQ populations around the world is sparse and can be argued to have little external validity. For one, the majority of available research is typically produced by the USA [1], thereby narrowing scope of research validity. However, the currently available research does touch on a few overarching topics including barriers to care as well as common risk factors, psychiatric pathologies, and comorbidities. It is notable to recognize the relative availability of research focused on LGBTQ refugees and transgender individuals.

Research points out numerous, mainly sociocultural and legal factors, that prevent adequate healthcare access for LGBTQ persons around the world. Regardless of sexual orientation, estimates for global psychiatric or substance-abuse disease burden are up to 15–20% with nearly 85% not receiving adequate treatment [10]. In many instances, gender remains a binary construct in the eyes of the law and culture. As such, the simple inability to recognize a third gender represents a barrier to care and resources (Thomas et al. 2017). The United Nations High Commissioner for Refugees [31] highlights the various forms of discrimination and resource exclusion experienced by LGBTQ persons around the world. These include, but are not limited to, exclusion from health care, protection, housing, education, employment, and social services [31]. Discriminatory laws, such as those in Uganda, instill structural violence and fear in LGBTQ individuals. Such hostile atmospheres not only reinforce the pre-existing local risk factors for psychiatric pathology (e.g., social isolation and trauma) but also deter LGBTQ individuals from coming forth for adequate health education and care [16]. As such, LGBTQ individuals may have to weigh priorities between personal safety and their health care when coming out publicly [16] or may not be as forthcoming about their healthcare needs [24]. Instances have been recorded where LGBTQ persons in such intimidating environments have been discouraged from seeking care [24].

It is clear that LGBTQ individuals are at risk for various psychiatric pathologies and comorbidities given the extensive list of psychosocial insults and/or trauma they tend to face and endure globally. A non-exhaustive list of trauma types includes physical, emotional, sexual, harassment, assault, resource discrimination, property damage, blackmail, extortion, forced prostitution, forced marriage, corrective rape, sexual orientation conversion, arbitrary arrests, and incarceration and even acts arguably described as torture [23, 30, 31]. With this in mind, it is important to note that these risk factors and experiences are not causal factors for same-sex practices. Studies indicate there is no evidence to suggest that men are more susceptible to have sex with other men in different parts of the world [6]. Additionally, any possible "causes" for sexual orientation or gender identity are unknown [7].

Much of the studies available focus on the prevalence of mood and trauma-related psychiatric disorders. With regards to mood disorders, it was observed there was no risk for depression that could be explained by homosexuality. However, both homosexuality and bisexuality are associated with increased risks for anxiety in certain statistical models [2]. Transgender individuals in certain populations showed a lower prevalence of depression [19]. It is important to note that sexual orientation was not, in itself, concluded to be a risk factor for mental illness [2]. Studies looking at trauma-based disorders consistently report cumulative, repetitive traumatic offenses towards LGBTQ persons leading to clinical pictures of "complex" or "insidious" trauma with an increased likelihood of psychiatric symptoms [7, 18, 23]. Substance use and abuse studies were limited and focused primarily on trans-gendered persons [19]. In addition, sexually transmitted infections (STIs), as a comorbidity to mental illness, were studied mainly in men who have sex with other men (MSM). These studies showed a growing STI burden in the MSM population. This pairs with the observation that gay men in urban areas are thirteen times more likely to engage in high-risk sexual practices and contract HIV [24].

Focused research attention was given to LGBTQ refugees and asylum seekers given the demand and current political atmosphere (*Rainbow Response* [17]). Some psychologically significant distinctions made for this community included the observation of stereotyped stressors as part of the migration process. Four core refu-gee stressors included traumatic, resettlement, acculturation, and isolation stress [14]. This included the asylum-seeking process in itself being both stressful and potentially re-traumatizing [18]. The LGBTQ refugee studies focused primarily on trauma and its relationship to PTSD, anxiety, and depression [14]. In addition to the previously cited conditions for non-displaced persons, common diagnoses included dissociative disorders, panic disorders, traumatic brain injuries, amnesia, somatiza-tion, and shame and despair [23].

JM is a 17-year-old female living in a suburban town outside Jakarta, Indonesia. Like many other young women in her community, she attends regular religious events and enjoys spending time with her friends. She has always found herself romantically uninterested in men and has, for many years, felt uncomfortable having breasts. She becomes particularly upset when she is menstruating. While researching online, she wonders if she is transgen-dered and has considered hormone replacement therapy. She is afraid to speak of this with her friends or a local gynecologist about this as she has heard about police brutality towards homosexual individuals in Jakarta. She intends to experiment with other women when she is on a school trip to Bangkok, Thailand.

Part Two: Challenges and Ethical Dilemmas

An obvious problem is the research itself. As always, research methods and the sociopolitical contexts in which the studies were conducted must always be consid-ered [19] when taking into account the validity. In many instances, LGBTQ global mental health research has been addressed from the standpoint of HIV, thereby con-flating sexual orientation and gender identity with disease status. Based off what studies are available, some might argue that LGBTQ global mental health, as an academic topic, is the study of gay men living with HIV, transgendered persons, and refugee settings. Even then, studies within these subsets, such as comparing trans-gender men and transgender women [9], remain limited. There is still a wide array of the LGBTQ population that is poorly understood, including lesbian women, those questioning their sexual orientation, and those who identify as pansexual. Other pertinent items that are sought after by researchers include mental health screening tools, the youth [24], psychotic disorders, personality disorders, gender transition and hormone use [9], and the influence of media and technology [15]. Clearly, the research in this field is not comprehensive, and there is much yet to learn about the mental health of LGBTQ persons around the world.

Though the concept of intersectionality may seem readily apparent to many LGBTQ persons, it is a social construct that may elude some. Coined in 1989, intersectionality looks at how the overlap of one's social identities (e.g., race, gender, socioeconomic class, and political views) may create specific means of discrimination [5]. In a Western paradigm, LGBTQ persons around the world may be categorized by their sexual orientation, country of origin, religion, political status, and mental illness. Each category and minority categorization combinations have their own associated inequities [22]. When it comes to marginalized identities, there may be an exponential effect of discrimination as opposed to an additive effect [15]. Though it is important to take into consideration in how one's identities play a role in their experiences and clinical findings [7, 12, 22], quantifying and operationalizing intersectionality as it pertains to LGBTQ global mental health are difficult [15].

One of the most challenging barriers to adequate mental health care for LGBTQ persons globally has to do with healthcare providers themselves. At a personal level, it is important for providers to remember their therapeutic role and set aside any personal prejudices that could hinder them from completing their roles. Mental health providers do not have the responsibility of encouraging an individual to "come out," reveal, or accept their sexual orientation. Though it is tempting to "free" the LGBTQ individual from the metaphorical closet, it is important to stray away from any savior complexes. Mental health providers can help LGBTQ individuals navigate the everyday challenges faced. However, how one navigates and handles their own internal and external struggles associated with their sexual orientation is not up to the care providers. It can be argued that a more proactive role could even be harmful and overwhelming. Revealing one's sexual orientation could be at odds with someone's personal morals or even alienate them, thereby potentially placing them in danger's way.

The provider should also be cognizant of the idea they may also have the potential to cause psychological harm by traumatizing or re-traumatizing LGBTQ individuals with their own alienating biases, assumptions, and practices [18]. How one understands, or rather misunderstands, the origins of non-heterosexual practices will influence how they perceive LGBTQ individuals and their care approaches. The conflation of non-heteronormative sexual practices and it being a "curable" illness are still recognized in a handful of countries and can be basis for involuntary psychiatric hospitalization [3]. As such, clinicians themselves can be seen as especially persecutory to an LGBTQ person who has faced trauma as a result of their sexual orientation. A psychiatric or psychological assessment could mimic traumatic interrogations and thereby have the potential to re-traumatize. Medical providers have also been cited for being involved in forced and clinically unnecessary anal examinations on MSM, thereby constituting physical harm and torture [4].

As care providers themselves need to be aware of their own implicit biases, presumptions, and attitudes, health care, as an institution, should also understand the heteronormative discourse it perpetuates [31]. Namely, this includes the idea that the LGBTQ population is a group of ill individuals or are distinct in being able to appreciate all aspects of the human experience, like marriage or parenting [1]. Simply because there should be an improved focus on LGBTQ global mental health, it is not to say there are no healthy, well-adjusted individuals.

How mental health clinicians approach psychotherapy can also present a significant challenge for this population. While therapy may be considered helpful for many individuals, the theoretical framework of therapy is often "Western" and focused on the emotional growth of the individual. Aside from the technical challenges of providing effective therapy in different cultural settings, the process of therapy and articulating one's emotions can be in conflict with one's beliefs and values [18]. In many cultures, openly speaking about emotions, especially for personal gain, is a foreign concept. Thus, efficacy of these modalities may be limited. On the contrary, the highly personal questions usually encountered during psychotherapy can mimic traumatic interrogations or asylum-seeking processes, thereby being seen as harmful. However, there can be a therapeutic role for certain populations like refugees [14].

One of the more obvious challenges faced by LGBTQ persons around the world is religion. While some organized religions have no explicit beliefs around sexual orientation or gender identity, religious texts and culturally associated practices are often used to isolate and discriminate against LGBTQ individuals. This includes religious excommunication of sex workers [20] leading to social isolation and media industries instilling homophobic Pentecostal ideologies [30]. Religious-based "conversion" therapies are still present in many other regions around the world [8]. As a recognized concern, only about 1.5% of United Nation member states have implemented bans on conversion-based therapies [3]. While personal faith may be seen as a protective factor against mental illness, religious beliefs undoubtedly remain a sensitive topic for some that is difficult to challenge.

While there are various challenges to adequately approaching mental health in LGBTQ individuals, the question arises of whether or not to treat the individual or the society in which they reside. As gleaned from the information presented, mental health issues faced by LGBTQ persons around the world are largely driven by societal and/or human rights factors. This thereby calls into question the role of the mental health provider. A human rights-based approach to helping such individuals may complicate a largely clinical field. While many sources suggest focusing on increasing support for rights-based community efforts (*The Lancet*), much of the training being provided to mental health providers in low- and middle-income countries (LMICs) is typically clinical and not focused around social change.

JG is a 24-year-old male from Guadalajara, Mexico and identifies as a homosexual male. Having been molested by a clergyman as a child, JG seldom attends church. He still identifies and lives by Christian values. He was beaten and kicked out of his home after his HIV medications were found among his belongings and refused to meet regularly with the clergyman who molested him as a child for his "sins". Since then, JG has found himself using more recreational heroin and subsequently finds it difficult to afford his rent and HIV-related medical bills.

Part Three: Considerations for Improvement

There are significant strides to be made to improve the mental health for LGBTQ individuals worldwide. Keeping the core ethical principles that drive health care in mind, there are generally three means by which mental health providers can improve the care they provide; education, clinical modifications, and advocacy. Beneficence and non-maleficence can be improved upon by educating mental health providers in the field as well as applying some alterations in clinical practice. Similarly, education and understanding varied cultural contexts and standards for patients may provide for improved recognition of one's autonomy or lack thereof. However, whether described as the principle of justice or social justice, most would say that it is an important component of bioethics. In the case of LGBTQ global mental health, advocacy is an important step to improve the lack of justice for this population.

Yet it is also pertinent to consider how one's culture colors the interpretation of medical ethics. The core ethical principles by which clinical mental health practices are based are arguably built from a modern Western social paradigm. While some care providers might find the process of psychotherapy helpful in addressing personal growth and autonomy, this may be at odds with the ethical values held by a patient based on their cultural background. This elicits the idea that although practicing LGBTQ global mental health guided by the principles of autonomy, beneficence, non-maleficence, and justice is ideal, it may not always apply or be plausible. Alternatively, the cultural background of the provider themselves, which includes what they have gathered and understood of LGBTQ individuals in their upbringing, may also affect care approaches. Issues arise with the mismatch of cultures between provider and patient. As such, understanding an individual's cultural context and personal ethical principles which is based upon their cultural background may be a more appropriate beacon for guiding therapeutic interventions.

Adequately educating mental health providers about the available research and unique challenges in LGBTQ global mental health is crucial. As mentioned earlier, starting this process early by introducing concepts in the curricula of health professionals will begin to prepare the upcoming generation of providers [1]. Certain countries are prioritizing research. Canada has funded the opening of a national research institute to focus on studies related to gender, sex, and health [26]. In particular, becoming familiar with the asylum-seeking and adjudication process allows providers to play a more supportive role for LGBTQ refugees with trauma [18, 23]. To this point, practical guides have been made to better assist mental health professionals given the increasing number of displaced individuals (*Rainbow Response* [17]).

However, education should go beyond facts, statistics, and patterns. Mental health providers should, in an attempt to better understand their patients, put efforts into educating themselves about the common LGBTQ subcultures and distinct risks of each group [31]. To accomplish this, providers should have a decent understanding of intersectionality. Just as important is maintaining a level of cultural competence and cultural humility requiring both professional and personal reflections to avoid making presumptive judgments of individuals [12]. The best educators are patients themselves, and it behooves mental health providers to be sensitive of what is and is not appropriate behavior when interacting with this population [31].

Possible clinical practices range from practical environmental changes to networking with community resources. Simply creating a welcoming, safe environment for this population can improve access to care [24]. This is especially important considering providers themselves can often be viewed as disciplinary or persecutory figures given past traumatic events [18]. This can be achieved by wearing a LGBTQ friendly pin on clothing or displaying the Pride flag somewhere visible. More importantly, being aware of any possible discriminatory attitudes and presumptions a provider might have and instead incorporating a welcoming attitude is crucial [1]. Safe spaces have also been created in the form group therapies specific to LGBTQ individuals from particular cultural backgrounds to promote a sense of community and peer support [18]. Alternatively, a safe environment may be achieved by bringing services into the patient's home with the option of telepsychiatry, an option which has potential to greatly increase access to care.

If individual providers do not feel they can meet the health and mental health needs of this patient population in culturally appropriate means, then they can refer patients to relevant community resources [14, 16, 31]. Both online and physical resources have been used. In Uganda, where there are prominent anti-LGBTQ laws, online peer networks for youths have been shown to improve education and health outcomes [24]. Programs like "Pehchan" in India mobilize the community to provide gender-affirming approaches to address health needs of the nation's transgender communities [21]. Similar such community partners are appearing in urban centers around the world.

Practicing LGBTQ global mental health invariably involves advocacy. There are innumerable examples of injustices and unethical practices faced by this community worldwide that providers have a role in ending by taking a stance against such practices [4]. In particular, laws that directly or indirectly discriminate against LGBTQ individuals perpetuate injustices and worsen upstream social determinants of health [10]. Thus, prioritizing political advocacy and community mobilization is of utmost importance to allow for the advancement of LGBTQ rights and health care [6, 13]. A top-down approach in policy change should, in theory, reduce oppression against LGBTQ persons worldwide and ultimately lead to an increase in mental healthcare utilization services [15]. However, a grassroots social movement may be what is needed to bring about social change. As seen in Brazil, new public health policies in the form of the "National Comprehensive LGBT Health Plan 2010" arose as a response to nationwide LGBTQ social movements [1].

The concern that follows is to discern who assumes the responsibility to bring about the aforementioned changes. Surely, mental health providers may have a significant impact in these arenas of change. However, it is important to think about barriers such as legal limitations abroad and the homophobic practitioner. From a clinical standpoint, supporting, training, and educating ancillary support workers in low- and middle-income countries will help mitigate the already evident lack of mental health providers worldwide [16]. Health organizations like the World Health

Organization should continue to pursue rights-based means to improve the mental health of LGBTQ persons [29]. Considering pre-existing historical post-colonial discourses and cultural barriers in place, those outside of health care in the humanities also have an important role in ushering change [25]. Still, it is of utmost importance to continue to involve and consult LGBTQ persons so as to give this population a means to voice and advocate for their views.

DB is a 48-year-old widow from Kampala, Uganda and is the mother of 2 college-aged children. She is struggling to come to terms with her son who has recently discreetly come out to her as gay. DB is being threatened by her intrusive neighbors to send her son away before they report him to the police for suspected homosexuality. She fears for her son's safety as he attends school.

At its current rate of interest and the evolving global atmosphere, there is a lot to look forward to in the field of LGBTQ global mental health. Care providers can look forward to more research as well as more academic discussion. This includes novel ways to acquire knowledge, such as the use of dating apps to discreetly recruit survey participants, as well as expansion of medical school and continuing education curricula. Today, social dating phone applications like Grindr now have corporate departments dedicated to social justice and harness these platforms and high user volume to educate and protect their users from oppression [11]. Beyond this, nuanced, targeted therapy modalities for this population may also be on the horizon using telepsychiatry or social media outlets [15]. These would all be to the effect of increasing access to mental health care and meeting the World Health Organization's agenda for 2030 in which no individual's mental health is left behind.

At large, however, though the field has much to look forward to and there is a sore lack of research to help drive change, there are larger more pressing issues faced by this particularly vulnerable community. Access to care, negative stigma, and even torture stem from the clear ethical violations of justice not being met. Without addressing these basic human rights issues enjoyed by more of the heterosexual community, there will continue to be a sore lack of knowledge to help LGBTQ persons worldwide. Like a nation unto itself, the LGBTQ community has a defined set of members, its own culture, its own language, and even its own flag that has evolved over time. It should be no surprise that this "nation" has its own unique mental health standards. It should be acknowledged in this new era that LGBTQ individuals around the globe struggling with mental health issues are not alone and there are indeed many around the world who understand their unique plight and the attention needed to adequately address their mental health.

AK is now 34 years old and has made significant progress in his mental health. He reports his PTSD and depression symptoms are adequately controlled with a combination of anti-depressants started two years after his initial visit as well as a bi-weekly group therapy run by a local Afghan community center. Though he still struggles with his sexual orientation, he notes he feels more comfortable around other men and intends to discreetly attend his city's upcoming PRIDE march with new friends he has made in his English class.

References

1. Alencar Albuquerque, G., de Lima Garcia, C., da Silva Quirino, G., Alves, M. J. H., Belém, J. M., dos Santos Figueiredo, F. W., da Silva Paiva, L., do Nascimento, V. B., da Silva Maciel, É., Valenti, V. E., de Abreu, L. C., & Adami, F. (2016). Access to health services by lesbian, gay, bisexual, and transgender persons: Systematic literature review. *BMC International Health and Human Rights, 16*, 2. https://doi.org/10.1186/s12914-015-0072-9.
2. Burns, R. A., Butterworth, P., & Jorm, A. F. (2018). The long-term mental health risk associated with non-heterosexual orientation. *Epidemiology and Psychiatric Sciences, 27*(1), 74–83. https://doi.org/10.1017/S2045796016000962.
3. Carroll, A., & Mendos, L. R. (2017). *State Sponsored Homophobia 2017: A world survey of sexual orientation laws: Criminalisation, protection and recognition*. International Lesbian, Gay, Bisexual, Trans and Intersex Association.
4. Cichowitz, C., Rubenstein, L., & Beyrer, C. (2018). Forced anal examinations to ascertain sexual orientation and sexual behavior: An abusive and medically unsound practice. *PLoS Medicine, 15*(3), e1002536. https://doi.org/10.1371/journal.pmed.1002536.
5. Crenshaw, K. (2015). Demarginalizing the intersection of race and sex: A black feminist critique of antidiscrimination doctrine, feminist theory and antiracist politics. *University of Chicago Legal Forum. 1989*(1). https://chicagounbound.uchicago.edu/uclf/vol1989/iss1/8.
6. de Vries, H. J. C., & Baral, S. (2017). Assessing the health and well-being of gay, bisexual and other men who have sex with men around the world. *Sexually Transmitted Infections, 93*(5), 303–304. https://doi.org/10.1136/sextrans-2016-052679.
7. Drescher, J., Roberts, L. W., & Termuehlen, G. (2019). Lesbian, gay, bisexual, and transgender patients. In *The APA publishing textbook of psychiatry* (7th ed., pp. 1185–1212). American Psychiatric Association.
8. El Feki, S. (2015). The Arab bed spring? Sexual rights in troubled times across the Middle East and North Africa. *Reproductive Health Matters, 23*(46), 38–44. https://doi.org/10.1016/j.rhm.2015.11.010.
9. Gooren, L. J., Sungkaew, T., Giltay, E. J., & Guadamuz, T. E. (2015). Cross-sex hormone use, functional health and mental well-being among transgender men (toms) and transgender women (Kathoeys) in Thailand. *Culture, Health & Sexuality, 17*(1), 92–103. https://doi.org/10.1080/13691058.2014.950982.
10. Gostin, L. O., Monahan, J. T., Kaldor, J., DeBartolo, M., Friedman, E. A., Gottschalk, K., Kim, S. C., Alwan, A., Binagwaho, A., Burci, G. L., Cabal, L., DeLand, K., Evans, T. G., Goosby, E., Hossain, S., Koh, H., Ooms, G., Roses Periago, M., Uprimny, R., & Yamin, A. E. (2019). The legal determinants of health: Harnessing the power of law for global health and sustainable development. *Lancet, 393*(10183), 1857–1910. https://doi.org/10.1016/S0140-6736(19)30233-8.
11. Harrison-Quintana, J. (2020). Sex and safety in the digital age. In *Bodies and barriers* (pp. 63–71). Oakland: PM Press.
12. Huminuik, K. (2017). Special competencies for psychological assessment of torture survivors. Transcultural Psychiatry, 54(2), 239–259. https://doi.org/10.1177/1363461516675561.
13. Lo, S., & Horton, R. (2016). Transgender health: An opportunity for global health equity. *Lancet, 388*(10042), 316–318. https://doi.org/10.1016/S0140-6736(16)30675-4.
14. Messih, M. (2016). Mental health in LGBT refugee populations. *American Journal of Psychiatry Residents' Journal, 11*(7), 5–7. https://doi.org/10.1176/appi.ajp-rj.2016.110704.
15. Muzyk, N. P. (2019). LGBT psychology and mental health: Emerging research and advances. *Psychiatry*, 1–6. https://doi.org/10.1080/00332747.2019.1565559.
16. Nagata, J. M. (2018). Challenges, health implications, and advocacy opportunities for lesbian, gay, bisexual, and transgender global health providers. *Global Health Promotion, 25*(3), 70–73. https://doi.org/10.1177/1757975916677504.
17. *Rainbow response: A practical guide to resettling LGBT refugees and asylees.* (n.d.) Heartland Alliance.

18. Reading, & Rubin, L. R. (2011). Advocacy and empowerment: Group therapy for LGBT asylum seekers. *Traumatology, 17*(2), 86–98.
19. Reisner, S. L., Poteat, T., Keatley, J., Cabral, M., Mothopeng, T., Dunham, E., Holland, C. E., Max, R., & Baral, S. D. (2016). Global health burden and needs of transgender populations: A review. *Lancet, 388*(10042), 412–436. https://doi.org/10.1016/S0140-6736(16)00684-X.
20. Scorgie, F., Vasey, K., Harper, E., Richter, M., Nare, P., Maseko, S., & Chersich, M. F. (2013). Human rights abuses and collective resilience among sex workers in four African countries: A qualitative study. *Globalization and Health, 9*(1), 33. https://doi.org/10.1186/1744-8603-9-33.
21. Shaikh, S., Mburu, G., Arumugam, V., Mattipalli, N., Aher, A., Mehta, S., & Robertson, J. (2016). Empowering communities and strengthening systems to improve transgender health: Outcomes from the Pehchan programme in India. *Journal of the International AIDS Society, 19*(3 Suppl 2), 20809. https://doi.org/10.7448/IAS.19.3.20809.
22. Shangani, S., Gamarel, K. E., Ogunbajo, A., Cai, J., & Operario, D. (2019). Intersectional minority stress disparities among sexual minority adults in the USA: The role of race/ethnicity and socioeconomic status. *Culture, Health & Sexuality*, 1–15. https://doi.org/10.1080/1369105 8.2019.1604994.
23. Shidlo, A., & Ahola, J. (2013). Mental health challenges of LGBT forced migrants. *Forced Migration Review, 42*, 9–10.
24. Silberholz, E. A., Brodie, N., Spector, N. D., & Pattishall, A. E. (2017). Disparities in access to care in marginalized populations. *Current Opinion in Pediatrics, 29*(6), 718–727. https://doi.org/10.1097/MOP.0000000000000549.
25. Spini, L. (2018). Ethics-based global health research for all, including women, children, indigenous people, LGBTQI, people with disabilities, refugees and other relevant stakeholders, especially in least developing countries and small island developing states in the global south. *Social Science & Medicine, 214*, 167–170. https://doi.org/10.1016/j.socscimed.2017.11.041.
26. Stewart, M., Kushner, K. E., Gray, J., & Hart, D. A. (2013). Promoting gender equity through health research: Impacts and insights from a Canadian initiative. *Global Health Promotion, 20*(1), 25–38. https://doi.org/10.1177/1757975913476903.
27. The History of Psychiatry & Homosexuality. (2012). https://www.aglp.org/gap/1_history/.
28. The Lancet, null. (2017). Advancing LGBTIQ rights. *Lancet. 389*(10085):2164. https://doi.org/10.1016/S0140-6736(17)31539-8.
29. Thomas, R., Pega, F., Khosla, R., Verster, A., Hana, T., & Say, L. (2017). Ensuring an inclusive global health agenda for transgender people. Bulletin of the World Health Organization, 95(2), 154–156. https://doi.org/10.2471/BLT.16.183913.
30. Winskell, K., Sabben, G., Pruitt, K. L., Allen, K., Findlay, T., & Stephenson, R. (2017). Young Africans' representations of the origins of same-sex attraction and implications for sexual and mental health. *Culture, Health & Sexuality, 19*(3), 366–380. https://doi.org/10.1080/1369105 8.2016.1225820.
31. Working with Lesbian, Gay, Bisexual, Transgender, and Intersex Persons in Forced Displacement. (2011). United Nations High Commissioner for Refugees.

The Ethics of Migration: Aspiring to Just Mercy in Immigration Policies

19

Suzanne Shanahan

We are all migrants through time.

—Mosin Hamid, Exit West

Introduction

Through a lyrical mix of magical realism and political fiction, Mosin Hamid's [1] *Exit West* makes clear the ubiquitous challenge of human movement. In every era, we tend to see the challenge as a unique crisis. But peoples always and everywhere have been on the move and other peoples have always and everywhere questioned their right to come, to stay, and to belong. If humanity is constituted by migration, it is also constituted by the impulse to exclude. Religious and legal traditions have over time and in different ways sought to either curb or reinforce that impulse. Borders have always been opening and closing.

Hamid, though, is making more than an empirical argument. He is making a prophetic and normative one as well. His novel reminds us that the human need for exit—to leave one's home in pursuit of a better, safer life—will become inevitable one day for all communities. Neither wealth nor education or opportunity can exempt us. All of us, you and I, our family, our friends will require understanding, compassion, and mercy when we are on the move. And make no mistake we will all be on the move one day, perhaps one day soon. Hamid asks us to consider this fact when we decide when and how we shut the door on another. Communities of senders will eventually all become communities of receivers. A world that does not recognize this fact is the dystopian nightmare world Hamid narrates in prosaic detail. Compassion

S. Shanahan (✉)
Kenan Institute for Ethics, Duke University, Durham, NC, USA
e-mail: suzanne.shanahan@duke.edu

© Springer Nature Switzerland AG 2021
A. R. Dyer et al. (eds.), *Global Mental Health Ethics*,
https://doi.org/10.1007/978-3-030-66296-7_19

for those exiting should be our point of departure in any policy prescription. When it comes to immigration, justice and mercy matter always and already.

Contemporary policy discussions about immigration present largely as political debates. We think of them as disagreements between right and left political perspectives. The standard characterization is that the political right advocates for more restriction and the political left advocates for less restriction. But immigration debates are always also ethical debates [2]. Debates are fundamental moral disagreements about what is right, just, fair, and good in liberal democratic states. Debates are not, in an of themselves, morally superior or inferior, they are just morally different. Immigration debates are also arguments about who we are and what we value. They are about what we ought to do and who we aspire to be. Public discourse on immigration is deeply personal and thus often more visceral.

This chapter explores the ethics of immigration and of contemporary immigration policies in Western liberal states. It puts in bold relief the moral arguments undergirding the current rancorous public debate on immigration policy globally. I argue first that by excavating the ethical principles implicit in the different poles of this debate, we might find a way forward that is consistent with principles of liberal democracy, that acknowledges the rights of individuals and states and that is fundamentally humane as well as just. I further argue, from a virtue ethics perspective, that if we start with a principle of compassion for the individual both open and closed borders can become more humane in practice. Compassion is about both what the policy is and how we implement it. To make this argument I draw heavily from the emergent literature on the ethics of immigration together with the work of two scholars in particular—Michael Blake [3] and Matthew Gibney [4].

This chapter is divided into three sections. The first outlines the challenge of contemporary immigration. The second provides an overview of the extant literature on the ethics of immigration. The third section advocates for a principle of compassion in immigration debates and policy. The chapter concludes with ethical wisdom from a 7-year old, Sudanese boy living in the United States under a temporary protected status visa. Compassion and kindness guide his decision making.

Contemporary Challenges of International Migration

Images of international migration—a child dead on the beach, boats filled with desperate families crossing the Mediterranean or the Timor Sea, frustrated crowds of migrants pushing at borders walls, children ripped from their parents' arms on the U.S. border—fuel the current debate about immigration. They also distort and misrepresent. The cynical rhetoric of swarms, invasions, floods, and armies of migrants misleads and frightens. Like the polarized public debate on immigration, media and political portrayals alternatively frame migrants as helpless innocents or job-stealing terrorists. Both formulations herald the impending global migration crisis and serve as a call to action. Both stereotypes belie the fact that orderly, legal migration is the norm and often a rather mundane part of daily life worldwide. Immigration is indeed everywhere.

So, what are the facts?[1] According to the UHCR's International National Migration Report [5], the number of international migrants (those who cross an international border) has almost doubled in the past decade. Today more than 277 million people live outside their country of birth. In 2019, forced displacement globally rose to almost 71 million [6]. And the total number of displaced persons grows by 37,000 daily. Refugees—individually fleeing their home country owing to a well-founded fear of persecution—constitute 25% of that increase. Europe hosts the largest number of international migrants with 82 million. The United States is the single largest country host to international migrants and India is the single largest source of international migrants. Women and girls comprise about 48% of the total. In this context, it is noteworthy that in 2019 when 111 countries were surveyed by UNHCR only 3% of countries had policies to lower current levels of legal migration. And almost 40% indicated a goal of increased migration. The majority favored policies to promote safe, orderly, and responsible migration.

In the United States, immigrants constitute almost 14% of the total population [7]. This percent has more than tripled since the 1970 record low of 4.7%. It is also slightly lower than the 1890 total of 15%. According to the U.S. Bureau of the Census, net immigration to the United States has been declining since 2016. While Mexicans are the largest foreign-born population at 25%, according to the U.S. Bureau of the Census, in 2018 China surpassed Mexico to become the largest sending country of foreign-born immigrants in the United States (U.S. Census Bureau). In 2019, the United States granted almost nine million visas, and in 2018 granted almost 40,000 asylum claims and admitted 22,405 refugees. The year prior the U.S. deported almost half a million individuals [8]. And according to the Brookings Institute (2019), the undocumented immigrant population in the United States is between 10 and 12 million or about 3.5% of the total population [9, 10]. Mexicans represent about half that total. And two-thirds of that population have resided in the United States for more than a decade.

In practice then it is hard to say we are experiencing a suddenly new and different wave of global migration. It would be fair, however, to say that "crisis" is the characterization most often employed in media and in public and popular discourse. The gap between what is actually happening in global migration and popular perception is rooted in two conceptual conflations and a third conceptual challenge in the evolution of international migration policy itself.

First, policy and practice are often conflated. Detaining young people who cross a border without documentation might well be legal. Indeed, detaining them in cages might also be legal. But for many people it is also unduly cruel and dehumanizing. In *Violent Borders* (2016), Reece Jones details the increasing fortification of, and growing violence around, borders. Jones himself challenges the legal and moral

---

[1] Note that I only discuss international migrants—or migrants who have crossed a national border. Within country migration or work or well-being is presumed higher than rates of international migration but is far less well documented. So while do have data on the more than 41 million internally displaced people and more than ten million stateless globally we do not have data on migrants within each country for a large sample of countries.

right of states to exclude migrants. But for many the concern is more limited. It is the violence that we see more and more around national borders that most people challenge, not the existence of the border itself [11]. It is the routine use of inhumane treatment and gratuitous violence as a migration deterrence strategy that so many find repugnant—unethical. The concern is often less with a policy that limits migration but more with the application of those limits—how they are enacted and enforced. Were boats full of desperate migrants not abandoned or turned around, were refugees not warehoused in uninhabitable offshore locations without basic amenities, were children not dying under trucks that carry them across borders, were soldiers not patrolling borders with lethal force the right of states to determine admission becomes far less controversial—at least in political debate and public discourse.

Second, distinct legal categories of migrants that matter significantly for the legal obligation they imply are conflated. The 1951 United Nations Refugee Convention emerged in the immediate post-war era to mark and detail the overwhelming international support for the protection of individuals, families, and communities fleeing persecution. Theorists, too, emphasized the special status of those fleeing persecution. Persecution for who you are and what you believe was understood to be fundamentally distinct from other human sufferings. Hannah Arendt most notably argued in *On Totalitarianism* [12] for the unique status of those migrating to escape persecution, "Man, it turns out, can lose all the so called right of man without losing his essential quality as man, his human dignity. Only the loss of polity itself expels him from humanity" (p. 297).

Since the 1951 United Nations Refugee Convention with more than 145 state signatories, most states continue to make both a rhetorical and a legal distinction between voluntary and forced migrants and those fleeing persecution in particular [13]. Voluntary migrants have a purported choice that forced migrants do not. The legal category has, over time, taken on moral significance. Forced migrants need and deserve compassion, voluntary migrants do not. This distinction is often cynically deployed by governments and media alike. To use the language of refugee is to invoke a worldwide legal and moral commitment. To use the language of migration does not carry the same legal or moral significance. The choice, for example, to use the language of the "migration crisis in the Mediterranean," is likely not unintentional [14].

Over time this distinction, however, has not been without critics and is often hard to maintain in practice. In recent decades, scholars and advocates have both criticized what they see as a false distinction. Pogge [15] makes one of the strongest cases, for example, that poverty and persecution are moral equivalents demanding a comparable treatment. This argument is echoed by the work of Kieran Oberman [16]. And others more recently have made clear the inextricable links between poverty and violence (See Cherem [17] for a discussion of analytic efforts to broaden the definition of refugee). Others still have argued that those fleeing the consequences of climate change should be considered refugees despite ongoing UN (2019) attempts to maintain the distinction [18, 19, 20].

For some, the greater moral claim can be made by not parsing the categories of migrants so finely. In *Home* (2015), Somali-British poet, Warsan Shire, also problematizes both the easy legal distinctions and popular misconceptions about the difference between forced and voluntary migration as well as the speciousness of distinctions between documented and undocumented migrants. Shire makes clear migration is really never anyone's first choice of life path.

> No one leaves home unless / home is the mouth of a shark.
> You only run for the border / when you see the whole city / running as well/

The third tension made manifest in the gap between perceptions and realities of migration is rooted in the relationship between the Refugee Convention and other post World War international legislation. The 1951 Refugee Convention is particularly significant because, unlike other international conventions relevant to the rights of migrants, this Convention details the rights of both individuals and states. These rights are reciprocal. That both the rights of states and of individuals are outlined in the 1951 Convention on Refugees and the absence elsewhere is part of the moral claim to inclusion for many. That is, Article 13 of the 1948 Universal Declaration of Human Rights upholds the freedom of movement as a human right noting that everyone has both the right to freedom of movement and residence within the borders of each state, and the right to leave any country, including his own, and to return to his country. The UDHR's affirmation of individuals' freedom of movement has an oft-cited flaw [21]: while individuals have the right to leave a country they do not have a parallel right to enter another country. Entry is the right of states. Except, of course, when you are fleeing persecution. Logically then there is an asymmetry between the right to exit and the right to enter and who arbitrates these rights—states or individuals. But there is a moral asymmetry as well. It is to this legal and moral asymmetry and how scholars have attempted to reconcile it that I now turn.

The Extant Literature on the Ethics of Immigration

I teach a course on immigration law and policy to first-year students at an American liberal arts college. And like many young people across the United States, the students generally decry the injustices of current restrictive immigration policies. And many impugn the ethical character of those developing the policies. The implicit argument is un-subtle. Bad people advocate for more closed borders and good people advocate for more open borders. Bad people are the reason parents need to risk the lives of their children crossing deserts in search of a better life; bad people are the reason we have people in indefinite detention in liberal democracies around the world.

There are three problems with this logic. First, it is a mistake to assume that it is the inherent malevolence of individuals and the inhumanity of societies that leads to these policies. There is little acknowledgment that closed borders like open borders are framed by ethical logic, a theory of justice, and an aspiration to do the right thing. Again, both make strong justice claims [22]. The second problem is that it confuses policy and practice. Children do not have to be in cages for immigration policies to be restrictive. And the third problem is that my students' perspective on immigration lacks context. There is a Kantian sensibility to their perspective. But when asked what they would personally sacrifice to maintain open borders the answer is usually "very little." And when asked if there should be broad exceptions for the health and well-being of citizens the answer is "of course." There are clear limits to their advocacy of open borders. Until pressed, the views of my students, like most public political debates on immigration, lack nuance.

David Miller [23] frames it thus: "the public debate on immigration generates much heart, but little light." The rhetorical sides are sharply drawn and push both camps to an unhelpful extremism. And here is where political theorists and moral philosophers have sought to fill the gap. The relatively nascent literature on the ethics of immigration illuminates and elaborates upon the normative assumptions we often and unconsciously make as individuals about immigration. If we can see the moral underpinnings might we be less dismissive?

In this section, I review this emergent literature on the ethics of immigration. Philosophical debates about immigration ethics are largely a late twentieth-century development. Indeed, the absence of earlier scholarly reflection or engagement with immigration is noteworthy [23]. Two early articulations appear in the work of Immanuel Kant (1795) and Henry Sidgwick [24] almost 100 years apart. In *Perpetual Peace* (1795) Kant writes of a natural right of hospitality and the need for those arriving in a territory not their own to be treated without hostility. But Kant limited his argument to those newcomers and strangers who were coming via commerce and not those coming to settle. Philosopher Henry Sidgwick spelled out an early states' rights perspective in a relatively brief discussion of the immigration question in his *Elements of Politics* (1891)

> A State must obviously have the right to admit aliens on its own terms imposing any such conditions on entrance or tolls on transit, and subjecting them to any legal restrictions or disabilities that it may deem expedient. It ought not, indeed, having once admitted them, to apply to them suddenly, and without warning, a harsh differential treatment: but as it may legitimately exclude them altogether, it must have a right to treat them in any way they see fit, after due warning given and due time allowed for withdrawal (Sidgwick [24]: 248)

Put differently, for Sidgwick states have no extant obligation to consider the interests of immigrants themselves.

Current scholarly engagement with the ethics of immigration owes its origin to the 1980s debate between Joseph Carens [25] and Michael Walzer [26]. It was here that the open versus closed border debate emerge and with it, the question of whose rights and interests—individuals or states—should prevail. In some sense, this debate was never a pure either or but rather a more or less. More individual and more open or more state and more closed. For Walzer, decisions about community membership are up to the community. Walzer argues that communities of character where there is a strong sense of common good, share history, and values demand more closure. Like Rawls [27], democracy thus demands a degree of closure. For Carens, the moral claim of states to their territorial integrity and the coinciding right to police their borders is far more limited. Again, for Carens and Waltzer like their more contemporary counterparts Wellman and Cole [28] "The argument is about rights, the state's right to control membership versus and individuals right to the freedom of international movement" (p. 7).

Simplistically, legitimate states possess the right to control their borders, deciding who enters and who does not. Legally, the right to sovereignty and territorial integrity remains fundamentally intact internationally as an operating principle. Whether and to what extent states ought rightly exclude continues to dominate the scholarship on the ethics of immigration. That is, according to Caspino and Lenard ([13]: 493) "Normative political theory over the recent decades has focused mainly on what ought to be done as far as migration policies are concerned. It faces a basic challenge, which seems from two competing, yet equally fundamental ideas underpinning liberal democratic societies: a commitment to moral universalism and the exclusionary requirement of democracy....how to reconcile state-based exclusion with a commitment to equal moral concern for all persons."

According to Blake [29], the so-called open borders position claims liberal states do not have the right to exclude unwanted outsiders or exert coercion or force in preventing migrants' entry [30]. For open border scholars, state borders are unjust, arbitrary, coercive, and reinforce inequality [3]. Three inter-related arguments are commonly cited [31, 32, 33]. The first argument is the symmetry argument positing that freedom of movement between states should mirror freedom of movement between states. For Carens [31] and others, there is a fundamental lack of consistency in upholding the liberal value on freedom of movement within states but not between states. In contrast for Blake [29] and Hosein [2], the freedom of movement is a privilege of membership not unlike voting.

The second invokes a more frequently cited moral asymmetry between the individual human right to exit and to enter [21]. Proponents of this argument note that the right to exit cannot be fully realized without the corresponding right to enter. So, if we are to respect the former, we must allow the latter. Christopher Heath Wellman (2011) makes a colorful analogy to counter this view ([28], p. 197–203). Wellman compares the right to exist to the right to marry. The latter right does not imply you have the right to marry anyone you choose. Similarly, for Blake ([29]: 525) there is an important distinction between exit and entry. Blake notes

....there is a rather important moral difference between my being unable to move because my government won't let me depart, and my being unable to move because some other government won't let me enter. Legitimate governments... are not allowed, consistent with their liberalism, to prevent subjects from leaving....The coercive act of exclusion is morally distinct from the coercion involved in the prevention of emigration.

The third argument for open borders is, for many, the most compelling. Indeed, for scholars like Javier Hidalgo [34], this global distributive justice argument serves as a powerful call to action and indeed civil disobedience. This perspective begins with the obvious fact that borders are, in some ways, arbitrary historical artifacts and a residue of colonialism. For Cole (2011), as colonial social constructions, they only maintain colonial privilege and are inconsistent with the prevailing universalism in contemporary liberal thought. State control of borders unjustly maintains global distributive injustice [35]. Thus, for Cole, justice both morally and practically demands the removal of barriers to entry. Skeptics worry open borders are only one cause of this injustice and likely only a weak and ineffective response to growing global inequality.

Hildago ([34]: 204) remains steadfast in the face of pragmatic critique instead calling forth the better angels of our nature:

> We can also situate our own actions to oppose unjust immigration restrictions in a bigger narrative of moral progress. Taking this broader perspective can help us to ward off despair. If we're part of a larger and progressive struggle against injustice, then this can motivate us to be steadfast, to refuse to participate in injustice, and to be for opportunities to effectively advance the ideal of open borders.

In this way, Hildalgo [34] appeals to both our sense of justice as well as the difference between who we are as a society and who we might aspire to become. I take up the question of justice and what we ought to do, in the next section.

Arguments in support of exclusion are also multiple and are based on an interpretation of the rights of individuals and the rights of states. Wellman (2011: 7) makes a multidimensional case for exclusion, noting "whether they [states] exercise this right rationally or not, it is their call to make." Wellman (p. 11) continues, "[I]n my view, legitimate political states are morally entitled to unilaterally design and enforce their own immigration policies, even if these policies exclude potential immigrations who desperately want to enter." His argument invokes both rights to self-determination and individuals' right to free association (including the right not to associate). States being made up of individuals possessing the right of freedom of association can refuse to admit certain immigrants. Self-determination means that legitimate states can determine their own path and that includes the right not to associate.

Similarly, Pervnick [36] makes an individual property right argument to bootstrap states' right to exclude. He argues that citizens have through their work and financial contributions to a state made possible state institutions and as such have property rights like claims to that state. Thus, in the same way that we can prevent a guest from coming to our home, we can prevent a migrant from entering the state in which we are as citizens.

In contrast, Blake [29] makes more of a jurisdictional argument about a states' rights to control the resources within their territory and how that leads to a states' right to exclude. Importantly, neither theorists understand this right to be absolute. For Blake, the relationship to human rights law is important noting the critical role states play in securing these rights. That is, they are rights largely operational within states.

David Miller [23] is probably the best-known proponent of states' rights to exclude. In his 2016 *Strangers in our Midst*, Miller frames his argument in terms of four principles. First, is a weak cosmopolitanism wherein all human beings are of equal worth but we invariably favor our fellow citizens. Of course, there are times where we must open our borders to fend off the most egregious of human rights violations, but in general, the needs and interests of citizens come first. The second principle is self-determination. Here, Miller [23] argues that citizens in any democratic society should have the right to decide on anything that might qualitatively alter that society—like immigration. The third principle is fairness. Would be immigrants need to be able to see and understand decisions and policies as reasonable. The fourth principle is probably the most controversial yet also most rooted in the legacies of Walzer [26] and Rawls [27]: social integration. Cultural cohesion is critical in any liberal democratic state, especially any welfare state. Expectations of integration and mutual cultural respect are pre-conditions for democracy.

What is most striking in the literature on the ethics of immigration is how ethically robust both the open borders and exclusion perspectives are in significant contrast to how they are characterized in political debate and public discourse.

When Law and Policy Are both Just and Merciful

Here in this third section, I try to explicitly move beyond the central duality— between open and closed borders—in the ethics of immigration literature. I argue that neither framework is, per se, good or bad, ethical or unethical. Both are rooted in a theory of justice. But justice alone is insufficient. Policy implementation must also be merciful. Indeed, I argue that a merciful practice is what makes for an ethical policy. To make this argument, I draw most centrally upon the work of Matthew Gibney [4] and Michael Blake [3].

In his work on refugee law and policy, Matthew Gibney [4] builds upon Miller [23] and others to note the ethical value of both more inclusive and more exclusive migration policies. Gibney offers a form of practical humanitarianism to guide state policy. To make this argument, Gibney asserts that states are always more partial (giving greater moral weight to the rights and needs of its own citizens) or more impartial (giving equal weight to the rights and need of citizens and non-citizens). The partial perspective, often shared by conservatives and nationalist alike, argues that the state's need for political and cultural autonomy morally justifies placing the interests of their own citizenry ahead of any other individuals. On the other hand, global liberal and utilitarian perspective support an impartial perspective. Here, states are obligated to consider the whole of humanity in making decisions about who enters and who does not. For Gibney where we ought rightly to land on this continuum is a place that is both ethical and practical. For any policy to be effective underlying ethical principles need to be actionable. For Gibney therefore, immigration policies can never in policy or practice be immutable we must always be attentive to the on-the-ground conditions—including the viability politically of any particular policy—before we lean fully one way or the other. One way is not always bad and the other way is not always good.

Blake's [3] call to mercy in immigration policy has parallels to Gibney's [4] insistence on context. In *Justice, Migration, Mercy,* Blake [3] builds on the ethics of care, to advocate for human decency in our immigration policy. Adherence to the law is insufficient.

> In ordinary life, we can be terrible people without actively violating rights. We can be cruel, callous, vicious, petty, and so on—and can do so without necessarily doing any actions considered unjust....I will use the concept of mercy here as a way of getting at the distinct moral virtue involved in doing more than simply failing to violate the obligations of justice. (p. 8).

In contemporary debates about immigration, it is in fact the policy *in practice* not the policy itself that often deeply offends. We may believe in rules for immigration, we may believe in limits to immigration, and still insist that those attempting to migrate be treated with respect and human dignity. We may believe in open borders, we may believe the rights of individuals within a state and beyond a state are identical, but we still want mercy to govern how these policies are deployed.

Blake offers a way of enacting policy, or practice if you will, that is applicable for both open or closed borders. "The state is defined as a moral agent most powerfully and directly by how it treats those to whom it has no particular obligations, and who themselves possess the least power to contest what is done... migration is an area in with we might find out a great deal about the character of wealthy states and the character of those who guide those states" (p. 209). Again, what I argue here is that both inclusive and exclusive policies can be the just and ethical path, the right thing to do, if merciful. But they can also be both the wrong thing to do if unmerciful.

Like Hildalgo's call for civil disobedience, Blake [3] invites us to consider a higher principle of being. He sets an aspirational standard for states using the language of a duty of care as well as for us as individuals and members of communities.

> I have defended the thought that a society ought to do more than simply avoid injustice. It should, instead, act in accordance with the distinct demands of mercy—which I understand to involve a principled reason to refrain from certain forms of hard treatment, even when one might engage in that harshness without injustice. The merciful act is done out of a recognition that the one who is vulnerable to us is human; her plans mean as much to her as ours do to us. The practice of mercy represents a way in which this fact is brought home to us, as citizens and as persons. It reflects the need to see human beings as valuable, as worthy of consideration—rather than as mere burdens, or as somehow morally unlike ourselves.... Mercy, in short, can help us come to grips with the ethics of policy, by extending our ethical toolkits beyond the concepts of justice and of the moral right. (p. 223).

But again, part of the current tension in the debate on immigration is that national policies implicate our collective ethos and our individual identities. We recoil at unjust national institutions because they reflect upon us that injustice. In a memoir about his lifelong advocacy for death row inmates, *Just Mercy* (2015), Bryan Stevenson, like Blake, advocates for a legal justice tempered by mercy for the individual. Stevenson makes clear we need both merciful institutions and merciful people. He like Hamid in *Exit West* reminds us we can follow the rules and still be wrong, unfair, unmerciful. "Finally, I've come to believe that the true measure of our commitment to justice, the character of our society, our commitment to the rule of law, fairness, and equality cannot be measured by how we treat the rich, the powerful, the privileged, and the respected among us. The true measure of our character is how we treat the poor, the disfavored, the accused, the incarcerated, and the condemned." ([37]: 5). The very same could be said of our immigration policies.

Conclusion

In this chapter, I have argued for a more compassionate, merciful approach to international migration policy and practice. The extant immigration debate in both public and in the scholarly literature, surrounding borders and inclusion is not a simple matter of right and wrong. It is a debate about competing theories of justice. Indeed, the debate is so hard to reconcile precisely because both inclusion and exclusion theorists and advocates make just claims [22]. In the case of inclusion, justice requires porous borders to ensure the rights of all humanity are protected and promoted. In the latter, justice demands exclusionary borders because citizens have legitimate claims over the exclusive use and enjoyment of their opportunities and advantages. Whether inclusion or exclusion frames state policy, the principle of justice obtains. Where policies err is when their deployment is unmerciful, when policies do not consider the particular implications of their application. We need always to consider, for example, the long-term human impact of a child held in a cage, separated from a parent, or an adult held in indefinite detention. If mercy is a virtue, then exclusive borders require it no less than inclusive one.

As I write this conclusion, we are amidst a historically unprecedented moment in the history of the modern liberal democratic state. A global pandemic has meant the closing of borders around the world and radical curtailing of the right to freedom of movement even within countries. The hard-fought open borders in Europe are closed. The once porous border between Canada and the United States is sealed. Even U.S. states are seeking to exclude individuals from other U.S. states. Billions of people globally are under stay at home orders. This moment puts in bold relief the precarity of our global migration regime. But it also affirms the importance of compassionate policies and practice that acknowledge different situations and circumstances. It seems surely trite to note that the way individuals and communities respond to crisis speaks to their values. The current "crisis" of migration is no different.

A 7-year old Sudanese refugee describes his birthday party plans and in doing so makes an astoundingly powerful analogy to immigration policy. He is having a big party. He is inviting his whole class to his birthday party not because they are friends but because it is the kind, humane thing to do. "Parties are like countries," he explained: "Sometimes you need to include people you don't really know or like because it is the right thing to do...." When asked what would happen if his parents therefore could not afford his vision of hamburgers and cake if so, many came he quipped back, "Then I guess we will only have cake." Sometimes doing the right thing takes personal sacrifice. And what if someone in the group was a bully to others, would they still get an invite? "No, then that's not fair to hurt someone else."

The virtues that matter are quite clear to a 7-year-old. And kindness, compassion, and mercy matter.

Malik and his family are in the United States on Temporary Protected Status visas—a non-permanent mechanism established by the U.S. Congress through the 1990 Immigration Act to offer time delimited refugee status to individuals from countries experiencing armed conflict, environmental disaster, or extraordinary and temporary conditions. Malik's parents are fighting deportation for having an "insufficient fear" of persecution in South Sudan. This, of course, Malik does not know.

References

1. Hamid, M. (2017). *Exit west: A novel*. London: Riverhead Books.
2. Hosein, A. (2019). *The ethics of migration: An introduction*. New York/London: Routledge.
3. Blake, M. (2020). *Justice, migration and mercy*. New York: Oxford University Press.
4. Gibney, M. J. (2004). *The ethics and politics of asylum: Liberal democracy and the response to refugees*. Cambridge: Cambridge University Press.
5. United Nations, Department of Economic and Social Affairs, Population Division. (2019). *International migration 2019: Report*. https://www.un.org/en/development/desa/population/migration/publications/migrationreport/docs/InternationalMigration2019_Report.pdf.
6. United Nations, High Commissioner for Refugees. (2019). Global trends. Forced displacement in https://www.unhcr.org/globaltrends2019/.
7. Capps, Randy, Kathleen Newland with Susan Fratzke, Susanna Groves, Gregory Auclair, Michael Fix, and Margie McHugh, Migration Policy Institute. (2015). The integration outcomes of U.S. refugees, https://www.immigrationresearch.org/system/files/UsRefugeeOutcomes-FINALWEB.pdf.
8. USA Facts. Immigration. (2019). https://usafacts.org/issues/immigration/?utm_source=google&utm_medium=cpc&utm_campaign=immigration&gclid=Cj0KCQjw6_vzBRCIARIsAOs54z4Uguf2ZfdOMdT8NKnfSjTgmn7v2a8ylvapFylgRZi45kcla2Nt-k7AaAmjlEALw_wcB.
9. Kant, I. (1970). Perpetual peace: A philosophical sketch. In H. Reiss (Ed.), *Kant's political writings*. Cambridge, UK: Cambridge University Press. pp. 93–130.
10. Kamarack, E., & Stenglein, C. (2019, Nov 12). *How many undocumented immigrants are in the United States and who are they?* Brookings Institute. https://www.brookings.edu/policy2020/votervital/how-many-undocumented-immigrants-are-in-the-united-states-and-who-are-they/.
11. Jones, R. (2016). *Violent borders: Refugees and the right to move*. London: Verso.
12. Arendt, H. (1966). *The origins of totalitarianism* (new ed.). New York: Harcourt, Brace & World.
13. Crispino, A. E. G., & Lenard, P. T. (2014). New challenges in immigration theory: An overview. *Critical Review of International Social and Political Philosophy, 17*(5), 493–502. https://doi-org.proxy.lib.duke.edu/10.1080/13698230.2014.919055.
14. Malone, B. (2015, Aug 20). Why Al Jazeera will not say Mediterranean "migrants." https://www.aljazeera.com/blogs/editors-blog/2015/08/al-jazeera-mediterranean-migrants-150820082226309.html.
15. Pogge, T. (1997). Migration and poverty. In V. Bader (Ed.), *Citizenship and exclusion*. Macmillan. pp. 12–27.
16. Oberman, K. (2011). Immigration, global poverty, and the right to stay. *Political Studies, 59*(2), 253–268. https://doi-org.proxy.lib.duke.edu/10.1111/j.1467-9248.2011.00889.x.
17. Cherem, M. (2015). Refugee rights: Against expanding the definition of a "defugee" and unilateral protection elsewhere. *Journal of Political Philosophy, 24*(2), 183–205.

18. Lonesco D. (2019, June 6). *Let's talk about climate migrants, not climate refugees*. United Nations. https://www.un.org/sustainabledevelopment/blog/2019/06/lets-talk-about-climate-migrants-not-climate-refugees/.
19. Wennersten, J. R., & Robbins, D. (2017). *Rising tides: Climate refugees in the twenty-first century*. Bloomington: Indiana University Press.
20. Kent, A. & S. Behrman. (2018). Facilitating the Resettlement and Rights of Climate Refugees. London: Routledge.
21. Fine, S., & Ypi, L. (Eds.). (2016). *Migration in political theory: The ethics of movement and membership*. Oxford: Oxford University Press.
22. Camacho-Beltran, E. (2019). Legitimate exclusion of would-be immigrants: A view from global ethics and the ethics of international relations. *Social Science, 8*(8), 1–19. https://doi.org/10.3390/socsci8080238.
23. Miller, D. (2016). *Strangers in our midst: The political philosophy of immigration*. Cambridge, MA: Harvard University Press.
24. Sidgwick, H. (1897). *The elements of politics* (2nd ed.). London: Macmillan.
25. Carens, J. H. (1987). Aliens and citizens: The case for open borders. *Review of Politics, 49*(2), 251–273.
26. Walzer, M. (1983). *Spheres of justice: A defense of pluralism and equality*. New York: Basic Books.
27. Rawls, J. (1993). *Political liberalism*. New York: Columbia University Press.
28. Wellman, C. H., & Cole, P. (2011). *Debating the ethics of immigration: Is there a right to exclude?*. Oxford: Oxford University Press.
29. Blake, M. (2014). The right to exclude. *Critical Review of International Social and Political Philosophy, 17*(5), 521–537. https://doi.org/10.1080/13698230.2014.919056.
30. Wilcox, S. (2009). Open borders debate on immigration. *Philosophy Compass, 4*(5), 813–21.
31. Carens, J. H. (2013). *The ethics of immigration*. New York/Oxford, UK: Oxford University Press.
32. Abizadeh, A. (2008). Democratic theory and boarder coercion: no right to unilaterally control your own borders. Political Theory, 36(10), 38–65.
33. Huemer, M. (2010). "Is there a right to immigrate?" Social Theory and Practice, *36*(3), 429–61.
34. Hildalgo, J. S. (2019). *Unjust borders: Individuals and the ethics of immigration*. New York/London: Routledge.
35. Sager, A. (2018). *Toward a cosmopolitan ethics of mobility: The migrants-eye view of the world*. New York: Palgrave Macmillan.
36. Pevnick, R. (2011). *Immigration and the constraints of justice: Between open borders and absolute sovereignty*. Cambridge/New York: Cambridge University Press.
37. Stevenson, B. (2015). *Just mercy: A story of justice and redemption*. New York: Spiegel & Grau.

Part VI

New Horizons and Ethical Considerations

Restorative Justice: Principles, Practices, and Possibilities

20

William M. Timpson

Restorative Justice, Core Principles, and Community Mental Health

Justice is a core principle in both ethics and law. The word "justice" has different connotations depending on the context. In its broadest sense, justice means fairness, impartiality. To someone who has been wronged, "justice" may mean seeing that the wrongdoer is punished. This form of justice is understood as "retributive justice" and will be distinguished here from "restorative justice," a process which emphasizes the need to repair the damage done through honest self-assessment, negotiation, mediation, and reparation. In both these forms of justice establishment and acknowledgment of the facts, the realities of the situation in question, is an important part of the process. In a criminal or civil court proceeding, this coming to the "facts" of the case depends on established standards of "evidence." In Restorative Justice, "the acknowledgment" of the reality is more personal at the level of the persons and communities involved.

Historically, Restorative Justice began in Canada in the 1970s and has gradually gained acceptance in the United States and elsewhere [2, 26]. In fact, many ancient traditions have stressed the importance of personal responsibility, community involvement, acknowledgment of the truth, and attempts at reconciliation. Globally, one could cite, truth and reconciliation processes employed in South Africa after the apartheid era, Rwanda after the 1994 genocide, where so many people were involved that the legal system was overwhelmed and community *gacaca courts* (people on a lawn, grass justice) assessed the testimony of people who were involved and wished

W. M. Timpson (✉)
School of Education, Colorado State University, Fort Collins, CO, USA
e-mail: william.timpson@colostate.edu

© Springer Nature Switzerland AG 2021
A. R. Dyer et al. (eds.), *Global Mental Health Ethics*,
https://doi.org/10.1007/978-3-030-66296-7_20

to make amends. Another notable example is Chile after the Pinochet atrocities [7]. Perhaps less well known, but no less significant, the City of Greensboro, North Carolina, employed a Truth and Acknowledgment commission to review the history of the 1979 "Greensboro Massacre", a clash between the Ku Klux Klan and a group calling itself the Communist Workers Party. Also, the Canadian government employed acknowledgment processes to review its own history of moving and isolating native Canadians to remote islands near the Arctic in order to claim that the islands were inhabited. These various movements draw on traditional cultures from Maori, to Native American (and Canadian) to Indian to Christian to maintain fairness and impartiality in systems of justice and in response to injustice. Principles of Restorative Justice have relevance at local community levels and at the level of international justice, conflict resolution, and peacemaking. In the international context, these processes are sometimes called "transitional justice" as a country moves from one phase to another.

By embracing these core concepts of restorative justice, mental health professionals and their allies, educators and social workers, legislators and government staff, church and community leaders, can shift from policing and courts to a much broader application that emphasizes responsibility, ethical decision-making, accountability, openness, and reconciliation for offenders and victims alike.

With a background in educational psychology, I have worked locally and internationally, in a variety of settings and with different emphases, to better understand those variables that help to explain why, when, where, and how restorative approaches can be successful. I draw from longstanding research and practice on the underlying learning and development theories, the role of motivation, how communication supports cooperation, critical, ethical, and creative thinking, and more with special attention to areas of compelling complexity like restorative justice, diversity, sustainability, peace, and reconciliation that can be addressed through case study analysis and other alternative approaches [12, 19, 21, 22].

Given that, I will identify this shift in emphasis from what happens in retributive justice, from a focus on punishment to a commitment to healing and learning, from fines and jailing to community service, from an ethic of avoiding arrest to one of accepting responsibility for illegal actions and societal impact.

Young people can get in trouble for any number of reasons. In my local community (Fort Collins, Colorado) I have worked most closely with those who have been caught shoplifting, but I have seen others arrested for stealing in schools or trespassing, for firing an air gun within city limits, and for setting off firecrackers on busy downtown streets. College students have been caught stealing traffic cones for their dorm rooms and for hosting parties that got out of hand. The same restorative principles that are in play locally can also be seen in a variety of international contexts, i.e., openness, responsibility, accountability, ethical decision-making, self-reflection, learning, healing, peacebuilding, and reconciliation.

Table 20.1 Outcomes for Criminal and Restorative Justice

Criminal Justice	Restorative Justice
Crime is a violation of the law and the state that have responsibilities to protect the innocent	Crime is a violation of people and the relationships that underlie community well-being
Violations lead to convictions	Violations create obligations and a need for healing
Justice requires the state to establish blame and impose punishment	Victims, offenders, and community work to address the damage done
Offenders get what they deserve and justice is served	The focus is on community identification of victim needs and offender responsibility

The Processes and Mechanics of Restorative Justice

Offenders have a choice when it comes to restorative justice, but that choice carries with it some clear criteria about responsibility. For example, in Fort Collins, Colorado, and in return for agreeing to the terms of their social contract, they can get a conviction for a criminal charge excused. The computer record for the arrest remains, while the notice of a conviction is eliminated. Before an RJ session begins, however, offenders must agree to the following (Table 20.1):

1. They must accept responsibility for their actions that caused harm.
2. They must participate in a circle that includes a trained facilitator, one or more peer representatives who have successfully completed the RJ Program.
3. When possible, the victim (individual, store, or agency representative) will also participate.
4. Others who may be represented in the circle are a community representative, someone from the store or agency, a police officer, a parent or guardian from someone less than 18 years of age.

Instead of handing these cases off to lawyers and judges to resolve, RJ emphasizes personal responsibility, face-to-face interactions between offenders and victims when possible, community involvement through different service commitments, accountability for fulfilling those contracts, and, in general, "healing the harm" done. When successful, restorative justice epitomizes what is possible when we balance the calls for justice and punishment with a move toward learning and an ethical common ground built on principles of positive mental health, when we face up to conflict and reconcile our differences through active engagement of local citizens and social contracting (Table 20.2).

The United States leads industrialized nations in percent of the population that is incarcerated. With enormously high recidivism rates, rehabilitation seems to be a failed concept in this context. While alcohol remains legal despite its risks, we continue to fill our jails with drug offenders. Among minority males living in impoverished areas with little in the way of gainful employment possible, the numbers of

Table 20.2 Questions for Criminal and Restorative Justice

Criminal justice	Restorative justice
What laws have been broken?	What is the law and who has been hurt?
Who did it?	What are the victim's needs? What motivates the offender? How can this relationship be healed?
What do offenders deserve?	Whose obligations do offenders have to help heal the damage done?

those incarcerated are staggering. Too often, minor offenses lead to criminal records that slam shut so many doors of opportunity.

Restorative principles and justice offer a proactive alternative that has proven successful in many different contexts. In a July 2016 report on the Public Broadcasting Service titled "States Consider Restorative Justice as Alternative to Mass Incarceration," it was noted that *"(instead) of fighting the charges in court, offenders selected for restorative justice agree to accept responsibility for their actions, meet face-to-face with victims and come up with a plan to repair the harm they've caused. Some jurisdictions are even using the strategy with adults, incorporating it into their probation for those who avoid prison time. Thirty-five states have adopted legislation encouraging the use of restorative justice for children and adults both before and after prison, though many local law enforcement departments have for years relied on local nonprofits to perform the sessions without an official blessing from the state. As states step back from mass incarceration, restorative justice is becoming more widespread and formalized."* (https://www.pbs.org/newshour/nation/states-consider-restorative-justice-alternative-mass-incarceration).

In these accounts punishment gives way to a learning that can directly help victims, that can help offenders better understand their motivations and actions as well as what they could do differently in the future. For example, when young offenders analyze their motivations, they often see the influence of certain "friends" who have been bad influences. One way forward for them is to begin the process of rethinking their friendships, identifying those who can be more positive influences in their lives. This becomes an issue of personal responsibility with the benefit of potentially long-lasting impacts.

I believe that restorative principles have the potential to help cut costs, heal the associated wounds and address our judicial and ethical abuses, using well-established principles of learning to replace an outmoded and destructive emphasis on punishment.

The Processes and Mechanics of Restorative Justice

As Restorative Justice is commonly practiced, there is an intake process where those arrested are presented with their options, i.e., a court appearance or a restorative "diversion program" where their acceptance of responsibility for the offense then allows them to commit to a community service requirement that supports accountability and healing. As evidenced by the success rate, offenders mature in their ethical thinking and behavior while communities can see a decline in conflicts and violence.

For the Fort Collins Restorative Justice Program, a circle session is scheduled for one to three offenders aged 10–22. When this convenes, the ground rules and procedures are explained. The emphasis will be on participation in the conference with the hope that offenders "will be able to move beyond the harm and impact caused by the incident toward healing and understanding." Everyone agrees to keep what is said in the circle confidential so that participants can have the trust needed to be open and honest. Everyone is assured that those in the circle are not there "to make judgments on whether the offenders are good or bad people" but instead to explore ways in which the harm could be repaired.

For individuals arrested for shoplifting, this initial circle session can last from 1.5 to 2.5 hours as they (1) describe the event, (2) comment on their thoughts and feelings about their actions, (3) consider the impact (i.e., "ripple effect) on others, (4) hear from others in the circle including the victim when possible, and (5) make a commitment to what they will do to repair the harm caused (i.e., they sign a contract that is legally binding and that will be evaluated by RJ personnel for compliance when completed in 1–2 months) (Table 20.3).

The Fort Collins Restorative Justice Program has developed a range of possibilities, each tied to core principles of learning and healing. Other programs might offer different options but the underlying principle is the same, i.e., connect a range of activities to the goal of increasing self-awareness, self-responsibility, and learning about the damage done and how it can be repaired.

- *Volunteering for a non-profit:* With many agencies in the area eager to have volunteers, there are many options available. Helping to care for rescued animals or to help at the County Food Bank are popular choices.
- *Apology letters* that can be sent to the victim or store manager, to siblings— younger children often look up to older siblings whose behavior can have a powerful influence on them—or to parents and teachers, and even to those no longer alive who may have been so very important in earlier years. These kinds of personal statements have long been used by mental health professionals as a vehicle for self-reflection.
- *Personal journal* that includes at least 15 entries which must focus on the offense, its impact, and the offender's thoughts and feelings.
- *Counseling sessions*—three are the minimum, arranged through the school, a public agency or private sources.

Table 20.3 Steps to Restorative Justice

1. *Preparation of victim(s):* Mentally, emotionally, ethically, consideration of forgiveness.
2. *Preparation of offenders:* Mentally, emotionally and ethically for learning, pragmatically (responsibility and accountability for fulfilling the community contract).
3. *The "circle" or "conference" or "meeting":* Deep listening, empathizing, noting the "ripple effect," options for healing the community.

- *Support group meetings* where, for example, an addiction to drugs or alcohol might be addressed.
- *A visit to a juvenile court* where offenders get to observe the formal court scene.
- *Family community serve* that goes above and beyond what is normally expected for chores at home.
- *Neighborhood community service*, for example, that would provide some help for someone in need.
- *Offer a creative activity that would be restorative.* For example, an offender can plan to assist a disabled relative or neighbor or provide day care for siblings who would otherwise require paid child care.

Because RJ staff and volunteers sit with offenders to evaluate the impact when everything promised has been completed, there are important elements of account-ability and responsibility within the system. RJ volunteers commonly ask about alternative behaviors and share their own stories about learning.

When parents are in the circle, we can often feel real healing and reconciliation occur as what had been a hidden pattern of behavior is now opened for all to see. The service offered by the offender can also help heal as individuals give back to the community. Effective communication is essential throughout this process so that underlying issues, in particular, can surface. Considered together, these impacts can help contribute to what could also be called "sustainable peacebuilding," i.e., those factors that contribute to the interconnected health of society, the economy, and the environment.

Key Sources for Implementing Restorative Justice

There are a number of sources that have proven popular with the staff and volun-teers who work with restorative justice programs. Amstutz and Mullet [1] have authored a widely read book that is a quick and easy guide to implementing restor-ative processes in a school environment. School discipline is a prevailing challenge for staff, students, parents, and other community members, especially when racial or special needs issues provoke tensions. In a similar vein, Bintliff [4] book offers research-based models that address social justice and diversity. The Claassens [6], in turn, offer lesson plans to help students learn, understand, and implement ideas for conflict resolution and peacemaking, the skills they will need in their roles as mediators. As in much of my own work, the emphasis for the classroom is highly interactive and experiential exploration of conflicts, in particular, in an effort to sup-port community mental and emotional well-being both within schools and beyond.

Llewellyn and Philpott [9] offer a framework for using restorative principles in peacebuilding. In their book, scholars from very different disciplines—transitional justice, relational theory, political philosophy, and international theory, including both secular and faith-based approaches—offer a multidimensional and holistic perspective. Here you can see the broader implications of restorative justice for other related fields and studies, efforts that call for interdisciplinary, even transdisciplinary, analyses that are ideal for case study analysis, inquiry, inductive, and other participatory and creative approaches.

Thorsborne and Blood [11] go further in explaining what has to happen in a school in order for it to become truly restorative. When successful, there can be positive outcomes for both students and teachers, including a deeper understanding of change and how best to manage it. Again, we see a call for engaging approaches that address both "head and heart" as Palmer [10] writes in *The Courage to Teach*. Umbreit and Armour's [24] book addresses victim-offender mediation, family-group counseling, peacemaking circles, and victim-offender dialogue in cases of severe violence.

Van Wormer and Walker [25] frame their analysis with a compelling critique of the present system of criminal justice and its heavy emphasis on harsh forms of punishment with little attention to the personal dimension. The authors insist that when contemplating restorative justice or its core principles, the more that is known about the failings of the criminal or retributive justice system the more attractive a restorative justice approach.

In two recent books, Zehr [27] calls for us to think differently about crime and justice. Drawing on a variety of sources, he examines the retributive justice system, then looks back at other models of justice in history and in the Bible. He then proposes a shift in the way our society thinks about justice from retributive to restorative justice. In another of his books, he [28] has provided help for educating new volunteers on the basics of restorative justice and restorative justice conferencing.

International Contexts

In what follows, I will offer case studies and examples from various international contexts—Northern Ireland, Burundi (East Africa), South Africa, South Korea, Israel and Palestine, the Ukraine, and Russia—where conflicts have erupted and where I have seen or helped establish restorative principles as part of a general healing and reconciliation peace process, i.e., to support openness, responsibility, accountability, ethical decision-making, self-reflection, learning, healing, and reconciliation. I follow the lead of Elise Boulding [5] and her arguments for looking past the media's preoccupation with war and violence for a deeper understanding about this peace process when it does take hold. Where successful these now stand in stark contrast to failed retributive justice practices of punishment, incarceration, and fines. When we examine the impact of restorative principles, the potential benefits for community mental health are clear: reduced violence in Northern Ireland since the signing of the Good Friday Peace Agreement in 1998, a similar reduction in violence in the region of Ngozi, Burundi after the signing of the Arusha Peace and Reconciliation Agreement in 2000.

Promoting Responsibility: Correcting Memories of Violence in Northern Ireland and South Africa

Applications of restorative justice can be quite broad in scope and serve as a foundation for a range of progressive innovations. We can emphasize core restorative principles and then link these to community-wide programs aimed at more generalized healing and transformation. In Northern Ireland, a grass-roots peace movement took hold after 400 years of conflict. In particular, the upsurge of violence from 1972 and the "Bloody Sunday" incident where British troops fired on protesters marching for civil rights led to an upsurge of a grassroots peace movement nationally and the signing of the Good Friday Peace Accords in 1998, a time period usually referred to as the "Troubles." Going into some depth with this example provides the background needed to see the role of restorative principles in helping a community heal from a violent past.

Despite the divisions, inequities, and suffering that were the legacy of British colonization of Ireland in the 1600s, the public—Protestant Loyalists eager to remain part of the United Kingdom and their Catholic Republican counterparts who longingly looked to join with Ireland to the south—had become tired of the conflict's underlying logic of "us or them," the "bombs and bullets" that the Irish Republican Army insisted would force the British to the peace table. Restorative principles of responsibility and accountability, of honest reflection and an emphasis on healing the wounds of the past, have proven vital in moving beyond this violent past and toward a peace that can also strengthen community mental health generally.

Alternative perspectives did exist as reference points. South Africa, for example, was moving toward democracy while it dismantled apartheid and its systemic subjugation of the black majority by the white minority. This meant a shift in self-reference to what Nelson Mandela and others referred to as the "Rainbow Nation," neither white nor black but a mix of every hue, background, and belief that resided there. Their Truth and Reconciliation Commission utilized restorative principles to heal the wounds of the past and propel the nation toward a new reality. In Northern Ireland, peace activists insisted that something similar could—and should—happen to define a way forward that would include Protestants and Catholics, Loyalists and Republicans, as well as every other citizen who resided there.

In Northern Ireland, I was able to interview former combatants, peace activists, and others who were deeply committed to finding restorative solutions to these historic conflicts. In the Spring of 2006, I held a Fulbright Senior Specialist Award that permitted me to spend 6 weeks at the University of Ulster's UNESCO Centre to address education for a people whose society was emerging from hundreds of years of conflict and violence over power, colonization, individual rights, respect, religion, opportunity, discrimination, sovereignty, and more, conflicts that pushed past conventional ethical boundaries and undermined community mental health for generations. Remarkably, in pursuit of peace, this small and divided nation of 1.5 million has had real success in disarming the militant wings while convincing the British to reduce their military presence and relieve some of what was undermining any sense of community well-being.

During my time there, I had an opportunity to see firsthand how memories, in particular, can distort reality and perpetuate violence, undermining the mental and emotional health of a community and region for years. From my home base in Port Rush at the tip of Northern Ireland, I took the train southwest to Derry, the walled city still celebrated by Protestant loyalists for resisting the siege of the Catholic King James in 1690. I went to hear a talk by Irish historian Kevin Whelan about memories, stories, and their role in healing. We met at a community relations resource center that sponsors various projects in an effort to address the violence of the past 30 years through storytelling and dialogue, listening, and empathizing.

The audience of some fifteen locals included one man in his 50s—I'll call him "Tom"—who was at the "Bloody Sunday" civil rights demonstrations in 1972 when British soldiers fired on a large group of marchers, killing fourteen and wounding another seventeen. Many nationalists quickly concluded that this attack on unarmed civilians discredited the very principles of nonviolence as used by Gandhi in India and then by Martin Luther King and the Civil Rights movement in the United States. Armed response was, accordingly, legitimized and deemed necessary by the militant wing of the Irish Republican Army (IRA).

After Professor Whalen concluded his remarks about the malleability of memory, how each of us constructs our worlds based on our recall of what we have experienced and been told, Tom recounted that he clearly remembered the bullets flying on Bloody Sunday and the British paratroopers with their distinguishing berets at that first barricade, something that nationalists are hard pressed to forgive. For them, to use elite combat troops against unarmed civilians was clear evidence of British brutality and the naiveté of nonviolence, reasons for the IRA to declare war on the British occupiers. Following bloody Sunday, the killings intensified and the bombings were even exported to England. Everyone suffered from this level of domestic terror.

But then Tom admitted that he had been wrong for all these thirty plus years. He told us that at a recent meeting on reconciliation, when the discussion turned to Bloody Sunday, someone had produced a photograph from 1972 of those infamous barricades. When Tom looked closely, he could clearly see that the British troops were all in helmets, not berets, the classic headgear for combat-ready paratroopers. Yes, there were paratroopers nearby and, yes, they did get involved and join in the shooting later, but it was a revelation for Tom to see something so different from what he distinctly remembered, and it is this personal responsibility that he was accepting, one of the core prerequisites for restorative justice. Individuals must be willing to be honest about their actions.

In the heat of any wild and traumatic moment, anyone can be forgiven for missing certain details. Yet Tom's memories had led him to embrace more extremist calls for reprisal, and he had become a celebrity as a fiery speaker about British oppression and brutality. Now, some 34 years later, he needed to admit his errors, rethink his positions and commit to healing himself and others, even though he had achieved a significant level of notoriety as an "eyewitness to this history."

As I observed and absorbed all this I began to reflect on events in the United States, and specifically what will be restorative for Americans about the Iraq War, for example, what memories would need to be revisited, what deceptions uncovered, and what lessons could be learned? Surveys at the time indicated that over 70% of the U.S. troops in Iraq fully believed that Sadam Hussein, the President of Iraq at that time, was directly involved in the attacks of September 11. That was not true and we later found no evidence of weapons of mass destruction, the threats we were told that drove our invasion. What will it take, intellectually and emotionally to confront the facts and reexamine the connections between their participation in that war effort and their own memories? How can the principles of restorative justice lead us to make amends and rethink our ethics, policies, and practices?

Burundi: Reclaiming Restorative Practices Through Case-Based Learning

In Burundi, "amahoro" is the Kirundi word for peace. After a century of colonial control and exploitation by Germans, and then Belgians, who put the minority Tutsi in power over the Hutu, independence in 1962 led to a predictable civil war that would last for nearly 40 years and push this nation of some 11 million people living in East Africa ever more deeply into poverty and pain. While the fighting would end with the Arusha Peace Accords in 2000 that Nelson Mandela helped to mediate, the trauma left by nearly a million dead and as many who fled as refugees continues to haunt the present and beg for restorative influences to help brighten the future.

Founded in 1999 with a commitment to reconciliation, the University of Ngozi (UNG) is eager to be a laboratory for peacebuilding and sustainable development. Through the fire of violence, Burundians here are forging a recovery and rebirth of spirit, a reconciliation of tribal rivalries imposed by colonial overlords to maintain control, a commitment to understand the truth of that past, and the resilience to rebuild their nation.

Stopping the violence was essential and the 2000 Arusha Peace Accords set the stage for that, what peace educators refer to as "peacemaking" or creating that policy framework for moving forward. After the last of the rebels signed a ceasefire agreement with the new government in 2008, Burundians could experience an essential "peacekeeping" function where combatants are finally separated. Now came the challenge of "peacebuilding," creating those restorative conditions that would help to heal the nation and allow for some hoped for peaceful progress and normalization. The University of Ngozi has taken a lead role in educating citizens of all ages about the ideas and skills that would be needed to develop a lasting or sustainable framework, and thus the focus on "sustainable peace and development," i.e., restorative principles and practices [14].

With such an ambitious beginning, the University of Ngozi has, in fact, proven to be an oasis of calm, welcome, and the restorative possibility for students in Burundi as well as many from Rwanda and the Democratic Republic of the Congo. Without any support from the national government, it began with modest contributions from local residents and a larger gift from the Catholic Diocese. Importantly, many of these students are quite poor themselves, their parents getting by on subsistence farming of small plots. Yet, so many are able to sacrifice and come to class full of hope, motivation, and potential.

Studies of Burundi reveal a complex mix of historical trauma with present-day resilience, a violent past with a current resolve that is echoed by so many at the University of Ngozi who want to use restorative principles to better understand the truth of the past, heal the damage, and prepare for the future. When we introduced principles of restorative justice into the curriculum of legal studies, students came to see connections with historic community practices before German and Belgian colonizers imposed Western European principles of retributive justice within the criminal codes of law.

In support of these endeavors, I used another Fulbright Specialist Award in 2011 to join with colleagues, student, and community members in Ngozi to propose the use *locally generated and regionally applicable case-based and project-based learning* to transform surface or memorized learning. With the support of two subsequent Global Grants from the Rotary Foundation, we are now working to extend these ideas out into schools and church communities.

Based on their work at the Harvard Business School where the case study method has been practiced and refined over many years, Barnes, Christensen, and Hansen [3] have laid out compelling reasons for this approach to instruction and learning. In evaluations of problem-based and case-based learning, it seems very clear that students appreciate the benefits of greater engagement, discovery, and relevance that are associated with problem- and case-based learning [8, 18].

A new model of restorative education, we believe, will aid the shift toward long-term stability and prosperity. Students will focus on real problems that beset their communities and then apply their skills to explore what solutions might be possible. Through this process, we believe that they will be developing their skills in communication and cooperation, critical and creative thinking. What proves viable in Burundi, East Africa and the developing world we believe could also have benefits for communities in the industrialized world that struggle with conflict, violence, polarization, and the costs of security.

Over the course of this project, we hope that the University of Ngozi will emerge as a viable on-going site and dissemination center for *research and development in sustainable peace and development* where restorative principles will be a central focus. We hope that leaders from around the world—in primary, secondary and higher education, from NGOs, government, business, churches, and other community groups—with content expertise and peace and reconciliation experience will join with UNG in these efforts [14].

Case Studies of Restorative Justice in Korea

Just 31 miles north of Seoul is the border with North Korea, the most heavily militarized in the world with large numbers of troops on both sides. In 2014 when I first arrived, there was an "incident" that got headlines that were widely reported here and abroad. As reported in *The Korea Herald* (Tue. Mar. 4, 2014): "North Korea on

Monday (March 3) fired two short-range ballistic missiles into the East Sea in its latest saber-rattling apparently to protest the South Korean-U.S. military drills, Seoul's Military Defense Minister said. Seoul called the move a 'provocative action' that further raised military tensions on the peninsula and violated a series of U.N. Security Council resolutions prohibiting any launch using ballistic missile technologies. The North fired four ballistic missiles last Thursday and four 'KN-09' rockets into the East Sea about a week earlier (1)."

I was serving that semester as a Fulbright Scholar at Kyung Hee University's Graduate Institute of Peace Studies (GIP) and teaching a class on peacemaking. GIP has its own campus in north Seoul with a dormitory, cafeteria, gym, library, and administration building with a separate mediation hall, all on meticulously mani-cured grounds. Every morning I would see students would gather for a brief talk, meditation, walk, and/or exercises.

Despite this "saber-rattling" from the north, few here seemed worried. They did not believe the North Koreans have the capacity to defeat the South and their American allies although they admit that, if it came to war, Seoul would be vulner-able. These threats from North Korea had been repeated so often that they had lost much of their ability to frighten anyone here.

One of my students was new to GIP. He had been in the army for 10 years and had achieved the rank of captain. Like others, he was not that worried about the North but was very appreciative of American sacrifices in fighting the Korean War and then providing troops—now at nearly 30,000—ever since to help secure the peace. Another of my students had completed his required military service and saw a real "weirdness" here. He remembered visiting China and being at the Beijing airport, waiting in line to board a flight to another city in China, when he noticed another line nearby for North Koreans on another flight. Here in China they could stand next to each other but never back home.

I had these questions: What would normalization and reconciliation require? What would be restorative? I am heartened by the interest of these active duty army officers who had enrolled in my class on peacemaking in the possibility of reunifica-tion of the two Koreas. They wanted to talk more about the reunification process in Germany instead of the sensational headlines about the latest missile launches from the north. Certainly their eagerness to study peacemaking aligned with Elise Boulding's [5] insistence that more people must commit to the study of peace if we are to make progress toward what is truly restorative. In a classic principle for restorative justice, learning takes precedence over punishment, healing over revenge.

Case Studies of Restorative Practices in Israel and Palestine

The Arab Association for Human Rights (HRA), founded in 1988 by lawyers and community activists, is an independent, grassroots, non-governmental organization (NGO), registered in Israel. HRA works from an international human rights per-spective to promote and protect the political, civil, economic, and cultural rights of the Palestinian Arab minority in Israel. I was there as part of a peacemaking study group in the summer of 2017. The description that follows illustrates a range of restorative principles from raising awareness to a commitment to networking to help heal, from analyzing data on impact to ongoing training.

HRA holds a unique position locally and worldwide as an indigenous organization that works on the community, national, and international levels for equality and non-discrimination, and for the domestic implementation of international minority rights protections. Over the years, HRA has conducted local community and international campaigns to raise awareness, understanding, and respect for human rights and democratic principles; monitored violations of human rights and published and distributed reports documenting abuses; initiated and participated in local NGO coalitions concerned with the rights of prisoners and administrative detainees, land, and housing rights, women's rights, and networking; facilitated community human rights education programs and events; advocated before United Nations and European Union bodies; and organized and participated in local and international training workshops and conferences.

By the mid-1990s, the HRA had formalized its goals, dividing its activities into three major fields: human-rights education, women's rights, and international advocacy—each of these restorative in its own rights. As an independent grassroots NGO, the HRA focuses on working with the local community. Its goal is to increase awareness of human rights among the Arab minority citizens in Israel, "since we believe that consciousness is the first step on the way to bring about constructive change. The second major strand of our activities involves international advocacy."

In 2003, the HRA expanded its activities to include a human-rights monitoring program, whose methodology relies on field research and interviews and legal analysis of the domestic and international human-rights laws. The idea of establishing a Research and Reporting program was first developed by the HRA in the wake of the events of October 2000, when 13 Palestinian Arabs (twelve citizens of Israel and one from the Occupied Palestinian Territories) were killed by state police forces. Since that time, a steady trickle of serious and often physical human-rights abuses against minority citizens means that the need for human-rights documentation and reporting of these abuses is more vital than ever.

When meeting with a touring group from the United States that I had joined in August of 2017, Muhammed Zeidan, Director of the HRA, offered a range of insights into Israeli and Palestinian issues. "While Israelis talk about the War of Independence in 1948, we Palestinians refer to it as the "Catastrophe." The majority of our people left and there were 530 villages from which they were evicted. The "Jewishness" of the state of Israel makes for discrimination. It seems almost impossible for Palestinians to convert to Jewishness. Currently, there is a military law in the occupied areas and civil law for Israel."

"Essentially we have an Israeli apartheid system" he continued. "Non-Jewish people must have permission to move around Israel. Many farmers have had their lands confiscated. Sixty percent of the Palestinians have faced eviction. Palestinians face four types of discrimination: (1) Legal and direct discrimination that favors Jewish ancestry; (2) Legal and indirect discrimination that favors those with military service where only five percent of Arabs have chosen to serve within Israel amid reports of the discrimination they face when they do apply; (3) Institutional policies and practices can reflect discrimination through funding; and (4) public discrimination, the most dangerous, reflects a culture of racism where, for example, Jews are discouraged from marriage with non-Jews." Like the HRA, many groups that work to promote peace in the Middle East are consistent in collecting and analyzing data about their own effectiveness.

While these are broad generalizations, I can see on display a number of restorative principles including an attempt at honest assessments of complex and conflicted issues, a commitment to accountability, and responsible actions in community healing. Hopefully, other principles of open communication, empathic, and respectful listening will help lead toward cooperative and constructive ways forward.

Case Studies in Ukraine and Russia

The killing fields in the former KGB grounds on the outskirts of Moscow are another illustration of the dangers of state secrecy on the mental and emotional health of the public as well as the importance of openness in healing when damage is done. I visited this site in mid-2019 as part of a Presbyterian Peacemaking study group. Parallel to what was happening in Spain in the 1930s, Stalin began purges that would lead to over twenty thousand secret executions and burials in Moscow alone, murders that lay buried for nearly 60 years.

It was only in 1995, some 40 years after Krushchev denounced Stalin for these and so many other abuses, that pressure from the families of the victims and their supporters forced an opening to examine this horror. Today, these killing fields are a public memorial with a stone wall that contains the names of the remains that have been identified along with two traditional village style church structures for mourners and visitors. The leaders and people of Russia who pushed for this recognize the restorative power of openness about the horrors of the past for finding new ways forward.

In 1985, former President Gorbachev's initiated a formal policy shift when he called for "Glasnost" or openness and helped to set the stage for this restorative transformation. Leadership is essential in promoting a restorative model since there are many moving parts, i.e., the interactions of offenders and victims, the need for an integrated "learning plan" that guides the offenders toward a deeper understanding of the healing process, of the ethical responsibility and accountability that must lie underneath.

Restorative Benefits of Forgiveness

Speaking the truth is one essential way for offenders to accept responsibility for their actions and begin to restore healing to their communities. It also becomes important for community members to heal themselves as they must hear and react to a range of tragedies and traumas. In the Postscript to his book, *No Future Without*

Forgiveness, Bishop Desmond Tutu concludes his description of the Truth and Reconciliation Commission's (TRC) work in South Africa to help heal the deep, bitter wounds left by apartheid, the oppressive policies and unethical practices that Whites imposed on majority Black Africans. Tutu writes, "At the beginning of our work on the commission our mental health worker on the staff gave us a briefing about coping with was to be a grueling and demanding task. We were advised to make sure that we had a soul mate or some such friend or counselor to who we could go to unburden ourselves; otherwise, we would be shocked by how easy it was to disintegrate, to become stressed, and even to suffer ourselves from posttraumatic stress disorder as we experienced by proxy the anguish and agony of those who came to testify before the commission" (pp. 285–286).

Summary and Conclusion

This chapter provides an overview of the core concepts that define restorative justice, a number of case studies where restorative justice (RJ), principles, and practices have been implemented to varying degrees as well as the evidence that has emerged about impacts on the mental health of individuals and communities. By embracing these core concepts mental health professionals and their allies can shift policing and courts, educators and social workers, legislators and government staff, church and community leaders beyond a narrow consideration of restorative justice into a much broader application that emphasizes responsibility, ethical decision-making, accountability, openness, and reconciliation for offenders and victims alike.

Restorative justice represents one powerful way to bring principles of healing, learning, and transformation into public viewing through the establishment of particular practices that can make it all very real. Those who volunteer with restorative justice can find regular opportunities to practice their skills at promoting responsibility and accountability among offenders, shifting the focus from incarceration to community service, from a limited focus on punishment to a concerted effort at learning. These principles and practices can then serve as laboratory for restorative ideals made real more broadly, building a foundation for improved community mental and emotional well-being.

References

1. Amstutz, L., & Mullet, J. (2005). *The little book of restorative discipline for schools: Teaching responsibility; creating caring climates.* Intercourse: Good Books.
2. Braithwaite, J. (2002). *Restorative justice & responsive regulation.* New York: Oxford University Press.
3. Barnes, L., Christensen, C. R., & Hansen, A. (1994). *Teaching and the case study method.* Boston: Harvard University Press.
4. Bintliff's. (2011). *Re-engaging disconnected youth: Transformative learning through restorative and social justice education.* New York: Peter Lang.
5. Boulding, E. (2000). *Cultures of peace: The hidden side of history.* New York: Syracuse University Press.

6. Claassen, R. (2015). *Making things right*. North Charleston: CreateSpace.
7. Diamond, Jarad, Upheavel, 2019.
8. Hmelo-Silver, C. (2004). Problem-based learning: What and how do students learn? *Educational Psychology Review, 16*(3), 235–266.
9. Llewellyn, J., & Philpott, D. (2014). *Restorative justice, reconciliation, and peace building*. New York: Oxford University Press.
10. Palmer, P. (1998). *The courage to teach*. San Francisco: Jossey-Bass.
11. Blood, P. (2013). *Implementing restorative practices in schools*. London: Jessica Kingsley.
12. Timpson, W., Yang, R., Borrayo, E., Canetto, S., Gonzalez, J., & Scott, M. (2019). *147 practical tips for teaching diversity* (2nd ed.). Madison: Atwood.
13. Timpson, W., Dunbar, B., Kimmel, G., Bruyere, B., Newman, P., Mizia, H., Birmingham, D., & Harmon, R. (2017). *147 practical tips for teaching sustainability: Connecting the environment, the economy, and society* (2nd ed.). Madison: Atwood.
14. Timpson, W., Ndura, E., & Bangayimbaga, A. (2015). *Conflict, reconciliation, and peace education: Moving Burundi toward a sustainable future*. New York: Routledge.
15. Timpson, W., & Holman, D. K. (Eds.). (2014). *Controversial case studies for teaching on sustainability, conflict, and diversity*. Madison: Atwood.
16. Timpson, W., Foley, J., Kees, N., & Waite, A. M. (2013). *147 practical tips for using experiential learning*. Madison: Atwood.
17. Timpson, W., & Holman, D. K. (Eds.). (2012). *Case studies of classrooms and communication: Integrating diversity, sustainability, peace and reconciliation*. Madison: Atwood.
18. Timpson, W., & Doe, S. (2008). *Concepts and choices for teaching: Meeting the challenges in higher education* (2nd ed.). Madison: Atwood.
19. Timpson, W. Canetto, S. Yang, R. and Borrayo, E. (Eds.). (2003) *Teaching Diversity: Challenges and Complexities, Identities and Integrity*. Madison, WI: Atwood.
20. Timpson, W., & Burgoyne, S. (2002). *Teaching and performing: Ideas for energizing your classes* (2nd ed.). Madison: Atwood.
21. Timpson, W. (2002) *Teaching and Learning Peace*. Madison, WI: Atwood.
22. Timpson, W. (1999). *Metateaching and the instructional map*. Madison: Atwood.
23. Tutu, D. (1999). *No future without forgiveness*. New York: Doubleday.
24. Umbreit, M., & Armour, M. (2011). *Restorative justice dialogue*. New York: Springer.
25. Van Wormer, K., & Walker, L. (2013). *Restorative justice today*. Los Angeles: Sage.
26. Walgrave, L. (Ed.). (2002). *Restorative justice and the law*. Uffculme, Cullompton, Devon, U.K.: Willan Publishing.
27. Zehr, H. (2015a). *Changing lenses: Restorative justice for our times*. Harrisonburg: Herald Press.
28. Zehr, H. (2015b). *The little book of restorative justice*. Intercourse: Good Books.

Community Response to Disaster: Hurricanes in the Caribbean

21

Vanessa Torres-Llenza and Jeremy Safran

> *"I believe that the community – in the fullest sense: a place and all its creatures – is the smallest unit of health and that to speak of the health of an isolated individual is a contradiction in terms."*
>
> —Wendell Berry in Health is Membership

Introduction: The Role of the Community in Disaster

It is not surprising when people are traumatized by disasters. Disasters overwhelm local communities' ability to cope. What is remarkable is the resilience people show when communities come together to address the needs of each other. In disasters, whether natural or human-made, government response is often lacking or insufficient. The responsibility then falls on communities to play an active role in disaster response [2]. Rather than succumbing to the role of victim, a community becomes an active participant in recovery and is engaged in logistics, planning, and implementation of services. The community becomes a major collaborative partner in the process of disaster recovery and resilience building [11]. As a result of global climate change and increasing political tensions, disasters are occurring with greater frequency, thereby highlighting the importance of community role in disasters.

V. Torres-Llenza (✉)
George Washington University Hospital, Washington, DC, USA
e-mail: VTorresLlenza@mfa.gwu.edu

J. Safran
Child and Adolescent Psychiatry Fellow at Children's National Hospital, The George Washington University School of Medicine, Washington, DC, USA

© Springer Nature Switzerland AG 2021
A. R. Dyer et al. (eds.), *Global Mental Health Ethics*,
https://doi.org/10.1007/978-3-030-66296-7_21

Finding Solidarity in Community

Community recovery begins with solidarity. *Solidarity* is defined as unity or agreement of feeling or action, especially among individuals with a common interest and mutual support. In looking for examples of solidarity, we are often humbled to find that even in the face of despair, humanity prevails. We see solidarity in organizations working with the homeless and migrant populations, and in protests around the world for a common cause such as human rights or climate change. Immediately after an earthquake with a magnitude of 7.1 in Mexico on September 2017, volunteers created a giant human-chain to rescue trapped victims. In Puerto Rico after Hurricane Maria, people began posting resources on social media where food and medications could be found.

Un buen correazo and Other Barriers Facing Puerto Rico

The archipelago of Puerto Rico (PR) consists of the Main Island and a number of smaller islands. Puerto Rico is a territory of the United States with commonwealth status. The Commonwealth establishes the islands' own system of government with administrative autonomy for internal affairs, but subject to US federal law and regulations. According to multiple estimates, more than 50% of the population in Puerto Rico has a mental health disorder. According to data from the Mental Health and Substance Abuse Services Administration (ASSMCA in Spanish), 800,000 people suffer a mental health disorder that could be described as moderate or severe. In 2003, 66% of those did not receive any mental health treatment services.

The lack of mental health treatment is not surprising given poor access overall, but significant stigma regarding mental health also leads to barriers in care. In Latino communities, it is not uncommon to hear, "he is just being *malcriado*," (misbehaved) or "all he needs is *un buen correazo*" (a good spanking). A common misconception is that one would only see a psychiatrist or psychologist if they are "being crazy." For those growing up in Puerto Rico, these sentiments are commonplace. They are also likely familiar in many other communities. Family members have described those struggling with drugs and alcohol as "*loco.*" Some families lack a support system and can even enable maladaptive processes to occur as a means of avoiding topics often not spoken about. Thus, at times neighbors, leaders, and organizations need to step in to educate and provide for a community in need of mental healing.

Vieques, a Small Island con un corazon grande

CrearConSalud is one such non-profit organization that focuses on mental health education in Puerto Rico. It began as the Mental Health Awareness Tour in 2015 funded by the US Substance Abuse Mental Administration Services Health (SAMHSA) Minority Fellowship Program through the American Psychiatric

Association in which one of us was an award recipient (Torres-Llenza, V). The goal was to provide mental health awareness and encourage students to pursue careers in mental health. Trips to Puerto Rico included a communications portion, going to radio stations and news channels, panels with local leaders, and going to different medical schools and high schools to promote science and mental health. A team of Puerto Rican psychiatrists with roots at home formed the group, CrearConSalud, and incorporated in August of 2017.

Much of the work at CrearConSalud has focused on the island of Vieques, one of Puerto Rico's 78 municipalities. Two of these municipalities are off the east coast, Vieques and Culebra. Vieques is an island town measuring 21-mile-long with a population of 10,000 and Culebra with a population of 1300. In order to get there, you have to take a ferry for 2 dollars or a small plane. The ferry is often late or full, which can be stressful for those who rely on it as their primary means for travel. Given the lack of access to health care, most Viequenses have to go to mainland PR, also known as '*isla grande*' or big island, for their treatment.

Vieques has proven to be an example of a resilient community, despite many hardships. The United States Navy acquired land in Vieques in the 1940s to use as a naval ammunition depot. The island suffered chemical dumps and ordinance drops, placing its inhabitants in harm's way. In 1999, David Sanes was killed by a bomb dropped by the military. His death led to mass protests to advocate for the removal of the Navy from their land. The military eventually left the island in 2003. Even so, many people there suffered high incidences of cancer and other illnesses as a result of chemical tests. An island deserving support was left damaged to heal on its own.

Vieques is a microcosm of the main island Puerto Rico. Often called a "colony within a colony," it encounters challenges in obtaining proper access to medical care, food, and transportation. The topics among Viequenses have included concerns regarding mistrust, privacy, and disruption in family relationships. After Hurricane María lashed Puerto Rico on September 20, 2017, the territory was plunged into complete darkness, and many areas were cut off from medical services.

"I was born and raised in Puerto Rico and lived there until 2009. My parents and many loved ones still live on the island. Although I was not there when the hurricanes hit, I felt their impact, perhaps not physically but vicariously Carissa Cabán-Alemán [13] a CrearConSalud member

---

The Virgin Islands Hit by the Same Storm

On September 6, 2017, Hurricane Irma tore through the British Virgin Islands. It was the first Category 5 hurricane ever to hit the islands. Although the islanders take pride at having built their homes strong, "like a Tortolan," this hurricane left four dead as well as buildings, roads, and homes in destruction. Just 2 weeks later, Hurricane Maria swept over the islands. One resident said, "Maria finished us off." Even after homes were rebuilt and roads repaved, debris and abandoned structures still litter the island. The government of the British Virgin Islands recognized that there was also another, less visible aperture in the wake. They sought assistance from the Pan American Health Organization and the Global Mental Health Program of the Department of Psychiatry and Behavioral Sciences at the George Washington University to conduct a series of Resilience Building workshops for medical and community leaders, first responders, teachers, clergy, and healthcare personnel. The workshops sought to provide a framework and context for anticipating issues that are likely to be encountered in the middle and long term and to provide tools to manage stress and trauma for the community [5]. The goal in working with the surviving community is to ensure human dignity, encourage participation, strengthen available resources, and capacity for holistic recovery [11].

Long Overdue

The British Virgin Island's first resident psychiatrist, Dr. June Samuel, came to the island in 1999. Dr. Samuel opened the workshop by reminding the group, "there's no health without mental health." She emphasized the importance and priority at times of mental wellbeing to a community that historically had not emphasized mental health. One participant described the role of a man as having to be "a rock," which meant both strength and a lack of emotion. Still, the group was able to engage in exercises in expressing emotions that were washed up by the storms.

The GWU Resilience Workshops

The GWU Resilience Workshops were designed to build resilience in humanitarian workers responding to the refugee crisis in Greece. It was originally organized for the American Embassy in Athens with the cooperation of the Greek NGO Metadrasi [12]. The workshops focus on building skills in self-care and caring for others through a series of didactic and interactive sessions as well as skill-building exercises. The core principles of the workshops are Psychological First Aid (PFA) and Compassionate Listening, Mindfulness-Based Stress Reduction, and Hope Modules. Hope modules are a series of strategies, developed at The George Washington University for dealing with the psychological impacts of acute and chronic illness, and now being applied to humanitarian emergencies. Hope modules focus not on feelings, but rather on behaviors, something that one does or learns to do, relying on coping skills that have already been acquired [9].

In the initial phase of these workshops, participants engaged in learning self-care and applying these core skills. The participants learned techniques to apply these skills in caring for others, caring for themselves, and then teaching the skills to others in a cascade model. In addition to workshops for community leaders and first responders, workshops were conducted for hospital staff and private sector medical participants. In each group, participants were asked to discuss where the island was in the journey of recovery (see Fig. 21.1).

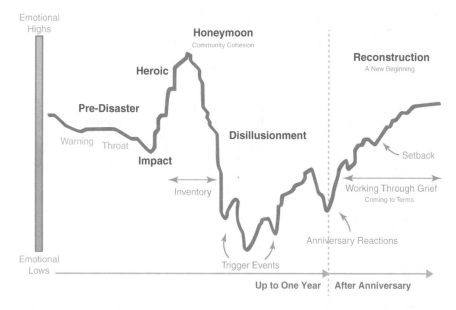

Fig. 21.1   Emotional stages, of disaster (Adapted from Zunin & Myers as cited in DeWolfe [6])

The Resilience Workshops Focus

The focus on resilience post-disaster is a recognition that, while both natural disasters, such as hurricanes, earthquakes, tsunamis, and wildfires, as well as human-made disasters, such as wars, conflicts, and complex emergencies, may be "traumatic" for everyone involved, the impacts are not necessarily manifestations of psychiatric disorder. Rather, they are the "normal reactions to an abnormal situation." Recovery after disaster involves the human connection and solidarity of supportive communities.

The resilience workshop format has been used previously in communities impacted by the Indian Ocean tsunami, the Great Sichuan Earthquake, the Japan Triple Disaster, the Haiti Earthquake, and further developed in response to the so-called "Syrian refugee crisis" in Greece (actually involving refugees from Iraq, Afghanistan, Northern Africa as well as Syria) [4, 5, 8, 14].

The format of the resilience workshops involves a series of didactic sessions, small group breakout sessions, and large group sharing sessions (see Table 21.1). This format utilizes recognized stages of group dynamics, a coming-together (inclusion), developing trust through openness and shared agenda setting (establishing group norms), and an opportunity to develop awareness of feelings and to share feelings as well as ideas (trust phase).

The didactic sessions not only provide information that may be useful to the groups (communities), but also serve to introduce the faculty to the larger

Table 21.1 General Format for a Resilience Workshop

Day 1 – Caring for Self	Day 2 Caring for self/caring for others
AM didactic session – Introduction to stress, trauma, and resilience – Mindfulness-based stress reduction	*AM didactic session –* Hope modules
Small group skills practice – Body scan, breathing exercises, tension reduction, mindful pausing, mindful eating	*Small group skills building:* Recognizing agency thinking and pathways thinking Identifying one's signature strengths: emotional regulation, relational coping, activating core identity, problem-solving, and goal setting
Large group – sharing session	*Large group* – sharing session
Lunch break	**Lunch break**
PM Didactic session – Psychological First Aid (PFA)	*PM – Didactic session –* Compassionate listening and goal setting
Small group practice session – Roleplay	*Small group activities* – Individual and organizational goal setting
Large group – sharing session	*Large group* session – Next steps

community. The small group activities facilitate skill development as well as contextualizing the skills in the local culture. The reconvening sessions provide an opportunity for community cohesion by presenting and sharing the work of the small groups and listening to others. In each half-day of a workshop, there is opportunity for a didactic session, small-group processing, then large group integration. As the cycle is repeated, the group develops an opportunity for community cohesion.

Developing a vocabulary to talk about emotional experience: "Stress," "trauma," "vicarious trauma," "burnout," and "resilience" are conceptualizations that help persons in groups in communities communicate and share the emotions they have experienced. The following schematic graph represents reactions that may be typical of what people experience in response to a disaster such as the Caribbean hurricanes.

The Different Emotional Stages of Disaster

After disaster, individuals within the community encounter different emotional stages that vary based on the time of the event and their experiences. The *heroic stage* includes processing the initial impact. Often it is the time where there is mobilization, high media focus, and a sense of urgency. In Puerto Rico, this stage was characterized by "Puerto Rico se levanta" translating to "Puerto Rico rises." The main goal is to establish a sense of security, shelter, food, and medical care.

After this stage, there is a *honeymoon period*. This phase is characterized by community cohesion after a shared experience. This phase occurs anytime from a few days to about 6 months after a disaster. In the past, some Puerto Ricans living on the island would express resentment toward those who had left. Those who stayed said "yo no me quito," or "I don't quit," implying that those who left had abandoned the land when in need. However, since the hurricane, everyone, inside and out of the island, has lived by "yo no me quito." There has been a reconnection with the Puerto Rican diaspora since Hurricane Maria. This crisis showed that it is possible to live outside the island and still carry with you the love for the land and the people – from wherever you are.

The *disillusionment stage* occurs when time continues to pass, but expectations for recovery do not match reality. At times during workshops, members described being in this emotional stage. They described being stuck in this stage due to a lack of government response, people leaving the island, and loss of employment.

The *reconstruction stage* can last several years after the original disaster. This stage can lead to the empowerment of a community if they can remain engaged and efficient. This can be seen in recent events taking place in Puerto Rico where protesters made their voices heard and reclaimed deserved leadership for their best interests.

One key emotional stage is the anniversary stage. An *anniversary reaction* can lead to a significant dip in emotional state and morale. Members who participated in workshops in Puerto Rico had expressed concern for the hurricane season and noted how increased worry might lead to re-experiencing previous reactions such as lack of sleep.

Teaching of emotional response to disaster was well-received. During workshops with community leaders, this topic led to in-depth discussions and increased awareness. It also led to a subjective sense of relief. In one group, some members felt they were in the heroic stage, while most felt they were still dealing with disillusionment. Others still felt they were in the reconstruction phase.

American Academy of Community Psychiatrists (AACP) Responds to Vieques

In January 2019, AACP held its winter board meeting in Vieques. Partnering with CrearConSalud, it led a forum for multiple nonprofit organizations. In Vieques, people came together to rebuild houses, make sure neighbors had transportation to healthcare, various churches stepped forward, and the humane society stressed the importance of looking after animals in the community. Dr. Michael Flaum, president of the AACP, pointed out that the community "despite power being out throughout much of the island for more than six months after Maria struck in September 2017, people from dozens of small agencies, churches, volunteer organizations, public entities as well as those working individually somehow continued going to work every day to help others, and then came home to deal with their own situations."

The different emotional stages among participants required attunement to one of many ethical considerations and responses. We had to meet participants where they were at, but also keep in mind that each individual was at a different stage in their emotional response to the disaster. Below are outlined other ethical considerations and responses when working with a community that has encountered disaster.

Ethical Considerations and Responses

Reflecting on the experiences of the BVI workshops, some best practices and group dynamics have led to the identification of a number of ethical principles for group facilitators that guide interactions.

Foster connection and communication when they may be at different stages of emotional response

- Fostering a discussion with an emphasis on how individuals feel rather than focusing on facts and discrepancy
- Redirecting participants from attributing feelings and stages of emotional response onto others (e.g., some participants began a discussion about what stage of emotional response the government officials were on, which led to disagreement and disconnect between group members)

First do no harm
- Avoid promises you can't keep
- Avoid dependency syndrome by engaging the community in pre- and post-disaster work. In this case, focusing on strengths to care for them themselves while caring for others in the event of another yet inevitable disaster
- *As an outsider to this island, do I risk harm by assuming I know what can be helpful? Am I callous if I just walk away?"*

Avoiding voyeurism while recognizing the importance of viewing the culture, resources, and devastation after the disaster

- Maintain an inquisitive attitude regarding topics participants engaged in
- Gave the participants an opportunity to speak openly
- Maintain privacy and established rules at the outset of the workshop regarding privacy
- Do not ask the participants to speak or elaborate on sensitive topics unless they wanted to

Avoiding exhibitionism in showcasing resources as well as clinical and mental health skills

- Use relevant examples and practical skills
- Utilize small groups to allow participants to apply skills to their own situations and stories
- Provide an atmosphere to allow participants to openly question and criticize techniques and principles

Maintaining sensitivity with all members of the group

- Attain background information regarding the participants' societal stressors and culture

- Listen first – before responding or lecturing, we gave the participants a setting to tell their stories and tell us about themselves and their communities
- *We listened – allowing people to reflect and connect around their thoughts and feelings of working and serving in Vieques.*

Recognizing the importance of religion and spirituality without alienating others

- Participants opened the workshop with prayer and were encouraged to discuss the role their religion had on their efforts to recover and rebuild
- Avoid keeping religion as the central focus in all discussions without disregarding its importance on the island
- Acknowledge and discuss the importance and power of faith without openly agreeing or disagreeing with religious focused comments

Understanding countertransference to improve our understanding of and relationship with the participants

- Shift projective identification away from that of someone who did not understand their culture (e.g., sharing stories from the United States and other countries with similar disasters)
- Avoid dependency on facilitators to give answers and solve issues, encouraged participants to problem solve and discuss stressors
- Avoid falling into a heroic role, which might be condescending and unhelpful

Assessing values rather than imposing them

- Discuss how mindfulness, hope, mental health, and resilience could be integrated into the British Virgin Island culture

Modeling self-care while providing as much support and information as possible

- Emphasize the importance of breaks and lunch
- Utilize humor when the workshop was behind schedule (e.g., we developed a running joke that we were always "ahead of schedule")
- We invited the participants to take a half-day for self-care on the final day of the workshop
- Can get pulled into overworking or exhausting self/others when the need for help is great

Mobilizing hope while avoiding the contrarian frame

- Meeting individuals where they were at prevented us from getting into a tug-of-war match between her despair and the proposed hope (can be viewed as redirecting sails rather than approaching despair straight on in an oppositional or contrarian frame)
- Working to break problems down into a manageable list to prevent them from feeling overwhelmed

Witnessing their story without being drawn into demoralization

- Utilize humor when appropriate
- Ask participants to describe past hopeless situations and what makes their situation so bad presently
- A key therapeutic component similar to narrative therapy
- Allowed participants to share their stories of demoralization and utilized hope modules to focus on strengths that helped them overcome these tragedies

Advocate without taking away the voice of those unheard

- Ensure all members of a group have an equal opportunity to speak in a variety of settings
- Utilize interpreters whenever possible
- Foster community autonomy

Finding common ground while also challenging the participants at times and providing new information

- Maintained an open mind with regard to differences in opinion (e.g., when a healthcare provider thought mindfulness was not relevant to her and could not be used with her patients, we asked her what kind of things she used to relax and regulate her emotions, which opened up the discussion)
- Validated the participants' experiences and stories
- Sang Do Re Mi (Doe, a deer) with the participants spontaneously
- Utilized a song about Galveston Texas and Hurricane Ike to connect with the participants
- Engaged with the participants in using humor at times while maintaining the importance and professionalism of the workshop
- We also provided support and educated participants on topics seemingly unrelated to the hurricanes. We learned no part of the island or its people went untouched by Irma's effects. These topics included faith/religion/spirituality, violence within the school system, sexism in the workplace, medication compliance and common mental health disorders, dementia/aging, income inequality, and housing crises.

After the Hurricanes Came a New Sense of Urgency: A Search for Opportunities

Community can include physical space, religious groups, sharing language, or being part of a team. Often geographical space defines a community. Many leave our home but do not leave the ethical obligation to respond when one's own is in need. The decision to leave one's home is never taken lightly. Reasons for leaving may include a search of opportunities, employment, education, a new life, security, and safety among other reasons. For some the moving is easy, buy a plane ticket and have the financial security of obtaining another roof quickly. But for others, the travel itself can be traumatic. Listening to immigrants and refugees share their stories of coming to the United States, gave me a sense of gratitude. One escaped his country seeking political asylum was detained for a month to do a credible interview and then released. Others who paid their hard work earned savings to coyotes, always fearful of their safety. Leaving an already unsafe environment only to struggle with challenges faced in travel.

The first aspect one misses is family and friends. Social connections that kept us safe and gave us a sense of community. One misses the music, the sounds of the environment, for example, "coqui." Panoramic views of the beach. At times even material things that hold emotional value such as a picture with grandparents. The weather, being away from family for the first time, away from our food, culture, everything I grew up with that made me who I was, certainly was challenging.

While also not feeling fully at home at the new geographic relocation. Unfortunately, for many it is more of geographic dislocation as they left, not because they chose to, but because they were forced to leave due to climate, resources, safety, or war. You are no longer part of one place and yet not fully at home with a new location. The process of denial occurs on many levels. Social denial rejecting the new local community ("I am not one of them"), psychological denial ("I don't have to grieve, I plan to go back"), and sensory denial ("I am not here; I am there") [1]. These sentiments are often transient when first moving, but may become heightened when hearing about events in one's home. They can become particularly heightened when hearing about a disaster that has torn through the place you once called home.

Survivors' Shame and Guilt

For those who were not on the islands or for whom Lady Luck spared their homes, along with the destruction came a wake of guilt. Many participants from the British Virgin Islands described feeling guilt that they were not on the islands during the hurricanes. Similarly, those who did stay on the island felt ashamed if they had not lost as much as their neighbor. One participant said, "Why do I feel pain when it wasn't so bad for me? Communal cookouts broke out among the island for whichever restaurant had their grill chained down by chance. A lone restaurant's refrigerator became a communal hub for medication and food. People came together to ensure the school reopened just 9 days after the hurricanes despite not restoring electricity on the island for 5 months.

Overcoming survivor's shame is the first step to reintegrating the community. Transcending survivor's shame is vital in that it allows altruism to thrive. If a portion of a community retains some resources through a disaster (physical and/or emotional), it is important that they are able to share their resources with their community. Often guilt and shame create barriers to care, which only further the disparities and perpetuate the cycle of survivor's shame. When a community can embrace one another and overcome this guilt, the survivors can rejoin their community and the community can utilize their complete resources. In this sense, survivors can return home (physically and emotionally) and with their arrival a community can rebuild.

Mobilizing Hope in a Community

During our workshops on the British Virgin Islands, one core skill of focus was hope mobilization. We taught hope mobilization by leading participants through an exercise on Hope Modules to highlight their own methods for mobilizing hope. These exercises provided the participants with a stage to tell their stories of despair and how they overcame their personal and community hardships. The Hope Modules are an evidence-based collection of brief psychotherapeutic interventions to counter demoralization [10]. They were designed to target daily stressors in chronically ill psychiatric patients, but have been expanded to integrate mental health into other healthcare platforms (primary care, emergency care, community health systems) and maintain utility in a variety of healthcare settings and patient populations in a cost-effective manner. Mobilization of hope accounts for 15% of the common factors of psychotherapeutic change [7]. Activating hope can also create a "domino effect" resulting in the mobilization of other common factors for change.

The Hope Modules are designed for the assessment, formulation, and intervention of an individual's core strengths and weaknesses in hope mobilization [10]. Assessment focuses on the core sectors of hope practices, which include Problem-Solving & Goal Seeking (2 core practices), Emotion Regulation (4 core practices), Activating a Core Identity (3 core practices), and Relational coping (6 core practices). Assessment typically begins with a question such as, "Can you remember any other time you felt like this?" The individual's response will indicate which core sector of hope practices the patient has utilized during previous moments of despair and which they may struggle to incorporate. Formulation includes identifying signature strengths and the category of hope mobilization, which represents the individuals' "strong suit." Formulation also includes identifying the hope practices that have been available in the past, if they are available currently, and if not, what obstacles are in the way. The final stage of formulation is identifying the strategy for hope mobilization that has the greatest likelihood for success and which objectives should be given priority. The intervention stage of hope mobilization includes intensifying or expanding the scope of signature strengths, strategizing how to overcome obstacles to accessing hope practices that have been available in the past, resurrect hope practices that have fallen in disuse or misuse due to demoralization, and adding novel hope practices (preferably from the category of the individual's "strong suit").

For our workshop, participants paired off and shared with each other one story of immense hardship. The listener then asked the storyteller how they responded to their hardship. The listener was asked to identify what chief methods the storyteller displayed in mobilizing hope. The two then switched roles. After they finished, we asked participants if they wanted to share their stories or have their partner share their stories with the group. One woman described her work at a distribution center. She struggled to provide for so many different people's needs. She struggled with emotional regulation at times due to the painful stories she heard and missing her daughter who was not on the island. She described how initially she felt overwhelmed, but would periodically remind herself that things were "okay" because there had not been a loss of life in any of the stories. She found solace in telling herself, "Things could have been worse." She also took time for herself before going to her distribution center, utilizing emotional regulation and self-care skills. Another skill she relied upon for hope mobilization was altruism. The distribution center itself allowed her to find hope in helping others.

Another woman on the island shared that she had actually been in three separate catastrophic events in her life. She found it helpful to reflect on her capacity to survive past events. She also utilized a strong core identity that reverberated within the community. She said, "In St Thomas, I went to a family friend's house who had built his home like a Tortolan." She noted how the Hope Mobilization exercises were helpful because although people use these skills all the time, there is empowerment in knowing you have the skills. She described emotional regulation and agency thinking through prayer and song. She sat with her children and sang with them to keep calm during the storm. When she found her kitchen was not harmed in the storm, she cooked for her family and her neighbors. She utilized three key features for hope mobilization in a community, relational coping, a collective identity, and altruism.

One man from Virgin Gorda asked his partner to tell his story to the group. The man came to Tortola to stay with a friend who had never been through a hurricane before. However, he had no contact with his family back in Virgin Gorda, so he was unable to utilize relational coping, possibly the most common method for mobilizing hope. He turned to emotional regulation and told himself that things were okay. He too relied on altruism to overcome the disaster by putting his focus on helping his friend. Lastly, he utilized agency thinking, telling himself the islanders had been through hurricanes before, so they can get through this.

Before, during, and after a disaster, emotion regulation can be difficult. Stimuli (sound and visual destruction) can be overwhelming and panic can ensue. One woman described her struggle in this regard. She described her panic when she discovered the category 5 hurricane was not downgraded. They had heard of category 5 hurricanes before, but in the past, they were always downgraded before hitting the islands. Her panic led to memory issues and confusion, which made it difficult for her to navigate after the storm. She did not leave her home for several days saying, "I did not want to see that this was Tortola." The only thing that got her out of her home was her dedication to her church community and a desire to be with her family.

Many people on the island had family members who lived far enough away that the journey took days to notify family members they had survived. One woman waited on her porch until her elderly brother's head showed itself on the horizon. Another man from Virgin Gorda could not get into contact with anyone due to the cell phone service being down, but he had a satellite phone and a knack for problem-solving. He called colleagues in London and asked them to publish the satellite phone number on Facebook. Suddenly he received a flood of phone calls from family members of those on the island who were checking on their loved ones. He was able to notify many members of his community that their loved ones were safe. He too was able to utilize problem-solving, altruism, and relational coping to mobilize hope in himself and his community.

Stories of Hope

Resilience and solidarity found in Vieques here are excerpts as recounted by members of AACP:

> *"I could see it in the eyes of a nurse at the makeshift hospital who explained how they were successfully able to transport a 25-week-old newborn to the main island for care. I could hear it in the voice of the EMT workers who choked up describing how he had to respond to a call for his own mentally ill mother. I could sense it in the determination of the stoic farmer: 'I am not alive to worry.' I could taste it in savory Mofongo and the sweet plantains unique to Vieques. I could feel it in the passion of the community organizer who checks in on her neighbors daily and rallies her fellow community leaders, asking 'What will happen to Vieques? Why aren't people here angrier?' What I experienced was the spirit of the people of Vieques who told their stories and are brave enough to stay and fight for their beloved island. Let us continue to remember, support, and advocate for our fellow Americans. ¡Todos somos Viequenses (We are all from Vieques)!"* (Deepika Sastry, MD, MBA)

> *'Were you here for the hurricane?' I ask. Maria. His smile wavers and suddenly he is watching the road. He was here... 'You are in your house,' he says, 'and everything is so dark.' 'You can hear the wind, and that sound, you cannot believe that sound, so loud. Then you can hear the trees cracking and falling and hitting the roof. You are with your family and you are trying to stay in the safest place and you are praying...then the next morning the wind is gone; so, you come out. And it is just ... see that green, those leaves, those trees over there. It was all gone. All no green, just mud and brown and broken things. And some of the houses are gone.'... How did people get through it? I ask. 'We are Viequesians!' ... 'I got water, I give you water. You got food, you give me food. We cut up the trees. We fix the houses if we can. We take care of the old people and the little kids.'... This is a beautiful place, I say; the people of this Island must be amazingly resilient. He looks away again. 'Yes,' he says, looking around him, 'but it is very hard.'* (Ann Hackman, MD)

A Storm on the Horizon
Although the workshop focused on resilience after a hurricane, much of our work touched on conditions that can be felt around the world. Not just in the wake of disaster. Throughout the workshops, we provided support and educated participants on topics seemingly unrelated (albeit significant) to the hurricanes. We learned that no part of the island or its people went untouched from Irma's effects. These topics included faith and spirituality, violence within the school system, sexism in the workplace, medication compliance, common mental health disorders, dementia and aging, income inequality, and housing crises. One anxiety that lingered in the shadows of the workshop was the precarious climate. Our conversations sometimes circled around the subject until it came too close for comfort. When participants mentioned the possibility of another hurricane or the impending annual hurricane season, the concerns were met with an invalidating and

uninformed reassurance that the island will never again be hit by another hurricane. At times the climate anxiety went unspoken or ignored, but it was ever present, like a storm on the horizon.

References

1. Akhtar, S. (2011). *Immigration and acculturation: Mourning, adaptation, and the next generation*. Lanham: Jason Aronson.
2. Barnett (2007) Patterson, O., Weil, F. & Patel, K. The Role of Community in Disaster Response: Conceptual Models. Popul Res Policy Rev 29, 127–141 (2010). https://doi.org/10.1007/s11113-009-9133-x
3. Candilis PJ, AR Dyer, F Noorani, M Ghabra, CS May, S Dhumad, E Kocher, (2018) The Hippocratic Oath for humanitarian aid workers The Pharos of Alpha Omega Alpha Summer 2018
4. Candilis PJ, AR Dyer, F Noorani, M Ghabra, CS May, S Dhumad, E Kocher, (2018) The Hippocratic Oath for humanitarian aid workers The Pharos of Alpha Omega Alpha Summer 2018.
5. DesMarias et al. (2012) Eric A. Des Marais, Subhasis Bhadra, Allen R. Dyer In the Wake of Japan's Triple Disaster: Rebuilding Capacity through International Collaboration Advances in Social Work Vol. 13 No. 2 (Summer 2012), 340–357
6. DeWolfe, D. J. (2000). *Training manual for mental health and human service workers in major disasters*. 2nd ed., HHS Publication No. ADM 90–538. Rockville: U.S. Department of Health and Human Services, Substance Abuse and Mental Health Services Administration, Center for Mental Health Services. (Adapted from Zunin & Myers).
7. Duncan, B. L., Miller, S. D., Wampold, B. E., & Hubble, M. A. (2010). *The heart and soul of change, second edition*. Washington, DC: American Psychological Association.
8. Dyer, A. R. (2016). Building Resilience for Humanitarian Workers, Athens, Greece. https://sites.google.com/site/gwresilienceworkshop/
9. Griffith, J. (2018). Hope modules: Brief psychotherapeutic interventions to counter demoralization from daily stressors of chronic illness. Academic Psychiatry, 42(1), 135–145. https://doi.org/10.1007/s40596-017-0748-7.
10. Griffith, J. L., Kohrt, A. B., Dyer, A. Polatin, P. Morse, M. Jabr, S. Abdeen, S. Gaby, L. M., Jindal, A. & Khin, E. K., (2017) Training Psychiatrists for Global Mental Health: Cultural Psychiatry, Collaborative Inquiry, and Ethics of AlterityAcad Psychiatry. Author manuscript; available in PMC 2017 Jul 3.Published in final edited form as: Acad Psychiatry. 2016 Aug;40(4): 701–706.Published online 2016 Apr 8. https://doi.org/10.1007/s40596-016-0541-z.
11. Bhadra, S., & Pulla V. (2014). Community interventions in disasters. In K. Goel, V. Pulla, & A. P. Francis (Eds.), Community work: Theories, experiences & challenges (pp. 103–117). Oxford: Oxford University Press.
12. Dyer, A., Dyer, A. R., Torres-LLenza, V., Cayetano, C., Posada, J., Safran, J., & Quesnell, C. (2019). Resilience training in the British Virgin Islands: An innovative program in the post disaster setting. publication pending. 2020.
13. Caban-Aleman, C. (2019). Puerto Rico Se Levanta ("Puerto Rico Rises"): From Denial and Passivity to Action and Hope. Psychiatric Times, July 30, 2019. https://www.psychiatrictimes.com/view/puerto-rico-se-levanta-puerto-rico-rises-denial-and-passivity-action-and-hope.
14. Kasi, S., Bhadra, S., & Dyer, A. (2007). A decade of disasters: Lessons from the Indian experience. Southern Medical Journal, 100 (9). https://doi.org/10.1097/SMJ.0b013e318145a5d5.

Global Mental Health, Planetary Health, and the Ethical Co-Benefit

Janet L. Lewis

Introduction

In my job as a psychiatrist, an exchange I have had with patients more than once has gone like this:

I'm drawing the patient's attention to some aspect of their situation that they are ignoring.

Then the patient says, only half-jokingly, "Hey, whose side are you on, anyway?"

And then I say, "I'm on the side of reality."

Our job in the mental health professions is helping people to function better and be more fulfilled within and in relation to reality. To do our jobs within the mental health professions, we have to understand both the patient and reality. We then help the patient deal with, influence, and hopefully thrive within reality.

Now we are all facing the question of what does it mean for our work, and what does it mean for the mental health professions, when reality includes human-made destabilization of the climate and other environmental degradation. This question has additional relevance when we consider global mental health.

Our Dilemma

It is now becoming urgently clear that global mental health is intimately connected to planetary health and that furthermore the biosphere which is our planet is experiencing ill-health, as a result of human activity. The burning of fossil fuels and animal agriculture are most responsible for the recent global heating which has destabilized our climate system. This is discussed at length by the Intergovernmental Panel on Climate Change and throughout respected medical journals (e.g., [18, 20]).

J. L. Lewis (✉)
University of Rochester, Penn Yan, NY, USA

© Springer Nature Switzerland AG 2021
A. R. Dyer et al. (eds.), *Global Mental Health Ethics*,
https://doi.org/10.1007/978-3-030-66296-7_22

Our understanding of climate change has an over century-long history [23]. In 1896, Swedish scientist Svante Arrhenius, as part of a theory designed to explain the Ice Ages, predicted that the burning of fossil fuels, by adding carbon dioxide to the atmosphere, would raise the planet's average temperature, in what we now call a "greenhouse effect." Whereas much solar radiation normally reflects off the Earth and back into space, carbon dioxide in the atmosphere traps the infrared portion of that energy, further warming the Earth. In the 1930s it was apparent that the Northern Atlantic and the United States had warmed, but it was thought to be part of a natural cycle. In 1960, very detailed measurements by C. D. Keeling showed that the level of carbon dioxide in the atmosphere was in fact rising. As the understanding of the complexity of the climate system and its feedback loops grew, it became apparent that small perturbations could prompt great shifts. It was also discovered that levels of methane and other "greenhouse gases" generated by human activity were rising. Then in the 1980s and 1990s data from the trapped CO_2 in Antarctic ice cores proved Arrhenius and the developing computer models to be correct. Carbon dioxide and temperature have been linked over hundreds of thousands of years, with a rise or fall in one corresponding to a rise or fall in the other. Simultaneously some corporations and individuals who opposed government regulation invested millions in advertising, lobbying, and scientific-looking "reports" designed to convince the public and lawmakers that global warming was not a problem. The link between human carbon emissions and rising global temperatures had been well established, however, two other factors, taken together, created room for nearly endless debate, delaying public acceptance of climate science. These were the complexity of climate science itself and the psychological difficulty inherent in accepting climate change.

Because of rising global temperature, the Intergovernmental Panel on Climate Change was formed and it issued its first report in 2001, which had to be cautiously phrased so no government representative would dissent, but which confirmed that it was very likely the world faces severe global warming. It is now scientific consensus that climate change is happening, is very serious, is largely human-caused, and that there are things we can do about it.

Climate change attributable to human greenhouse gas emissions is causing and predicted to cause worsened:

- Disasters – storms, floods, heat waves, wildfires, droughts, sea level rise
- Food and water insecurity
- Migration of vector-borne diseases, increased harmful algal blooms
- Forced migrations and violence
- Resultant increased psychological trauma from all of the above

Heat itself is now associated with both violence and suicide [1, 6]. Furthermore, we can expect the transgenerational transmission of these traumas, whereby the progeny of those affected can, by various psychological, social, epigenetic, and hormonal mechanisms, also be affected [2, 19, 25, 26].

In examining planetary health it becomes clear that manifestations of planetary ill-health, most urgently climate change, but also plastics in the oceans and other ecosystems, air pollution, pesticides, and other toxins, the massive die-off of insects, the sixth mass extinction we are currently undergoing, are all symptoms of a more overarching issue which is essentially relational. Therefore, our understanding of and approach to planetary health must be layered, much like a clinical case of an eating disordered patient whose potassium level is so dangerously low her heart might stop. We would recognize her overarching issues as behavioral, cognitive, and relational, even as we most urgently focus on correction of the life-threatening potassium. Similarly, with regard to planetary health, we are most urgently concerned with climate change because it threatens planet-wide catastrophe if not immediately addressed. However, we know all planetary health issues are related. We know we are not facing a choice between focus on the elimination of greenhouse gas emissions, preparation for climate change impacts, or better orienting ourselves to our real relationship with the living biosphere. Rather we recognize the nested nature of these problems.

The pediatrician and psychoanalyst Donald Winnicott famously said there is no such thing as an infant, there is only a mother and an infant [22]. Similarly, we now see there is no such thing as a human being; there are only humans being embedded in the living biosphere, "Mother Earth," inextricably connected both to Her and through Her to each-other. It is now clear that we are all in the same boat. In order to address climate change, developing countries must skip over fossil fuels, countries with rain forests must be economically capable of preserving them, and so all of us must concern ourselves with distant others. The overarching relational issue of planetary health is about the quality of humanity's relationship with the natural world and it is about the quality of humanity's relationship with itself.

The Ethical Co-benefit and Climate Inequity

In addition to layers of problems, there are also layers of co-benefits in the addressing of these problems. Health co-benefits of addressing climate change are now widely discussed. These include the elimination of diseases due to air pollution and better health from more active transport (walking, bicycling) as well as improved mental health and resilience resulting from necessary coming together in community for climate adaptation work (e.g., [27]).

Could an additional co-benefit of addressing climate change be an ethical one? Many systems of moral development recognize expanding circles of concern as the hallmark of moral development. In order to successfully address and prepare for climate change, an ultimately world-centric focus is now not only ethical. It is practical.

Whereas much mental health discussion about climate change discusses defense mechanisms and becomes a discussion about climate denial and what is wrong with us, we can benefit much more from a discussion about what is right with us. Almost all humans care for others beyond themselves and also have the capacity to even further extend that care. In addressing climate change and other manifestations of planetary ill-health, we are aiming for a future that has these advantages – a coming together to work for our collective health and the ability to attend realistically to our relationship with the natural world. Recent climate communications research indicates that, in addition to valuing scientific and economic advancement, the public values a more moral and caring community as a potential outcome of climate work [3].

As many writers discuss, we are all currently emerging from various degrees of denial about climate change (e.g., [21]). Part of what we are awakening to is a disturbing situation of inequity wherein the burdens of climate change are being, and are expected to further be, disproportionately borne by the populations of the world who have been least involved in the generation of greenhouse gases (Fig. 22.1).

The first map above illustrates regional carbon dioxide emissions for the years 1950–2000, illustrating the large contribution to atmospheric CO_2 by developed nations. The second map describes the estimated distribution of climate-related increase in mortality from diarrhea, malaria, inland and coastal flooding, and malnutrition from 2000 to 2030. The relative size of each region represents the increase in fatalities from these causes attributable to climate change for each region during

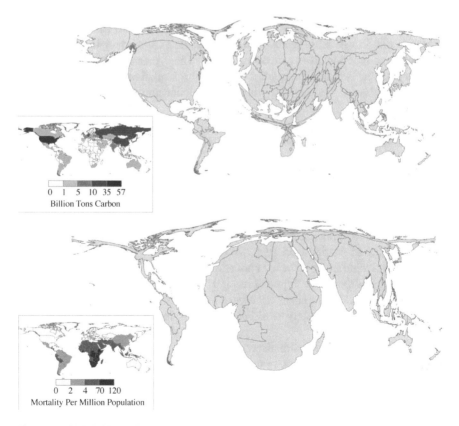

Fig. 22.1 Global CO_2 Emissions and Health Impacts

that period, illustrating the vulnerability of resource-limited regions to climate health effects. (Reprinted with permission from Patz et al. [15])

Extending our care more consciously to global health will create a beneficial feedback loop. Opening to "them" is opening also to the reality of us, the reality of what we are all facing. If we take more seriously the suffering in developing countries, we would act more quickly on climate change which would ultimately be beneficial to all of us. Climate awareness produces ethical awareness which produces greater climate awareness. (repeat) It has been said that people either come to be concerned about climate change because of social justice awareness or they come to concern about social justice because of environmental awareness [16]. In either case, one's circle of concern is expanded, which can be seen to be an ethical co-benefit.

Mitigation and Adaptation/Resilience

Literature in all fields relating to climate change describes two crucial aspects of our healthy response to climate change – mitigation and adaptation.

Mitigation is reducing the severity of something, it is *avoiding what can be avoided*.

NASA defines mitigation as "Reducing emissions of and stabilizing the levels of heat-trapping greenhouse gases in the atmosphere" [14] (https://climate.nasa.gov/solutions/adaptation-mitigation/).

Why should mental health professionals work on mitigation in our activities? There are two reasons. In the 1960s, cigarette companies had ads that depicted doctors smoking. When clinicians act as though it is business as usual and do not change their own behavior, it sends the implicit message that the behavior is not really a health issue. Even though one's own behavior is easily thought of as a drop in the bucket, it has additional power because it helps to change culture. The second reason is directly practical, in that the carbon footprint (greenhouse gas production) of the mental health system is not insignificant. This has been documented in data from the UK National Health Service [13], where the largest portion of the mental health system's carbon footprint is found to be attributable to pharmaceuticals. Mitigation strategies there include efforts at reducing medication wastage and more use of social and nature-based treatments.

Adaptation means becoming better suited to one's environment; it is *adapting to the unavoidable, and reducing vulnerability*. NASA defines adaptation as "Adapting to the climate change already in the pipeline [14]." Greenhouse gases have long residence times in the atmosphere and keep producing increased heat long after they have been emitted. According to the Intergovernmental Panel on Climate Change, methane stays in the atmosphere for 12 years. Carbon dioxide stays in the atmosphere for varying lengths of time dependent on conditions, but generally for many decades. Therefore, we are now experiencing the results of greenhouse gas emissions from decades ago and we can expect increased global heating effects even if we rapidly become carbon neutral in our activities. Adding to the seriousness of our situation are feedback loops in the climate system, such as loss of the albedo effect with ice melt and the release of methane from melting permafrost, that create accelerations in heating beyond what would be expected from the presence of the greenhouse gases themselves. The term adaptation encompasses all activities that help us to prepare for and be less vulnerable to these effects.

Out of concern for adaptation has grown a particular focus on the notion of *resilience.*

Resilience is defined in many ways. I like this definition by the Rockefeller Foundation. *Resilience is "the capacity of individuals, communities and systems to survive, adapt, and grow in the face of stress and shocks, and even transform when conditions require it"* [17] (https://www.rockefellerfoundation.org).

Resilience is a useful concept, but some controversy surrounds it.

Those expressing wariness of the concept of resilience cite the multiple implicit meanings that the word resilience can have. Resilience can mean *resisting change, accommodating change, or directing change* [9]. Critics express concern that in practice apparently resilient behaviors could actually be maladaptive as people double down on rebuilding in the same old individualistic, high consumption ways. People can unconsciously consider survival to mean survival of lifestyles with which they are identified. Another pitfall is that encouraging resilience of affected groups can distract from, and be used as a substitute for, addressing the systemic issues that perpetuate their vulnerability. It is more convenient to engage in "resilience training" of affected populations than to advocate legislatively for measures that will reduce poverty, improve education, enhance security, and in those ways strengthen communities. Nevertheless, it is crucial that the activities of resilience training and social justice work be seen as both/and responses rather than as mutually exclusive.

First Person Narrative

People who are between disasters have responsibilities as I have learned from disasters I have experienced in my own life. Talk of one's own difficult experience is often a projective identification, where one is simply projecting one's own trauma-related feelings in talking about something terrible, with a lack of useful digestion of that experience. What I hope to provide here is useful digestion, useful reflection on the implications of multiple disasters. I do this because the reality of multiple disasters is an important part of what we confront with climate change. I have been through some disasters, which I describe here as background to explain principles with which I have emerged. I have been through a hurricane – Hurricane Hugo in Charleston S.C. During that hurricane, I was a psychiatry resident on call in the County hospital near the water. The building shook all night; the first floor flooded, we lost power and water and telephones. It really did feel as though the building might crumble. I have also had my house burn down, killing my cats who I was unable to rescue. I had flooding in the basement of my office in a "freak storm" a year and a half after the house burned down. A year after that I had flooding in the basement of my next home, in another "freak storm".

Here is what I have come to believe:

- *We are either within or between disasters;*
- *therefore those between disasters have a responsibility:*

Even under fortunate circumstances of financial security and extensive social support, a disaster is enormously disruptive. A lot of time and attention goes into maintaining and rebuilding. There is the dirty work of attending to possessions, and there is the displacement which highlights one's dependence on all the particular places and routines undergirding a life. There is grief, the processing of which typically gets delayed in the immediate disaster aftermath. There is also cognitive dissonance as one deals with systems that march on unaffected by disaster and with others who are not in the disaster. With the flooding of my basement, I one day went straight from wringing muddy water out of my clothes to sitting in my office listening to someone who was excitedly describing small details of their perfect new house. Not only is disaster disruptive, but it also sets one apart socially. When an entire community goes through a disaster, as I experienced with Hurricane Hugo, there is a comradery in the initial phase of heroically pulling together, but it is followed by more difficult phases.

It became clear to me that, because of the attention-intensive disruption caused by disaster, people in the midst of or in the immediate aftermath of disasters are not able to be working on necessary mitigation and adaptation to climate change. That means it is incumbent upon the rest of us to be doing this work. I refer to "the rest of us" as those who are between disasters. Disasters are becoming more frequent and severe. Clearly, no part of the country or the world is immune from the increasing disasters related to sea level rise, wildfires, increasingly intense storms, heat waves, and toxic algal blooms. Nobody is now immune. Therefore, in doing the work to address climate change we must function like a flock of geese, where the head goose, tired by the brunt of the wind will drop back and somebody else will take the lead, allowing others to ride in their draft. I credit my daughter with this lovely metaphor. This is what will need to happen across neighborhoods and across the world as areas in the midst of and aftermath of disasters will be unable to do as much for themselves and will certainly be unable to initiate necessary large programs for the addressing of climate change. Therefore, those less affected must do the work. Since no one is immune, the practical logic of this should be apparent.

Respect for Autonomy, in the Context of Disasters, Can Be Inappropriate

Because people in the midst of disasters must attend to so much, they are not in the best position to know what they need. I cannot tell you how many people sincerely said, "Let me know if there is anything I can do," after my house burned down. I was in no position to figure out what others might do. My family and I were best helped by those who took it upon themselves to do things or give us stuff. Analogously, it makes no sense, and is neglectful, to wait for those most affected by climate change to educate us about climate change or to tell us what they need.

Waking up and Mobilizing Requires Varieties of Containment

Around the time of my second flood experience, I was at an Integral Theory conference, where climate change was being discussed. This gathering dealt with complex metamodels of reality and was also spiritually oriented, so the environment of the conference was open, intellectually curious, and supportive. My suitemate there was distressed by the climate change information. In contrast to the equanimity of most attendees, she spoke to me with agitation, looking me in the eye and saying, "The bottom line, Janet, is that we might be able to adapt to 2 degrees. But right now we are on track for over 4 degrees, and that will create an Earth we would not recognize." Even though I had heard these things before, in that instant the information penetrated me and it was immediately clear to me that this was the most important thing happening and I must work on it. In short order, I reflected on what I could contribute and set about finding like-minded colleagues. I credit the *containing* environment of that conference with my waking up and mobilizing. Climate change evokes many fears which are then unconsciously defended against, interfering with awareness and engagement [21]. However, we have many means of bearing difficult information. The term containment was notably used in the psychotherapeutic literature by Bion [5] to refer very specifically to the process whereby an infant's emotional distress is taken in by the mother and modified into a bearable form within the mother and through the mother's communications back to the infant. Since Bion, the term containment has also been used more broadly. I use it here to refer to all things which allow us to bear difficult information and feelings. In that moment at the conference, I was contained by intellectual frameworks, relationships, and spirituality. From that point on I have also been contained by my own agentic work in concert with other people. The particular meanings granted to the natural world and to human struggle from the cultures and religious traditions that influence me are easy to take for granted, but I am coming to also recognize their profoundly containing effects.

Waking up to and engaging with climate change and our larger environmental dilemma requires varieties of containment [12]. Therefore part of the project now before us requires the cultivation, and the provision, of these kinds of containment – relational, cognitive, spiritual, and agentic, as well as kinds of containment available in systems of meaning-making and support inherited or adopted from cultural and religious traditions. These containing activities are often subsumed under the notion of resilience, or of "transformational resilience." However, as I mentioned earlier, there are connotations of resilience that are problematic. Therefore, because of the importance of containment, I believe it is useful to appreciate and consider the need for containment separately.

Global mental health will be supported by work on the various forms of containment that can allow for clear thinking and action among those who are not in the immediate aftermath of disasters. Therefore, the promotion of these forms of containment can be recognized as important to global health.

Complex Systems and Wicked Problems

Cognitively, an important containing framework for understanding our situation is that of complex systems. There is a technical difference between a complicated system and a complex system.

A complicated system is like the workings of an analog watch. There are many gears, multiple moving parts in contact with other moving parts. However, if you know the math and physics and the size and placement of the gears, you can determine precisely what the effect of any intervention will be in the system. This is a complicated system.

A complex system is different. Climate is a complex system. Those working in mental health and in global health also have experience with complex systems, because human beings are complex systems. With a complex system, you cannot predict precisely what the effect of any intervention will be. Here are some other characteristics of complex systems [7]:

- System memory/history
- A diversity of behaviors
- Elements interact dynamically
- Level of interaction is fairly rich
- Interactions are nonlinear
- There are loops in the interconnections
- Complex systems are open systems
- Complex systems operate under conditions far from equilibrium
- Individual elements are ignorant of the behavior of the whole system within which they are embedded
- Chaos (the butterfly effect) and self-organization (emergence, evolution)

I am describing the nature of complexity for three reasons.

- The first is that it is important to understand that with which we are dealing.
- The second is that there are some hopeful features of complex systems that can be usefully taken to heart, like "the butterfly effect" and "emergence" of higher levels of organization. Because of complexity, anyone's actions could have important repercussions (the butterfly effect). Because of complexity, we can look beyond even extensive and painful environmental degradation to the possibility of new workable patterns/systems coming into being, the characteristics of which cannot be entirely predicted ahead of time (emergence). The creation of these new structures would involve the participation of all parts of the planetary system, which includes us.
- The third reason is that complex systems produce implications, believe it or not, for the appropriateness of our involvement with climate.

Problems involving many aspects of complex systems get called "wicked problems." The term *wicked problem* was first coined in 1967 in discussions about social policy. Climate is a wicked problem. The geosciences involved are enormously complex. Additionally, with climate, beyond the complexity of the geosciences, there is now involvement of all the human factors – human systems, human cultures, the functioning of the psychology of individuals – all of these factors are influencing climate.

Many theorists in various disciplines have been grappling with the question of what is the best approach to a wicked problem such as climate, where there are so many moving parts and we cannot know with certainty what the effect of an intervention will be. Two things have been concluded.

The first is that there must be interdisciplinary and what is now being called transdisciplinary work. The second is that there must be continual reassessment of our situation and of the effects of interventions [4, 8, 10].

So not only is it easily argued that our involvement with the climate change emergency is appropriate because of our obligations to work for public health. It also makes sense for us to be involved because the very nature of the wicked climate problem *calls for* interdisciplinary response and action.

Defries and Nagendra describe two "traps" in work with the wicked problem of climate – falsely assuming a tame solution and inaction from overwhelming complexity. There is not a tame solution to a complex problem. A complex wicked problem calls for work from multiple angles. Given the emergency that is this problem, it can be easily argued that it calls for all hands on deck.

There are three facets of mental health systems' relationship with climate change, all of which now have developing literature. The first two, mitigation and adaptation, are described above. The third is what can be called "Reckoning with reality."

Reckoning with Reality Is an Ongoing Task, As Essential as Mitigation and Adaptation

In reckoning with reality, the complexity and emotionally charged nature of climate change material make it difficult to psychologically hold. As a result, almost prismatically, a constellation of dialectics arises as one considers climate change. Examples of these dialectics are hope–despair, certainty–uncertainty, scientific climate reality–social reality, individual agency–collective agency, nature as comfort–nature as a threat, collapse–evolving civilization. It can be tempting to constrict one's attention to only one pole of these dialectics, but, for the purposes of learning and creative response, it is important to hold dialectics open, exploring the poles and the tensions between them [12].

Many psychoanalysts are describing individuals being in degrees of disavowal in relation to climate change. Disavowal is a defense mechanism wherein one can know and not know something at the same time [21]. Because of degrees of ambivalence about climate change, people can appear as though they are from different tribes when they may be at different stages en route to acceptance or acknowledgment. Data from the Yale Climate surveys [11] support this supposition. They divide the population into the so-called "Six Americas," consisting of "the Alarmed," "the Concerned," "the Cautious," "the Disengaged,", "the Doubtful," and "the Dismissive." However, the Yale surveys document increases in the proportion of Concerned and Alarmed over time, with decreases in the proportion of Dismissive, Doubtful, and Cautious. They also document that even among less concerned Americans, significant minorities endorse feelings of fear and helplessness about global warming. So it can be argued that even those who appear less concerned are in some stage of a process of reckoning with reality (Fig. 22.2).

Reckoning with reality involves respecting our actual relationship with the natural world. We cannot just objectively assess and then decide what to do, though

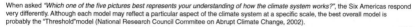

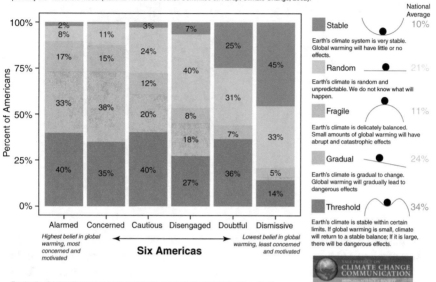

Fig. 22.2 Climate Stability as understood by global warming's six Americas [24]. (https://climatecommunication.yale.edu/publications/climate-stability-as-understood-by-global-warmings-six-americas/)

objective assessment is important. An approach of only objective assessment would be instrumental; it would be objectifying. It would not be appreciating the real relationship we are involved in. Our relationship with the natural world is like any relationship – always unfolding, ultimately uncertain, influenceable by us, influencing of us, and eliciting our own feelings and reactions which in turn influence our attitudes and our responses. Some categorize this kind of reflection as part of adaptation or resilience. But given our tendency to ignore our real relationship with and our embeddedness in the natural world, the ongoing need for reckoning with reality is too easily overlooked. Therefore I recommend we consider it a separate category. We, our individual lives, all of our cultural inheritances, our systems, and institutions, have all been created within a relatively stable climate system which is now dramatically changing. We are necessarily inside that which we are now seeking to understand and influence. We are completely dependent upon that which we are seeking to understand and influence. These factors challenge us practically, intellectually, and emotionally, making the necessary reckoning, and the fruits which can emerge from it, very easy to ignore or gloss over. Ongoing reassessment of our situation, our values, and our goals will necessarily be a process of continuous revelation, just as in any healthy long-term relationship. Reckoning with reality on an individual level means time for deep reflection and processing of thoughts and feelings with others.

Fig. 22.3 Addressing Global Mental Health within Planetary Health

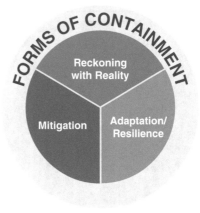

Addressing Global Mental Health within Planetary Health

Reckoning with reality at the global scale means understanding and lending one's advocacy to policies such as those in the Paris agreement, and understanding the evolving recommendations of the Intergovernmental Panel on Climate Change (IPCC). It also means deciding how in one's own personal and professional life, one can best contribute and finding allies in doing so. There are no sidelines on which to sit. We are by definition all included in the problems and solutions of planetary health (Fig. 22.3).

Recommendations

The Importance of Focusing on Less Affected Areas for Education

It is the populations who are not in the aftermath of disasters that can bear more of the headwinds.

Those who are wringing muddy water out of their clothes, grieving lost loved ones, figuring out new routines in alien households, or migrating to more hospitable locations are not in positions to be devoting attention to the influencing of necessary policies and cultural attitudes that can support mitigation and adaptation to climate change.

Populations less affected should be targeted for the processing of planetary health information and for the cultivation of forms of containment that can assist with the processing of this information and the taking of action to mitigate and adapt.

Both/and Thinking

Climate change easily elicits seeming polarities that should be held in dynamic tension. Ongoing aggressive work is needed on multiple fronts within the three domains of mitigation, adaptation, and reckoning with reality. Because of the multifaceted nature of the problem and solutions, everyone has things to contribute and different people will play different roles. We should use care not to exclude some avenues as we pursue others. Wicked problems require work from multiple angles.

Remembering Containment

Given the challenging nature of reckoning with this reality and its dynamic uncertainty, means of containment should be kept in mind and promoted – cognitive containment, relational containment, spiritual containment, containment provided by cultural and religious traditions, and perhaps most importantly agentic containment. All those working in the field of mental health should be prepared to transmit the containing understanding that though we traverse tumultuous times, within complex systems new stable patterns can emerge. However, no one is on the sidelines of that emergence, and urgent change is now required, for the living systems of the planet and for ourselves. Before you go back to what you were doing, take a moment to think deeply about what you can do.

References

1. Anderson, C. A. (2001). Heat and violence. *Current Directions in Psychological Science, 10*, 33–38.
2. Baider, L., Peretz, T., Hadani, P. E., et al. (2000). Transmission of response to trauma? Second-generation Holocaust survivors' reaction to cancer. *The American Journal of Psychiatry, 157*(6), 904–910.
3. Bain, P. G., Milfont, T. L., Kashima, Y., Bilewicz, M., Doron, G., Gardarsdottir, R. B., et al. (2016). Co-benefits of addressing climate change can motivate action around the world. *Nature Climate Change, 6*(2), 154–157.
4. Berry, H. L., et al. (2018). The case for systems thinking about climate change and mental health. *Nature Climate Change, 8*(4), 282–290.
5. Bion, W. (1962). *Learning from experience*. London: Karnac Books.
6. Burke, M., González, F., Baylis, P., Heft-Neal, S., Baysan, C., Basu, S., & Hsiang, S. (2018). Higher temperatures increase suicide rates in the United States and Mexico. *Nature Climate Change, 8*(8), 723–729.
7. Cilliers, P. (Ed.). (2007). *Thinking complexity: Complexity & Philosophy, volume 1*. Marblehead: ISCE Publishing.
8. Defries, R., & Nagendra, H. (2017). Ecosystem management as a wicked problem. *Science, 21*, 265–270.
9. Fisichelli, N. A., Schuurman, G. W., & Hoffman, C. H. (2016). Is 'resilience' maladaptive? Towards an accurate lexicon for climate change adaptation. *Environmental Management, 57*(4), 753–758. https://doi.org/10.1007/s00267-015-0650-6.
10. Galway, L. P., Parkes, M. W., Corbett, K. K., Allen, D. M., & Takaro, T. K. (2016). Climate change frames in public health and water resource management: Towards Intersectoral climate change adaptation. In F. W. Leal, H. Musa, G. Cavan, P. O'Hare, & J. Seixas (Eds.), *Climate change adaptation, resilience and hazards. Climate change management*. Cham: Springer.
11. Leiserowitz, A., Maibach, E., Rosenthal, S., Kotcher, J., Ballew, M., Goldberg, M., & Gustafson, A. (2018). *Climate change in the American mind: December 2018*. New Haven: Yale University and George Mason University. Yale Program on Climate Change Communication.
12. Lewis, J., Haase, E., & Trope, A. (2020). Climate dialectics: Holding open the space between abyss and advance. *Psychodynamic Psychiatry, 48*(3), 271–294.
13. Maughan, D. (2015). *Sustainability in psychiatry. Occasional paper 97*. London: Royal College of Psychiatrists.

14. National Aeronautics and Space Administration. https://climate.nasa.gov/solutions/adaptation-mitigation/. Accessed 9/15/19.
15. Patz, J. A., Gibbs, H. K., Foley, J. A., Rogers, J. V., & Smith, K. R. (2007). Climate change and global health: Quantifying a growing ethical crisis. *EcoHealth, 4*(4), 400.
16. Ray, S. J. (n.d). My favorite lecture: Coming of age at the end of the world. Accessed at https://www.khsu.org/post/my-favorite-lecture-coming-age-end-world, 9/15/19.
17. Rockefeller Foundation. https://www.rockefellerfoundation.org/blog/investing-right-now-tomorrow/. Accessed 9/15/19.
18. Salas, R. N., Malina, D., & Solomon, C. G. (2019). Prioritizing health in a changing climate. *The New England Journal of Medicine, 381*, 773–774.
19. Volkan, V. D. (2001). Transgenerational transmissions and chosen traumas: An aspect of large-group identity. *Group Analysis, 34*(1), 79–97.
20. Watts, N., Amann, M., Arnell, N., et al. (2018). The 2018 report of the Lancet countdown on health and climate change: Shaping the health of nations for centuries to come. *Lancet, 392*, 2479–2514.
21. Weintrobe, S. (Ed.). (2013). *Engaging with climate change: Psychoanalytic and interdisciplinary perspectives*. London/New York: Routledge.
22. Winnicott, D. W. (1960). The theory of the parent-infant relationship. *The International Journal of Psycho-Analysis, 41*, 585–595.
23. Weart, S. (2008). *The discovery of global warming: Revised and expanded edition*. Cambridge, MA: Harvard University Press.
24. Yale Project on Climate Change Communication. https://climatecommunication.yale.edu/publications/climate-stability-as-understood-by-global-warmings-six-americas/. Accessed 7/15/2020.
25. Yehuda, R., & Bierer, L. M. (2009). The relevance of epigenetics to PTSD: Implications for the DSM-V. *Journal of Traumatic Stress, 22*(5), 427–434.
26. Yehuda, R., & Bierer, L. M. (2008). Transgenerational transmission of cortisol and PTSD risk. *Progress in Brain Research, 167*, 121–135.
27. Younger, M., Morrow-Almeida, H. R., Vindigni, S. M., & Dannenberg, A. L. (2008). The built environment, climate change, and health: Opportunities for co-benefits. *American Journal of Preventive Medicine, 35*(5), 517–526.

Part VII

Conclusion

Arriving at the Ethics of Global Mental Health

23

Philip J. Candilis

The Variety of Ethics Approaches

It may be clear by now that the ethics of global mental health requires an appreciation of the many perspectives that inform the work. Whether it is the cultural sensitivity required of mental health staff, aid-workers, and policy-makers who work with people from all over the world, or the accountability required of organizations and funders, the language of perspective is omnipresent. Stakeholders each have a unique viewpoint that affects their choices – viewpoints that require more than a claim to objectivity, right, or principle.

Nowhere is this issue more poignant than in the distribution of scarce resources. With mental health services neglected in even the wealthiest nations [1], recent population shifts as a result of war and drought only make matters worse. 2015 marked monumental economic and public health challenges as a historic migration from the Middle East and Africa flooded Asia Minor and Europe. The 2017 educational installation, Forced from Home, on the National Mall in Washington DC asked visitors to choose which critical items to give up as they made their way through the refugee experience. Like refugees, would the visitors choose to give up their money at some stage of their passage, their valuables, their papers, their bodies?

Families, aid agencies, and governments all experience limitations to their resources, whether for their well-being, for a trip to the clinic, or for funding a program of psychological support. In 2018, Medicins sans Frontieres (MSF), the prominent Swiss-based non-governmental organization, spent 542 million Euros in the ten most disadvantaged countries on their roster, providing 11.2 million outpatient

P. J. Candilis (✉)
Department of Behavioral Health, Saint Elizabeths Hospital, Washington, DC, USA

Department of Psychiatry and Behavioral Sciences, The George Washington University, Washington, DC, USA
e-mail: philip.candilis@dc.gov

© Springer Nature Switzerland AG 2021
A. R. Dyer et al. (eds.), *Global Mental Health Ethics*,
https://doi.org/10.1007/978-3-030-66296-7_23

consultations, 2.4 million treatments for malaria, 74,000 inpatient feedings for severely malnourished children, and 25,000 medical treatments for people experiencing sexual violence [2]. The MSF's own public filings are clear that this falls substantially short of assisting the families and individuals that seek their help; indeed, the number of MSF projects working with displaced people alone has more than doubled since 2012 ([2], p. 6).

The question for students of both ethics and global health is what the idea, rule, or standard must be for applying scarce funds, medicines, and staffing. Does one prioritize the neediest or most vulnerable, each family or individual equally, those who apply first, or those who can make it to established centers? Which is most effective? Is that the same as what is right? Are these mutually exclusive? Each option requires an ethics decision before families, budget officers, or governments can make appropriate choices.

The good news is that there are numerous choices among ethics frameworks for deciding moral outcomes – many of them reviewed in previous chapters. There are arguments for the greatest good for the greatest number (consequentialism/utilitarianism), for doing one's duty (deontology, Kantian ethics, religious imperatives), for being virtuous (Aristotle, virtue ethics), for following specific guiding principles (especially justice as fairness), for using processes suited to a specific community (communitarian or liberal democratic ethics), and many more. It is heartening to policy-makers and clinicians alike to have so many tools for analyzing the global challenge of insufficient mental health resources. There is strength to approaches that can choose among theories to fit the unique human requirement of disparate settings [3].

The problem is that such choices themselves require guidance, so that balancing one principle or theory against another (say, balancing international support and national sovereignty), or setting one *above* another (ideas of fairness over the economic realities of transporting supplies to rural areas), may result in highly imperfect solutions that violate other dearly held standards. Tying foreign aid to internal political changes or setting eligibility requirements for individual benefits is a time-honored yet controversial strategy for setting external standards over national or personal autonomy.

For those who weigh classic principles against each other by balancing or ordering (rather than choosing a single unifying idea or set of ideas), scholars have found ways to minimize the damage. Ethicist James Childress [4], for example, is among those who counsel that the infringement of a valued principle or rule must carry a realistic prospect of attaining the moral objective; the infringement of the principle must be necessary in the circumstances, the infringement must be the least possible to achieve the primary goal, and the actor must seek to minimize the negative effects of the infringement.

As satisfying as this classic treatment can be, a consensus has developed in much of ethics that this too may be insufficient (e.g., [5, 6, 7]). The narratives of families, nations, and peoples may be ignored by applications of principle that are taken out of context or that ignore situational influences, especially oppressive ones. Ignoring the story of how a crisis arose is as harmful as ignoring the patient's unique experience of illness. Philosopher John Arras [8] is among those who recognize that ethics was never about principles without narrative. Stories provide not only symptoms, but also perspective and meaning – the moral context to any ethics decision.

The story of the individual Syrian who is physically and psychologically devastated by civil war matters in this richer framework, and may yield a different ethical claim than that of the local hospital or international aid agency struggling to provide assistance in a warzone. How strenuous is the obligation for a person to reach the hospital for a family member, or for a supply truck to reach a safe zone? Does the story change if the family member is a child, or the truck holds the last of the penicillin? Of course it does.

In an evolving global ethics that rarely views truth as absolute, competing principles like "Help thy neighbor" or "To each his own" are enriched by story-telling knowledge. The individual's personal trajectory toward a mental health or humanitarian crisis is as much part of the analysis as any political history that resists it (i.e., anti-psychiatry or anti-immigration movements), or that created it in the first place (e.g., domestic violence or proxy wars).

The story or narrative brings perspective to difficult moral work, and everyone has a perspective. Philosopher Thomas Nagel [9] in his seminal work was surely right when he argued that there is no "view from nowhere": one cannot help being influenced by one's upbringing, education, and experiences. Although multiple perspectives may confound objectivity, they enrich the moral view of complex problems.

Consequently, a contemporary combination of principles and narrative may be more helpful than classic theories that struggled with the condition of societies divided by class, economics, and cultural identity. If one recognizes how scholars often thought about the obligations between people one may see the advantage of a narrative-enriched ethics.

Much of the development of ethics is found in role theory – the idea that expectations derive from one's status in society. It is an idea that is evident in cultures across history, from India and Japan's caste systems, to the propertied classes of England and Iran. Nineteenth-century British philosopher F.H. Bradley [10], who exemplified this approach in the West, located moral understanding in the cultural and historical particulars of his time – especially in class distinctions and social constraints. For Europe, *noblesse oblige* was a common social construct of the day: the occasion of noble birth and status generated certain obligations to the less fortunate. This is a far cry from modern views of the United Nations or World Health Organization that honor (in the main) the perspective, identity, and culture of their constituents regardless of historical origin, wealth, or geography.

An ethics of global mental health that incorporates cultural narratives alongside fundamental principles may consequently be a richer, more robust, framework for the dire mental health consequences of war, famine, and economic catastrophe. The combined approach can do more moral work, distilling complex ideas into recognizable short-cuts and themes. Stories matter, and they can be governed by some basic heuristics: peace is better than war, health is better than illness, life is better than death [11]. This hybrid starting point can be tested at any level of ethical discourse. Targeting the needs of the few can be a clearer choice when preventing a camp epidemic segregates people by infectivity rather than the more common sex, ethnicity, or age. A recent analysis struggled with exactly this problem: how do public health officials respond when burial rituals in the Ebola crisis increase the risk of infection [12]? Grounding biosafety in the context of local cultural narratives by including family members in burial teams was far more successful in controlling infection than any unadorned principle of quarantine alone.

The Theoretical Level: Finding a Unifying Justification

Bringing ideas together may be the richer option for those working with complex problems. Instead of being helpful, the variety of theories can result in a conceptual and empirical confusion as policy-makers and scholars try to parse out all the potential outcomes and their values. This "problem of multiple ethical criteria" as it has been called (e.g., [13], citing JS Mill) leads to impossible algorithms of choice where every decision-point is laden with moral and cultural perspectives. Unifying ideas may be more powerful and effective.

Middle East conflict resolution expert Donna Hicks [14, 15] uses narrative to take a satisfying step toward a unifying theme for the ethics of global health – mental or otherwise. In a classic story-gathering fashion, she interviewed people from across the globe. Her respondents identified critical elements of a unifying idea that had to be present for them to function well as individuals and in groups: dignity.

Hicks' research into this unifying theme uncovers important elements like acknowledging others' identity, being fair, and taking responsibility – elements echoed by advocates for minority or non-dominant groups, by philosophers advocating theories of justice, and institutional leaders espousing transparency and social responsibility. Hicks is not alone in emphasizing dignity as the moral driver of human interaction. Human rights theorists and advocates had been using dignity as the cornerstone of international treatises and declarations for centuries.

Traceable for some to the American Declaration of Independence [16], or, for others, to the United Nations Universal Declaration of Human Rights [17], policy-makers and governments alike recognized some kernel of value inherent to all persons. From our contemporary perspective, it was a value much needed for a world that commodified people as slaves, treated outsiders with contempt, and held women and children as chattel. Some ethical model was required for nations and individuals that did not wish to suffer a life that was, in the words of the seventeenth-century's Thomas Hobbes [18], "nasty, brutish, and short."

Harvard professor Michael Rosen [19] finds this cardinal concept of dignity in luminaries Thomas Aquinas and Immanuel Kant, thinkers who molded centuries of Western thought. Both found intrinsic value in one's mere existence. For Aquinas, a Catholic theologian of the thirteenth century, the value was dependent on God's creation – a good thing in and of itself. If something occupied a proper place in Creation, it had intrinsic value.

Kant did not require a religious origin for dignity, finding it innate in humanity. Dignity was independent of God, yet raised above all else – a value that was intrinsic, unconditional, and incomparable ([19], p. 21). Setting aside the similarity to Aquinas (and indeed to other prominent philosophers as well), Rosen centers Kant's view of dignity on the capacity for morality – the capacity for internal law-giving, mutual respect, and aspiring to who one ought to be. The capacity for morality was, in Rosen's modern analysis, the essence of dignity, of inherent value. Recognizing rules and aspirations would be a powerful influence on future writers seeking dignity in one's self, one's behavior, and in one's work.

From such auspicious beginnings, dignity came to be associated with the celebrated term "inalienable." Thomas Jefferson's Declaration of Independence – bathed in the era's radical anti-monarchist thinking – is known for describing persons endowed "with certain inalienable rights: life, liberty, and the pursuit of happiness." Celebrated thinkers like Thomas Paine, Jeremy Bentham, and John Stuart Mill all wrote in a similar manner: there are rights or conditions that simply cannot be taken or even given away (e.g., JS Mill, On Liberty) [20]. The United Nations Declaration too [17], in the very first words of its Preamble, found something inalienable in humanity's inherent value:

"Whereas recognition of the inherent dignity and of the equal and inalienable rights of all members of the human family is the foundation of freedom, justice and peace in the world…"

And then again in Article 1:

"All human beings are born free and equal in dignity and rights."

The inherent worth of individuals could not be a clearer marker for those seeking justification for the application of global resources to mental healthcare shortages worldwide. Just as for Jefferson and the United Nations, rights sprang from the idea that everyone had worth. These were claims arising from one's inherent value: claims to liberty, health, and peace. In an equation universally taught to ethics students, rights give rise to duties: if there is a right to something, there must be a related duty to provide it. It was no accident that dignity gave birth to the international human rights movement and its claims on governments, agencies, and the global community.

These aspirations notwithstanding, there is no more sobering influence on universal ambitions than the reality of catastrophe. In modern times, health crises have overwhelmed borders and agreements that were never intended to manage global threats like HIV (with its associated depression and dementia), Ebola, and sexual violence. Gender-based violence, already pandemic according to the UN and its WHO [21], has now been reported as a military strategy everywhere from Bosnia and Colombia to the Democratic Republic of Congo.

Ironically, many of Europe's pre-2015 agreements to facilitate trade and the movement of workers (e.g., the Common Market, the European Union, the Schengen Borders Agreement), could not respond to the structural needs of devastated neighboring nations, their migrants, refugees, and asylum seekers. Functioning outside the usual international accords, the inherent value – the dignity – of those living in and fleeing war, drought, and famine were not prioritized as social programs ground to a halt and international borders slammed shut in the face of the world's largest global migrations since World War II.

The Practical Level: Operationalizing the Theory

In the face of such realities, where can one begin to operationalize a unified understanding of an ethics for global mental health? How does an aspirational idea like dignity apply among the grim realities of scarcity?

The world already finds itself at a certain unsettled equilibrium of international policy and collaboration – a starting point for this exploration. There are international agreements between nations, often adjudicated by the international tribunals at The Hague or in international parliaments like Europe's. These follow broad principles of international law and liberal democracy. There is a United Nations, with its High Commissioner for Human Rights and special rapporteurs (experts) on healthcare access. These espouse universal access and human rights. There are international and regional councils to address an entire continent's Ebola and famine catastrophes. These seek fairness in the distribution of resources. There is a World Health Organization committed to the highest attainable standards of physical and mental health [22]. What practicalities do the common aspirations of these bodies require of nations, professionals, and citizens?

For the unifying idea of dignity to be useful, attempts at collaboration and co-existence must follow some kind of generalized practice. Are we required to practice the "effective altruism" of philosopher Peter Singer [23]: choosing problems that affect many and are most influenced by targeted resources. Or to practice allocating resources as if we did not know where we would be in the world. This was John Rawls' famous idea, considering justice as fairness with resources distributed from behind a "veil of ignorance" [24]. Where does one allot resources to improve opportunities for everyone without being influenced by one's own situation? Rawls would not go so far as to force contributions from those already endowed with resources, but his idea of fairness of opportunity is one of the most influential concepts of the twentieth century.

Political economist Amartya Sen [25] puts a somewhat finer point on Rawls, requiring fairness of outcome (reflecting capability and choice) rather than mere opportunity: it is not enough simply to offer opportunity; one must include the values of those affected and provide some assurance that the outcome itself is acceptable. Sen effectively uses historical narratives of famine to advance the requirements of political accountability and social justice. More recently, Sam Harris [26] extended the idea of what constitutes an acceptable outcome by requiring human fulfillment or well-being as the primary goal of human endeavor – a kind of modern utilitarianism.

These universal calls for altruism, justice, and well-being all use the major ethics theories (i.e., consequentialism, principlism, narrative) to establish obligations that global health already recognizes. They build on the centuries-old search for how people should act and interact. If dignity of the person can be the unifying theme that generates global ideals of human rights like those from Thomas Jefferson and the United Nations, how does it work? If all are equal and have equal dignity, one may simply be reverting to the question of whether distributing resources equally is ethically sufficient, or even effective.

It is not. Georgetown University philosopher Terry Pinkard in his classic lectures on justice famously invoked US baseball star Pete Rose to emphasize the inherent unfairness of social and cultural existence. How does Pete Rose attain fame and fortune merely by saying, "Throw that ball at me and I'll hit it with a stick one out of three times" [27]. The idiosyncrasy and good fortune of this culmination of social accidents is recognizable more broadly. Geographer Jared Diamond [28] found it in Europe's unique combination of guns, germs, and steel – a combination that allowed it to dominate cultures across continents. Others find it in the presence of a civilization-building fertile crescent around Ancient Egypt, or in fortuitous geographic barriers protecting Japan and the United States. Idiosyncratic developments arise in cultures that strike inventive lotteries (e.g., sub-Saharan languages, Assyrian weapons, Egyptian irrigation, Greek and Arabic mathematics, Chinese compasses). Such accidents allow some to thrive while others starve, or submit.

Because there is no inherent justice – or dignity for that matter – to winning a series of lotteries, claims can legitimately be made against them without violating the dignity or related rights of resource-rich groups. Winning the lotteries of birth, good health, and geography distinguishes patients from clinicians and hosts from beneficiaries in ways that create a starting point for operationalizing the ethics of the haves and have-nots. Nations already practice this form of distributive ethics by placing tariffs or quotas on their trading partners, or taxing their citizens by status, purchase, or behavior (e.g., taxing businesses, cars, and luxury purchases). Governments may incentivize other behaviors by dropping trade barriers or encouraging personal and business choices with educational, environmental, or healthcare rebates. Prioritizing values and goods in a way that is good for the community is not a new idea, but in the face of a growing mental health burden it may be time to push it further.

For some studying professional ethics in the United States, the work of ethicists at the American Medical Association (AMA) offered a unique opportunity to prioritize and operationalize values. Matthew Wynia and Ezekiel Emanuel were among those moving medicine's understanding of its professional role beyond traditional virtues, characteristics, or competencies [29, 30]. The importance of addressing medicine's moral basis was not lost on writers who worked in academic and public health. After all, advocating for healthcare access, public health, and anti-poverty initiatives are the very currency of medical and public health groups.

In terms recognizable to ethicists and economists alike, this group would define professionalism "as an activity that involves both the distribution of a commodity and the fair allocation of a social good, but that is uniquely defined according to moral relationships. Professionalism is a structurally stabilizing, morally protective force in society." They go on to argue for a professionalism that "protects not only vulnerable persons but also vulnerable social values" ([29], p. 1612).

Understanding healthcare as a commodity may not be satisfying to those like the authors of this text who see healthcare as a right, but finite budgets, resources, and political will do ultimately provide limitations. And economic metrics like those surrounding commodities are historically translatable across regions and cultures. It is the fair allocation of this limited commodity that invokes the familiar idea of justice as fairness – the powerful moral idea that Rawls and his school espoused. Distribution of healthcare through a professional's work had to be done in an equitable manner. Although the authors do not yet define what they mean by "fair," the use of professionalism to do the practical work of a moral healthcare is set.

What may resonate strongly for those considering their obligations to strangers from faraway places is defining ethics in terms of moral relationships – those fundamental connections between people and groups that ground their interactions. If each person has dignity, the obligation to honor that dignity may now extend quite broadly. In an interconnected modern world where the new coronavirus, COVID-19, moves from one place to another because of air travel, where fires in the Amazon affect the planet's oxygen cycle and biodiversity, where industrial plastics and exhaust affect entire bodies of water and global air circulation, and local downturns in popular goods like coffee and tea affect international trade networks, the relationships between distant moral actors grow tighter and tighter.

Although early ethics may have been defined by its cultures of origin (Aristotle and Confucius had different views of the good life for example), recognizing that distant people and nations are connected to each other by mutual concerns is no longer a moral stretch. This connection consequently incurs both the obligations *and* accountability we have seen in our pursuit of a unifying idea for global mental health. Individual consumers may be obligated to make globally sound economic and healthcare choices just like governments. Wide-ranging water use, antibiotic, and recycling efforts are but the tip of the iceberg.

The ethicists from the AMA next define professionalism as a structurally stabilizing, morally protective force. Here is a way to inject dignity into the professional foundations of healthcare delivery across the globe. Acting to be structurally stabilizing and morally protective operationalizes theoretical dignity in a way that makes conceptual discussions far more practical. Decisions can now be made in ways that prioritize stability and protection over transience and vulnerability. Developing policies and interventions that improve or sustain local capabilities (e.g., by stabilizing transportation or mental health delivery systems), and providing assessment tools that translate across nations and cultures are firm examples of these values. Such sustainable practices underscore stability and morality.

Because patients are vulnerable in specific ways – weakened by their condition, their worry, and their lack of medical knowledge – the appeal to vulnerable people and values is recognizable as well. For the purpose of operationalizing dignity, the prioritization of vulnerable persons is particularly meaningful. It is a method for triaging resources in a traditional manner: resources to the neediest, the most vulnerable first; not simply an equal share for all.

What then are the vulnerable *values* in our dignity construct for global mental health? Respect (and attendant respectful behavior) would seem a likely choice. Elena Cherepanov [31] is among those who worry that the global mental health workforce could use more robust training and professional development. Recent scandals of sexual exploitation by aid-workers are a stark reminder of the need for behavioral standards and strong hiring practices [32, 33].

Cherepanov's advocacy for developing professional competencies of knowledge, attitude, and self-care resonates strongly for those seeking to overcome the public health burden of mental illness – a burden that could cost the world 16 trillion US dollars by 2030 [1]. Her call for "deep accountability" ([31], p. 144), reverberates throughout a field that has been criticized for failing to seek community consent, avoid exploitation, or assure proper training.

Resilience that prevents burn-out among clinicians and aid-workers must be a vulnerable value as well. The literature is rife with reports of Posttraumatic Stress Disorder (PTSD) among volunteers and professionals alike, with rotations lasting as little as 3 months in some humanitarian theaters [34, 35, 36]. Burn-out is prevalent among physicians in their home countries as well, with physicians as a group being less likely than the general public to access needed care; they are more likely to self-diagnose and self-treat [37, 38, 39, 40]. Protecting vulnerable clinicians who experience similar symptoms as their patients honors their worth while extending the life of their expertise.

Representation of those affected is a value that has been similarly neglected in recent years. If dignity is to have any meaning at all it must honor the perspective of those affected by mental health initiatives. Consider the perspective of one Rwandan talking to writer Andrew Solomon [41]:

> We had a lot of trouble with Western mental health workers who came here immediately after the genocide and we had to ask some of them to leave.
>
> They came and their practice did not involve being outside in the sun where you begin to feel better. There was no music or drumming to get your blood flowing again. There was no sense that everyone had taken the day off so that the entire community could come together to try to lift you up and bring you back to joy. There was no acknowledgement of the depression as something invasive and external that could actually be cast out again.
>
> Instead they would take people one at a time into these dingy little rooms and have them sit around for an hour or so and talk about bad things that had happened to them. We had to ask them to leave.

This is not merely a claim for honoring cultural narratives, but an appeal for including those with a stake in the outcome. "Nothing about us without us," is a time-honored maxim with origins in politics, research ethics, and more recently disability and mental health rights (e.g., [42]). From the American Revolution's "No taxation without representation," to calls for the inclusion of research participants in the design of clinical research, inclusiveness has been a vulnerable value for many resource-poor communities, not the least of which is mental health.

Similarly, in the global migration's registration camps, promoting internal leadership and social support networks improves or prevents psychological symptoms [43]. Creating councils comprised of refugees encourages their application of community values in deciding camp matters for themselves.

Conclusion

This summative chapter began by declaring that perspective matters. Why it matters derives from the dignity inherent in all people. It is a concept built on centuries of thinking about the obligations between both individuals and groups. Dignity has been an established way for governments, agencies, and communities to justify the inclusion of others and to honor their views, especially when they have been marginalized by history, stigma, or catastrophe.

Finding value in all persons is therefore a legitimate justification for articulating a global mental health ethic. People deserve the attention and resources that may not otherwise be available because of accidents of history or birth. Found in the seminal work of philosophers, politicians, and organizations, dignity gives the field a core reason for involvement and advocacy.

Dignity in turn gives rise to rights and duties. What is the point of a justification if it does not validate an action or claim? Initially avoiding the question of whose duty it is to provide the right of access and health, a Justice-colored view of lotteries arrived at the answer: it is the lottery-winners with resources who have the duty to provide help. It is not fair simply to be born into success; fairness requires some recognition of the idiosyncrasies that led to the outcome. And if that success is achieved on the backs of those less fortunate, the obligation grows.

Next, resources must be provided to the most vulnerable first. I have left aside other models of triage, only because the concept of vulnerability is such a powerful one. When communities decide what vulnerability means, the ensuing quest will be for which vulnerabilities best respond to which interventions and at what cost. Happily, there is already a literature on triage and cost-effectiveness [44].

If the dignity of the person, with its attendant rights and duties, works at the theoretical level to provide justification for an ethics of global mental health, it is professionalism that puts it to work. This is a classic structure for ethical theories: one idea functions as an overall justification while another operationalizes it. Operationalizing dignity or making it practical means protecting vulnerable values just like vulnerable people. Professionalism is then the means for articulating specific behaviors: prioritizing education and training, avoiding exploitation, overcoming stigma, obtaining consent and input, being culturally sensitive, and acting in a sustainable, stabilizing way. Together, dignity and professionalism can be the structural components that anchor an ethics of global mental health.

References

1. Patel, V., Saxena, S., Lund, C., Thornicroft, G., Baingana, F., Bolton, P., et al. (2018). The Lancet Commission on global mental health and sustainable development. *Lancet, 392*(10157), 1553–1598. https://doi.org/10.1016/S0140-6736(18)31612-X.
2. MSF. (2019). *International activity report 2018 | MSF*. Retrieved from https://www.msf.org/international-activity-report-2018.
3. Kipnis, K. (1997). Confessions of an expert ethics witness. *The Journal of Medicine and Philosophy, 22*(4), 325–343. https://doi.org/10.1093/jmp/22.4.325.
4. Childress, J. F. (1997). *Practical reasoning in bioethics*. Bloomington: Indiana University Press.

5. Candilis, P., Martinez, R., & Dording, C. (2001). Principles and narrative in forensic psychiatry: Toward a robust view of professional role. *The Journal of the American Academy of Psychiatry and the Law, 29*(2), 167–173.
6. Chambers, T. (1999). *The fiction of bioethics: Cases as literary texts.* New York: Routledge.
7. Nelson, H. L. (1997). *Stories and their limits: Narrative approaches to bioethics.* London: Routledge.
8. Arras, J. (1997). Nice story, but so what?: Narrative and justification in ethics. In H. L. Nelson (Ed.), *Stories and their limits* (pp. 65–89). London: Routledge.
9. Nagel, T. (1986). *The view from nowhere.* Oxford: Oxford University Press.
10. Bradley, F. H. (1988). *Ethical studies.* Oxford, UK/New York: Clarendon Press/Oxford University Press.
11. Beauchamp, T. L., & Childress, J. F. (2019). *Principles of biomedical ethics* (8th ed.). New York: Oxford University Press.
12. Mokuwa, E., & Richards, P. (2020). How should public health officials respond when important local rituals increase risk of contagion? *AMA Journal of Ethics, 22*(1), E5–E9. https://doi.org/10.1001/amajethics.2020.5.
13. Benicourt, E. (2004). Contre Amartya Sen. *L'Economie Politique, 23*(3), 72–84.
14. Hicks, D. (2011). *Dignity: The essential role in resolving conflict.* New Haven/London: Yale University Press.
15. Hicks, D. (2018). *Leading with dignity: How to create a culture that brings out the best in people.* New Haven/London: Yale University Press.
16. Archives, United States National. (2015). *Declaration of independence: A transcription.* Retrieved from https://www.archives.gov/founding-docs/declaration-transcript.
17. United Nations. (1948). *Universal declaration of human rights.* Retrieved from https://www.un.org/en/universal-declaration-human-rights/index.html.
18. Hobbes, T., & Malcolm, N. (2014). *Leviathan.* Oxford: Clarendon Press.
19. Rosen, M. (2012). *Dignity: Its history and meaning.* Cambridge, MA: Harvard University Press.
20. Mill, J. S. (2002). *On liberty.* Mineola: Dover Publications.
21. United Nations Population Fund. (2019). *Gender-based-violence.* Retrieved from https://www.unfpa.org/gender-based-violence.
22. World Health Organization. (2006). *Constitution. WHO Basic Documents* (45th ed., Supplement).
23. Singer, P. (2015). *The most good you can do: How effective altruism is changing ideas about living ethically.* New Haven: Yale University Press.
24. Rawls, J. (1971). *A theory of justice.* Cambridge, MA: The Belknap Press of Harvard University Press.
25. Sen, A. K. (2010). *The idea of justice.* London: Penguin Books.
26. Harris, S. (2012). *The moral landscape: How science can determine human values.* London: Black Swan.
27. Pinkard T. Personal communication, January 6, 2020.
28. Diamond, J. M. (1997). *Guns, germs, and steel: The fates of human societies.* New York: W.W. Norton & Co..
29. Wynia, M. K., Latham, S. R., Kao, A. C., Berg, J. W., & Emanuel, L. L. (1999). Medical professionalism in society. *The New England Journal of Medicine, 341*(21), 1612–1616. https://doi.org/10.1056/NEJM199911183412112.
30. Wynia, M. K., Papadakis, M. A., Sullivan, W. M., & Hafferty, F. W. (2014). More than a list of values and desired behaviors: A foundational understanding of medical professionalism. *Academic Medicine, 89*(5), 712–714. https://doi.org/10.1097/ACM.0000000000000212.
31. Cherepanov, E. (2019). *Ethics for global mental health: From good intentions to humanitarian accountability.* New York: Routledge.
32. Inter-Agency Standing Committee. (2002). *Report of the Task Force on protection from sexual exploitation and abuse in humanitarian crises.* Retrieved from https://www.unicef.org/emerg/files/IASCTFReport.pdf.

33. Inter-Agency Standing Committee. (2012). *Sexual exploitation and abuse by UN, NGO and INGO personnel: A self-assessment*. Retrieved from https://odihpn.org/magazine/sexual-exploitation-and-abuse-by-un-ngo-and-ingo-personnel-a-self-assessment/.
34. Connorton, E., Perry, M. J., Hemenway, D., & Miller, M. (2012). Humanitarian relief workers and trauma-related mental illness. *Epidemiologic Reviews, 34*, 145–155. https://doi.org/10.1093/epirev/mxr026.
35. Lopes Cardozo, B., Gotway Crawford, C., Eriksson, C., Zhu, J., Sabin, M., Ager, A., et al. (2012). Psychological distress, depression, anxiety, and burnout among international humanitarian aid workers: A longitudinal study. *PLoS One, 7*(9), e44948. https://doi.org/10.1371/journal.pone.0044948.
36. Thormar, S. B., Gersons, B. P. R., Juen, B., Marschang, A., Djakababa, M. N., & Olff, M. (2010). The mental health impact of volunteering in a disaster setting: A review. *The Journal of Nervous and Mental Disease, 198*(8), 529–538. https://doi.org/10.1097/NMD.0b013e3181ea1fa9.
37. Benkhadra, K., Adusumalli, J., Rajjo, T., Hagen, P. T., Wang, Z., & Murad, M. H. (2016). A survey of health care needs of physicians. *BMC Health Services Research, 16*(1), 472. https://doi.org/10.1186/s12913-016-1728-4.
38. Candilis, P. J., Kim, D. T., Sulmasy, L. S., & ACP Ethics, P. a. H. R. C. (2019). Physician impairment and rehabilitation: Reintegration into medical practice while ensuring patient safety: A position paper from the American College of Physicians. *Annals of Internal Medicine, 170*(12), 871–879. https://doi.org/10.7326/M18-3605.
39. Chiu, Y. L., Kao, S., Lin, H. C., Tsai, M. C., & Lee, C. Z. (2016). Healthcare service utilization for practicing physicians: A population-based study. *PLoS One, 11*(1), e0130690. https://doi.org/10.1371/journal.pone.0130690.
40. Steffen, M. W., Hagen, P. T., Benkhadra, K., Molella, R. G., Newcomb, R. D., & Murad, M. H. (2015). A survey of physicians' perceptions of their health care needs. *Occupational Medicine (London), 65*(1), 49–53. https://doi.org/10.1093/occmed/kqu145.
41. Dyer, A. (2019). *Global mental health: Ethical principles and practices*. George Washington University Department of Psychiatry Grand Rounds, November 21, 2019.
42. Charlton, J. M. (1998). *Nothing about us without us: Disability oppression and empowerment*. Berkeley: University of California.
43. Hobfoll, S. E., Watson, P., Bell, C. C., Bryant, R. A., Brymer, M. J., Friedman, M. J., et al. (2007). Five essential elements of immediate and mid-term mass trauma intervention: Empirical evidence. *Psychiatry, 70*(4), 283–369. https://doi.org/10.1521/psyc.2007.70.4.283.
44. Dyer, A.R. (2021). Global mental health through the lens of ethics. In A.R. Dyer, Kohrt B.A., Candilis, P.J. (Eds.), Global mental health ethics (pp. xx–xx). London: Springer.

Index

Printed in the United States
by Baker & Taylor Publisher Services